The Self and Its Pleasures

Carolyn J. Dean

THE SELF
AND ITS
PLEASURES

*Bataille, Lacan, and
the History of the
Decentered Subject*

Cornell University Press

Ithaca and London

First published 1992 by Cornell University Press.
First printing, Cornell Paperbacks, 1992.
Second printing 1994.

International Standard Book Number 0-8014-2660-X (cloth)
International Standard Book Number 0-8014-9954-2 (paper)
Library of Congress Catalog Card Number 92-52748
Printed in the United States of America
Librarians: Library of Congress cataloging information appears on the last page of the book.

♾ The paper in this book meets the minimum requirements of the American National Standard for Information Sciences—Permanence of Paper for Printed Library Materials, ANSI Z39.48-1984.

To my parents

Harriet Katzman Dean
Albert Robert Dean

Contents

Acknowledgments   ix

Introduction   1

PART ONE   Psychoanalysis and the Self   11

    1. The Legal Status of the Irrational   17
    2. Gender Complexes   58
    3. Sight Unseen (Reading the Unconscious)   98

PART TWO   Sade's Selflessness   123

    4. The Virtue of Crime   127
    5. The Pleasure of Pain   170

PART THREE   Headlessness   201

    6. Writing and Crime   205
    7. Returning to the Scene of the Crime   221

    Conclusion   246

    Selected Bibliography   253

    Index   265

Acknowledgments

I thank the University of California at Berkeley and the Andrew W. Mellon Foundation for providing the funds and leave time necessary to undertake the writing and research of this book.

I am especially grateful to Mary Gluck, David Joravsky, and Sarah Maza, who graciously read various portions of the manuscript. I am also indebted to Mark Poster's criticism and to Michael Roth, whose close reading of the final draft helped me clarify and sharpen my argument.

I owe my most profound intellectual debts to Denis Hollier, Lynn Hunt, and Martin Jay, without whose encouragement, criticism, and commitment this book might never have taken the direction it did. Martin Jay guided and commented on this work at every stage of its unfolding, and it is to him that I owe the deepest gratitude.

John Ackerman, Judith Bailey, and the editorial staff at Cornell University Press helped prepare the final manuscript and offered invaluable assistance. Gretchen Schultz and Brigitte Mahuzier advised me on translations and helped me relax. For everything else, I thank my colleagues and friends Elizabeth Barnes, Laird Boswell, Julie Greenberg, Laura Hein, Walter Hixson, James Beale, Michael Sherry, Jennifer Terry, and Sharon Ullman. And a special thank you to Michael Polignano, Laurie Bernstein, Robert Weinberg, and Nicole Albert.

One portion of this book has appeared in different form in *Representations* 13 (Winter 1986).

C. J. D.

The Self and Its Pleasures

Introduction

In 1966 the historian Michel Foucault declared that the concept of man "would be erased, like a face drawn in sand at the edge of the sea."[1] Foucault's dramatic declaration represented the culmination of nearly a century of philosophical and aesthetic commentary that questioned whether "man" was in fact a unitary, transcendental, rational, knowing subject. Indeed, French modernists, existentialists, phenomenologists, structuralists, and now poststructuralists have "decentered" the self in radically different ways since the late nineteenth century. They have developed the idea that the self no longer masters the world through its reason but is mired in and constituted by culture. This book is about the development of one contemporary form of self-"dissolution," whose different and most recent manifestations have often been termed structuralist or poststructuralist. But it is above all an attempt to *account* for the idea of a decentered self as it has been articulated primarily in the works of two French thinkers who were friends as well as contemporaries: Georges Bataille (1897–1962) and Jacques Lacan (1901–1981). I use their work to frame three interrelated questions: Why, quite simply, has France been the home of the most influential theories of self-dissolution? How, then, is the decentered self historically and culturally specific? And how do we account for rather than just describe what Judith Butler has called the "regulatory fictions" that constitute it?[2]

Why, first of all, Bataille and Lacan? Intellectual historians and

---

[1] Michel Foucault, *The Order of Things* (New York: Vintage, 1970), p. 387.
[2] Judith Butler, *Gender Trouble: Feminism and the Subversion of Identity* (New York: Routledge and Kegan Paul, 1990), p. 33.

others usually place them in different categories. Scholars consider Lacan a structuralist (or a poststructuralist in disguise). No one calls Bataille a structuralist, since he never implicitly or explicitly used Saussurian linguistics to ground his thought. Instead, Jürgen Habermas places him first in a line that leads from "Bataille via Michel Foucault to Jacques Derrida,"[3] implying that Bataille is closest to poststructuralist thinkers. There have in fact been several recent attempts to see Bataille as a forerunner of poststructuralism, and one critic claims that Bataille's work constitutes an "urtext of deconstruction."[4]

This effort to understand their work by reference to theories of the decentered subject helps us place Bataille and Lacan in the history of ideas. It tells us to whom they demonstrated intellectual affinities or allegiances, and it accounts for the significance of their contributions to the development of structuralist psychoanalysis or poststructuralist literary theory. But while it may be true, for example, that Lacan was Foucault's structuralist contemporary (insofar as the early Foucault was seen as a structuralist), and Bataille his proto-poststructuralist predecessor, this kind of assertion still begs the question of the historical meaning and relevance of structuralism and poststructuralism (not to mention the difficulty of pinning down Foucault). I have chosen Bataille and Lacan because they are each slippery enough to defy easy categorization and yet important enough in the history of French (and Western) theories of the self to be considered predecessors, founders, or exemplars of particular schools of thought. So, what if we were to conceive their formulations of the self as local, historical practices rather than in terms of broad, shifting paradigms of subjectivity?

---

[3] Jürgen Habermas, "Modernity—An Incomplete Project," in Hal Foster, ed., *The Anti-Aesthetic: Essays on Postmodern Culture* (Seattle: Bay Press, 1983), p. 14.

[4] Allan Stoekl, *Politics, Writing, Mutilation: The Cases of Bataille, Blanchot, Roussel, Leiris, and Ponge* (Minneapolis: University of Minnesota Press, 1985), p. xiii. Other attempts are Michèle Richman, "Introduction to the *Collège de Sociologie*: Post-structuralism before Its Time?" *Stanford French Review* 12 (Spring 1988), 79–95; Jean-Michel Heimonet, *Politiques de l'écriture: Bataille/Derrida: Le Sens du sacré dans la pensée française du surréalisme à nos jours* (Chapel Hill: University of North Carolina Press, 1987); and Julian Pefanis, *Heterology and the Postmodern: Bataille, Baudrillard, and Lyotard* (Durham: Duke University Press, 1991), pp. 3, 9–58. Pefanis warns us to resist calling Bataille a poststructuralist or postmodernist "in order to avoid the easy retrospective projection of Bataille into a seminal prehistory of these two categories" (p. 40). Nevertheless, he proceeds to analyze Bataille more or less in those terms.

In this book I seek to account for Bataille's and Lacan's formulation of decentered subjectivity as part of a cultural crisis in interwar France in which all the criteria defining what makes a self and what gives it legitimacy were perceived as having dissolved. In the chapters that follow, I look at the relationship between this self and changing constructions of the other in order to account for what makes the French interwar critiques of the subject—in particular the works of Bataille and Lacan—culturally specific. More precisely, I try to document the process through which, in France, all psychoanalytic and literary attempts to rescue the self after the Great War led instead to its dissolution, and all attempts to stabilize the self in new theoretical terms reiterated its instability.

This approach requires treating ideas as historical practices. Yet what it means to do so is far from clear. Other scholars have written the history of how the decentered self emerged prior to structuralism and poststructuralism in terms of a complex meshing of intellectual influences facilitated by cultural, spiritual crises. Most trace decentering to a general philosophical recognition of the other.[5] Beginning in the nineteenth century, philosophers and members of literary movements in particular effected a shift away from a rational or empirical to what might be called an intuitive model of the sources of subjectivity: from seeing as a primary mode of cognition to an emphasis on being which rejects the supposed neutrality or passivity of the observer.

Abandoning the pose of the neutral recorder of experience, philosophers, including Edmund Husserl and Henri Bergson, engaged in a common effort to save the self from a world they perceived as

[5]Jürgen Habermas, *The Philosophical Discourse of Modernity* (Cambridge: MIT Press, 1987); Michael Theunissen, *The Other: Studies in the Social Ontology of Husserl, Heidegger, Sartre, and Buber* (Cambridge: MIT Press, 1984), p. x. Habermas links this "post-Cartesian turn to Otherness" to Nietzsche and Heidegger, who problematized in a specific way the religious foundations of truth. He argues that the Judeo-Christian notion that truth is always located in an only indirectly accessible other (God) formed the premise of traditional Western metaphysics in which truth was guaranteed because built on a religious foundation. Nietzsche and Heidegger set this otherness loose from religion, Habermas says, and, in so doing, "point[ed] into the domain of radical experiences that the avant-garde has opened up." The redefinition of self as other thus represents a modern, secularized reworking of the Western metaphysical tradition (pp. 182–84). For a discussion of Lacan's Christian "ethics" which reiterates Habermas in a different way, see Michel de Certeau, *Heterologies: Discourses on the Other* (Minneapolis: University of Minnesota Press, 1986), pp. 47–64.

being dominated by technology and consumerism and hence by the hegemony of instrumental reason. In distinct ways, they looked to lived experience, intuitively known, transmissible, and not reducible to mechanical laws, as recourse against that hegemony. Thus, the French philosopher Henri Bergson emphasized the power of intuition and insisted that experience could not be explained in purely mechanistic terms. Bergson, whose lectures influenced a generation of French intellectuals, facilitated the theoretical turn away from the Cartesianism still evident in French positivism and naturalism at the turn of the century.

With and after Bergson, French thinkers and especially French artists and writers sought to uncover what Habermas has called the "unthought and hidden foundations of performing subjectivity."[6] In other words, they tried to locate and retrieve the sources of the self. They looked to the other of the instrumental reason that they believed dominated the world—to the authentic, original self, now conceived as hidden or obscured. The Great War most dramatically brought the question of the self to the fore and made many French thinkers, many of them war veterans, ever more receptive to ideas touting the power of the irrational and calling for spiritual renewal through the exploration of the nether regions of the soul. For the first time, psychoanalysis found French adherents, above all in the surrealists, who looked to Freud's teaching for inspiration in their own effort to recover the so-called true self. And while the surrealists also paid tribute to the post-Cartesian German dialectician Hegel, it was not until the 1930s that Hegel was afforded a broad French reception.[7]

The most influential interpreter of Hegel in France was the Rus-

---

[6]Habermas, *The Philosophical Discourse*, p. 263.

[7]See Vincent Descombes, *Modern French Philosophy* (Cambridge: Cambridge University Press, 1980), p. 3. See also Michael Roth, *Knowing and History: Appropriations of Hegel in Twentieth-Century France* (Ithaca: Cornell University Press, 1988), esp. pp. 81–146; Judith Butler, *Subjects of Desire: Hegelian Reflections in Twentieth-Century France* (New York: Columbia University Press, 1987), pp. 63–79. On French Marxism (which requires an analysis of the reception of Hegel), see Arthur Hirsch, *The French New Left: An Intellectual History from Sartre to Gorz* (Boston: South End Press, 1981); Mark Poster, *Existential Marxism in Postwar France* (Princeton: Princeton University Press, 1975); Michael Kelly, *Modern French Marxism* (Baltimore: Johns Hopkins University Press, 1982). On the relationship between the Great War and the avant-garde, see H. Stuart Hughes, *Consciousness and Society: The Reorientation of European Social Thought, 1890–1930* (New York: Vintage, 1961). One literary critic has written that the development of nonmimetic

sian émigré Alexandre Kojève (Kozhevnikov), who studied in Germany from 1921 to 1927 under the influence of Heidegger. From 1933 to 1939, Kojève presented his phenomenological-existentialist reading of Hegel in a course on *The Phenomenology of Mind*, which drew some of the most notable intellectuals of the era, including Bataille, Lacan, Pierre Klossowski, Maurice Merleau-Ponty, and Jean-Paul Sartre. This émigré philosopher, to whom both Bataille and Lacan paid homage, conceived the dialectic as a struggle for recognition illustrated above all in Hegel's analysis of the master-slave conflict. He focused on *The Phenomenology of Mind*, instead of Hegel's other texts, and stressed the existential forces of desire, lack, and struggle over Hegel's more metaphysical emphasis on reason, totality, and knowledge. He thus participated in a more general rejection of rationalism by focusing on the paradoxes and indeed the violence implicit in Hegel's account of the dialectic. In other words, Kojève focused on the other side of reason, on struggle rather than on synthesis, and hence turned Hegel's positive dialectic of self-recognition into a negative one. He pointed to what one philosopher has called the "unreasonable origins of reason."[8]

Bataille and Lacan drew in different ways on both surrealism and Kojève's lectures on Hegel, and used them to frame their other interests in anthropology, sociology, philosophy, and psychoanalysis. They both participated in the general attempt to rescue the self from reification, and both assimilated Kojève's reading of Hegel in terms of a negative dialectic. Together and yet separately, they redefined the relation of desire to culture and aesthetics and, in so doing, constructed the foundations of a new theory of subjectivity that extended and transformed modernist and psychoanalytic thought. Both conceived the true self to be an other. But closer to Kojève (and in Bataille's case, to Nietzsche) than to the surrealists, Husserl, or Heidegger, they did not see the self as simply cut loose, alienated from its origins; they believed these origins to be irretrievable. Bataille and Lacan thus conceived the "true" self, paradoxically, as an unsymbolizable and hence inaccessible

---

art was symptomatic of a world deprived of referents. The "void" of language, he claims, mirrored in complicated ways the abyss symbolized by the power vacuum in French politics during the 1930s. Heimonet, pp. 33–51.

[8] Descombes, p. 14.

other. In so doing, they separated truth from knowledge in a new and radical way. The self, in their view, is impossible to locate either metaphorically underneath (in the unconscious as Freud conceived it) or above something else (it perpetually "falls").

Historians and literary critics insist through this kind of narrative that the self is culturally and ideologically constructed; they generally agree that it is constructed of a new interest in otherness, but they seldom specify how and why the relationship between self and other is constructed the way it is. Even the philosopher Jacques Derrida, who has contributed significantly to our understanding of the constructed nature of reality, and the historian Michel Foucault, who has demonstrated to what extent ideas are constructs of discourses of power, have been less successful in helping to explain why and how concepts are constructed the way they are. In their work, an emphasis on historical processes, and hence a concern to account for the formation of concepts, is methodologically irrelevant. Derrida asserts that there is no reality outside the text.[9] Foucault analyzes discourses as constitutive of power. Both, that is, emphasize the primacy of language over historical actors and thus conflate language with history, so that ideas—writing, concepts—are always already historical practices. Questions about how and why ideas are generated by specific social relations are neglected in favor of locating contradictions immanent in texts (Derrida) or of providing brilliant descriptions of how power works but no explanation of why power works the way it does (Foucault).

For example, most of the voluminous literature on Lacan locates the originality of his work in its new synthesis of Freud, phenomenology, and structuralism. And much of this work is solely concerned with the internal coherence or explication of Lacan's text itself.[10] Most historical studies of Lacanian psychoanalysis

[9] Jacques Derrida, *Of Grammatology*, trans. Gayatri Chakravorty Spivak (Baltimore: Johns Hopkins University Press, 1976), p. 158.

[10] The list of works about Lacan is endless. See, among others, Mikkel Borch-Jacobsen, *Lacan: The Absolute Master*, trans. Douglas Brick (Stanford: Stanford University Press, 1991); Shoshana Felman, *Jacques Lacan and the Adventure of Insight: Psychoanalysis in Contemporary Culture* (Cambridge: Harvard University Press, 1987); Jane Gallop, *Reading Lacan* (Ithaca: Cornell University Press, 1985); Alain Juranville, *Lacan et la philosophie* (Paris: Presses Universitaires Françaises 1984); Anika Lemaire, *Jacques Lacan*, trans. David Macey (London: Routledge and Kegan Paul, 1977); François Roustang, *Lacan: De l'équivoque à l'impasse* (Paris: Minuit, 1986); Slavoj Zizek, *The Sublime Object of Ideology* (London: Verso, 1989).

hail Lacan as the man who saved Freud from the deviations of French psychoanalysts still beholden to Cartesianism. Jean-Pierre Mordier and Elisabeth Roudinesco have both argued that French psychiatry and psychoanalysis represented a "deformation" of Freud's thought until Lacan revived a more authentic version of Freud, "returned" to him.[11] Some recent works do insist on the connection between Lacanian analysis and the historical context in which it emerged, but they do not go beyond Lacan's reading of Kojève to explain why he may have read Kojève the way he did.[12]

Discussions of Bataille have been largely confined to monographs or conventional intellectual histories. One recent work does attempt to go beyond conventional notions of "genesis" and "impact," however.[13] In his analysis of Bataille and other interwar writers, Allan Stoekl proposes an essentially Derridean evaluation of the so-called otherness of modernist texts. These texts are subversive, he suggests, less because of what they represent than because they call their own representations into question. Thus, Bataille, Michel Leiris, and Maurice Blanchot (among others) have been excluded from literary histories because they "necessarily fall between its cracks," not because they "lack importance but because of a subversiveness that can never be erected and displayed as a law of the land."[14] But here Stoekl fails to resolve the question about the historical meaning of these works because he conflates the product (the "discourse" or the "text") with the process that produces it. He takes otherness out of the world and roots it in language itself.

[11] Jean-Pierre Mordier, *Les Débuts de la psychanalyse en France, 1895–1926* (Paris: Maspéro, 1981); and the most important study of French psychoanalysis to date, Elisabeth Roudinesco, *La Bataille de cent ans: Histoire de la psychanalyse en France,* vol. 1 (Paris: Ramsay, 1982); and *Jacques Lacan and Co.: A History of Psychoanalysis in France, 1925–1985,* trans. Jeffrey Mehlman (Chicago: University of Chicago Press, 1990). The latter is a translation of the second volume of Roudinesco's history. For a critique of Roudinesco's view of French psychoanalysis, see Paul Bercherie, "The Quadrifocal Oculary: The Epistemology of the Freudian Heritage," *Economy and Society* 15 (February 1986), 39, 66.

[12] See David Macey, *Lacan in Contexts* (London: Verso, 1988), and especially Borch-Jacobsen, *Lacan.*

[13] For a discussion of this trend as it affects intellectual history, see Dominick LaCapra's essay "Rethinking Intellectual History and Reading Texts," in LaCapra and Steven Kaplan, eds., *Modern European Intellectual History: Reappraisals and New Perspectives* (Ithaca: Cornell University Press, 1982), pp. 47–85.

[14] Stoekl, *Politics, Writing, Mutilation,* p. xiv. In his book politics constitutes the "other" of the text. Stoekl makes this argument most forcefully in "Nizan, Drieu, and the Question of Death," *Representations* 21 (Winter 1988), 117–45.

This book is not an effort to see theory and history as continuous with each other. Nor do I insist on a clear conceptual boundary between theory and history in which history would by itself account for or function as the background of textual production. In order to analyze why the self was constructed as an irretrievable other, I focus on how the relationship between texts and contexts was formulated rather than on one realm or the other. I analyze the process by which the self comes to symbolize an other. In other words, I try not to privilege either history or theory or to conflate the two. Instead, I look at how theory and history are implicated in each other or, more specifically, how theory represents, symbolizes, and hence constructs history, makes it "mean" (in this case, certain things about the self). I do not mean to argue simply that theory is infused with history and vice versa but to describe and account for a specific process of cultural symbolization, for why and how the self is produced the way it is, for its "regulatory fictions." My focus, then, is on the process by which meaning is constructed as meaning: it is an effort to account for why one story was told about the self and not another.[15]

Each part of this book focuses on the criminal as a metaphor for an other self that interwar psychiatrists, psychoanalysts, and avant-garde writers sought to rescue. And each traces symmetrical and overlapping movements aimed at self-renewal: the mental hygiene movement, French psychoanalysis, and surrealism. Together they explore how these various attempts to rescue the self laid the foundation for its unraveling. The first part examines how psychiatrists' and psychoanalysts' efforts to rehabilitate criminals led to Lacan's earliest revisions of Freud. In the second part, I focus on how the recovery of the marquis de Sade's work shaped new literary and psychiatric constructions of the self. In it I also seek to establish a common ground on which medical and avant-garde discourses meet. The third part explores how the surrealists' commitment to rescuing the self shaped Bataille's concept of literary production.

All three parts show how the self is "replotted"[16] after the Great

[15] On history as a kind of storytelling with no ontological status, see Lynn Hunt, "History as Gesture; or, The Scandal of History," in Jonathan Arac and Barbara Johnson eds., *The Consequences of Theory* (Baltimore: Johns Hopkins University Press, 1991), pp. 102–3.

[16] I am borrowing Malcolm Bowie's particularly apt term from "Jacques Lacan," in John Sturrock, ed., *Structuralism and Since* (Oxford: Oxford University Press, 1979), p. 131.

War and how Bataille, Lacan, and others dissolved the self by trying to rescue it from dissolution.[17] The chapters are thus layers of shifting and interrelated themes whose unity is determined by a coherent, if complicated, dialectic. I use the blurring of the boundaries between self and other as perceived and constructed by medical experts and writers as one particular expression of interwar anxieties, concerns, and politics. My focus is on how the representation of political and cultural threats as deviance both reinforced and dissolved conventional distinctions between self and other; I emphasize locally constituent moments at the expense of other, broader contextual and also textual referents.

At issue here is the stake these thinkers have in metamorphosing the self into an irretrievable other, for in discovering why this transformation is so important, we may begin to explain why France has been so hospitable to the most radical forms of it. To the extent that Bataille—as well as such writers as Pierre Klossowski—has begun to be seen as a forerunner of poststructuralism, this book is about its prehistory. That is, it seeks to explain the history of poststructuralist thought by reference to a context other than structuralism, phenomenology, and existentialism. This book bears out the insight, implicit in many recent critical works, that structuralism and poststructuralism are convenient rather than historically accurate categories.[18]

What follows is a poststructuralist history of the cultural origins of (what we now call) poststructuralism. This may be perceived as a rather paradoxical (if not impossible) procedure, but I hope to make a case for its usefulness. I understand poststructuralism here not as a form of pan-textualism but rather as the assumption that meaning can never fully reside in either texts or contexts.[19] I hope this book begins to assess under what conditions self-fragmentation can be conceived as part of a radical politics; to assess, for the time period discussed here, whose selves were at risk and why, and why those who put the self at risk did so. That is, if the self was and still

[17] For a discussion of this dynamic in a literary context, see Leo Bersani, *The Culture of Redemption* (Cambridge: Harvard University Press, 1990).

[18] See, among others, Stoekl, *Politics, Writing, Mutilation*, p. xiii; Jonathan Culler, *On Deconstruction* (Ithaca: Cornell University Press, 1982), 8–9; Macey, pp. 4–5.

[19] On this point (in reference to deconstruction), see Martin Jay, "The Textual Approach to Intellectual History" in Gisela Brude-Firnau and Karin J. MacHardy, eds., *Fact and Fiction: German History and Literature: 1848–1924* (Tübingen: Franke Verlag, 1990), pp. 77–86.

is at stake, and if dissolving its boundaries or reshaping its contours was conceived as a meaningful, even subversive, gesture, it is essential to figure out precisely what that act meant. It is essential to know how theory may be specific to history and culture, how theory always refers to something outside its conceptual boundaries.

PART ONE

PSYCHOANALYSIS
AND THE SELF

In a most annoying manner, M. Lacan says "the constitution of
reality" instead of simply "reality."
—Edouard Pichon,
   "La Famille devant M. Lacan," 1939

The reception of psychoanalysis in France is usually said to
have been rather inhospitable. Freud's version of the unconscious
was allowed in only through the back door—by way of the literary
avant-garde.[1] Although at least one medical periodical, *l'Encéphale*,
was receptive to psychoanalysis, in general the discipline had no
official embodiment in France until 1926, when twelve men and
women—Marie Bonaparte, René Laforgue, Edouard Pichon, Adrien
Borel, Angelo Hesnard, Raymond de Saussure, Charles Odier, René
Allendy, Georges Parcheminey, Rudolph Loewenstein, Eugénie

---

[1] See Pamela Tytell, *La Plume sur le divan* (Paris: Aubier, 1982); and Roudinesco,
Lacan and Co., pp. 22–25. Here, I address only the advent of psychoanalysis in
France as it relates to French psychiatry and certain of Lacan's texts. I omit a
discussion of Gaston Bachelard and Georges Canguilhem, who were instrumental
in dissolving the distinction between normality and pathology. But as Roudinesco
has pointed out, they had little relation to French psychoanalysis (*Lacan and Co.*, p.
xx). For general histories of the movement, see, above all, Roudinesco, *La Bataille*,
vols. 1 and 2; Mordier; Victor N. Smirnoff, "De Vienne à Paris: Sur les origines
d'une psychanalyse à la française," *Nouvelle Revue de Psychanalyse* 20 (Autumn
1979), 13–58; Marcel Scheidhauer, *Le Rêve freudien en France, 1920–1926* (Paris:
Navarin, 1985).

Sokolnicka, and Henri Codet—formed the Société Psychanalytique de Paris.

At the time, Freud's theories were so controversial that the society's members debated whether to place his name on the cover of the new *Revue Française de Psychanalyse*. Most French commentary on Freud and translations of his work were inadequate at best and erroneous at worst, and thus helped mar his reputation. In 1913 the great psychiatrist Pierre Janet offered a critique of Freud filled with what the scholar C. M. Prévost calls "the most narrow and vulgar clichés that have circulated about psychoanalysis for the last half-century."[2] Janet believed incorrectly that Freud's theories about dreams were archaic, in part because they neglected interpretative techniques drawn from French psychopathology, especially Janet's own teachings.[3] Furthermore, the first important medical article to appear on Freud in *L'Encéphale*, "Le Doctrine de Freud et son école" by Emmanuel Régis and Angelo Hesnard, represented an entirely adulterated version of his thought.

Sherry Turkle believes that psychoanalysis was received with skepticism in France because professional establishments, and psychiatry in particular, were wedded to a strong Cartesian tradition intrinsically hostile to Freudian assumptions about human irrationality. Moreover, France had its own hero in Janet, often touted by the French as the "real" father of psychoanalysis. Finally, Germanophobia and anti-Semitism led to the rejection of psychoanalysis as a foreign and "Jewish" theory incompatible with "le génie latin."[4]

[2] C. M. Prévost, quoted in Scheidhauer, p. 71. Janet had developed a model of the psyche in which a hierarchy of different levels maintained a dynamic equilibrium of psychic "forces," conceived of as physiological. Pathology, in this view, resulted from a "lack of psychological force," which could be remedied by regulating psychic energy. He used hypnotism for this purpose and suggested that the neurotic individual modify his or her environment—work patterns, food and alcohol intake—or transform mental agitation by engaging in "useful" activity. Janet was, therefore, a functionalist. For an excellent overview of Janet's work, see Henri Ellenberger, *The Discovery of the Unconscious: The Evolution of Dynamic Psychiatry* (New York: Basic Books, 1970), pp. 331–417.

[3] Paul Bercherie has noted that "Freud's first model was constructed with conceptual instruments which seemed archaic compared to the modernity of Janet or [Henri] Bergson. For a long time, associationism . . . was dominant in Germany; . . . [German psychiatry] was not influenced by the evolutionism and functionalism which marked the development of both the French and the Anglo-American currents" at the turn of the century and defined their sophistication. Bercherie, p. 67n.

[4] Sherry Turkle, *Psychoanalytic Politics* (Cambridge: Harvard University Press, 1981), p. 39.

In France, nevertheless, as in most European countries and in the United States after World War I, the increasing recognition of the psychological origin of pathological symptoms was linked to psychoanalytic insights into unconscious motivation. Yet whereas elsewhere psychoanalysis rescued the rational subject, the self, from the domination of the unconscious,[5] in France it was tied in with the dissolution of the self, a dissolution that the psychoanalyst Jacques Lacan made the organizing principle of his work.

How and why, then, did French psychoanalysis contribute to the dissolution of the self? Here I concentrate primarily on texts Lacan wrote before the advent of Lacanian analysis in 1953.[6] I analyze how Lacan's work both reflected and recast in new, psychoanalytic terms the dissolution of conventional boundaries between normality and pathology after the Great War. Of course that dissolution was itself the product of and a response to cultural perceptions, in particular the psychiatric perceptions of criminals, the New Woman, and other "deviants" who threatened the return to normalcy after the unprecedented upheaval of that "great" war. I focus on the relationship between those perceptions and three aspects of Lacan's work: his analyses of criminality, the patriarchal family, and schizophrenia, which are connected, if freely, to the categories Lacan later termed the imaginary, the symbolic, and the real, respectively. This triad loosely corresponds to Freud's ego, superego, and id, though Lacan's concept of the role of these psychic agencies is by no means equivalent to Freud's.

The content of Lacan's categories shifted between the 1950s and the 1970s as they were developing, and a full elaboration of these shifts is outside the scope of this book. Instead, I use them as a sort of retrospective frame to give coherence to my argument. It seems necessary to employ them in this way if I am to preserve a clear

[5] American ego psychology is a case in point. It was "founded" by Heinz Hartmann in 1958. He based his own work, *Ego Psychology and the Problem of Adaptation*, on Anna Freud's 1936 book *The Ego and the Mechanisms of Defense*. As Bercherie has remarked, ego psychology easily infiltrated the American analytic community because of its compatibility with functionalism, even though its origins were Viennese. Many proponents of ego psychology were Austrian analysts who emigrated to America before and during the Second World War. Bercherie, pp. 46–47, 67n.

[6] This was the year Lacan gave his famous talk "The Function and Field of Speech and Language in Psychoanalysis," often known as the Rome Discourse. The talk was given at the Rome Congress of the French Psychoanalytic Society, which had split from the Société Psychanalytique de Paris in 1952 and been expelled from the International Psychoanalytic Association.

focus and a clearly defined context, and permissible to do so as long as I do not project a "final state"—an ahistorical, idealized conception of his corpus—onto Lacan's early writing.[7] Thus, I recognize that his earlier work anticipated such shifts (and I often refer to them), but I focus on a specific historical context before 1950. (I make an exception in Chapter 3, which I hope the reader will deem justifiable). No doubt Lacan scholars will find my focus too narrow and reductive and historians will find my focus too general, but such are the perils of interdisciplinary scholarship.

Lacan rejected the post-1920 Freudian topography outlined in *The Ego and the Id*, wherein Freud conceived the ego as an agent of adaptation, integration, and synthesis—of reality—and theorized sexual identity more generally as constituted by the normative regulation of unconscious drives through oral, anal, and genital stages. Lacan rejected both the ego's adaptive role and Freud's model of sexual maturation. Instead, he used Freud's earlier writing on narcissism—one's desire to be recognized and, ultimately, to be desired—as a model for ego formation. He believed that sexual identity was dependent not on innate or instinctual structures but on the mediation of others. That is, as Fredric Jameson has put it, "a previously biological instinct must undergo an alienation to a fundamentally communicational or linguistic relationship—that of the demand for recognition by the Other—in order to find satisfaction."[8] While the psychic agencies perform the same analytic work for Lacan as for Freud, Lacan sees identity as constituted through the mediation of others, through, paradoxically, a process of self-alienation, so that the psychic agencies' operations are determined by, conceal or reveal a lack, an other (as Lacan called it) at the very heart of the self.

In his discussion of the imaginary, the symbolic, and the real, Lacan theorized the different ways in which this other constitutes the self. But what precisely is the other? In Lacan, it refers to the forces that shape the unconscious (on both primary and secondary

[7] The term "final state" is Macey's, pp. 1–25. Macey demonstrates to what extent Lacan's admirers (and even his critics) present all his work as if it were always already in its "final state." He argues that in so doing they dehistoricize his writing.

[8] Fredric Jameson, "Imaginary and Symbolic in Lacan: Marxism, Psychoanalytic Criticism, and the Problem of the Subject," in Shoshana Felman, ed., *Literature and Psychoanalysis: The Question of Reading: Otherwise* (Baltimore: Johns Hopkins University Press, 1977), p. 367.

levels) and is defined in so many ways that it seems infinitely "convertible" and difficult to pin down. For example, the imaginary other may be the mother with whom the child first identifies. The symbolic other is the father, who represents the language that organizes unconscious (imaginary) perceptions. The real other, however, according to Lacan, is impossible to symbolize.[9]

In the chapters that follow, I attempt to pin down the other in its various incarnations by reconstructing the process through which it came both to symbolize and structure the unconscious, the locus of the Other, our "real" self. Yet my emphasis is not exclusively on theory but on history: How are these "others" constructed as other and how, then, does the self come to be constructed as an-other?[10] How did interwar culture generate the structures of the unconscious? Chapter 1 focuses on Lacan's reconstruction of the criminal other, Chapter 2 on the female other, and Chapter 3 on the psychotic, the other side of reason. The story, however, does not begin with Lacan.

[9]Anthony Wilden argues that "it is not possible . . . to define the Other in any definite way, since for Lacan it has a functional value." Later he suggests that "one is led to suspect that the substitution of the words 'the unconscious' for 'the Other' in many of Lacan's formulations will produce an adequate translation." Anthony Wilden, in Jacques Lacan, *The Language of the Self: The Function of Language in Psychoanalysis,* ed. and trans. Wilden (Baltimore: Johns Hopkins University Press, 1968), pp. 264–66. Lacan also introduced a "small other object" (object a) that represents the cause of desire displaced onto a substitute object (e.g., the phallus).

[10]Theory has been admirably emphasized by Juliet Mitchell and Jacqueline Rose in their introductions to Jacques Lacan, *Feminine Sexuality,* trans. Rose (New York: Norton, 1985) pp. 1–57; and in Bowie, "Jacques Lacan," pp. 116–53. See also Bice Benvenuto and Roger Kennedy, *The Works of Jacques Lacan: An Introduction* (New York: St. Martin's Press, 1986); Elizabeth Grosz, *Jacques Lacan: A Feminist Introduction* (New York: Routledge, 1990); and Lemaire. One of the best theoretical accounts of Lacanian analysis is Ellie Ragland-Sullivan, *Jacques Lacan and the Philosophy of Psychoanalysis* (Chicago: University of Illinois Press, 1987). The only limitation of the book is the author's virtually uncritical assessment of Lacan.

Chapter One

The Legal Status
of the Irrational

After about 1860, the criminal body came to be taken as evidence of deviance, and the function of law was to survey and repress criminals who presented a social danger. Scientists measured and minutely detailed the deviant's physique, trying to localize deviance in physical anomalies. The criminal body and criminal behavior were conceived as transparent expressions of a deviant soul, so that the causes and symptoms of deviance were conflated in a physical mark that by its very presence testified to the perversity of the moral will and explained deviance simply by making it visible. Dr. Emile Laurent described the criminal as "a being apart," as "a vulgar type, a cool temperament, average height, a low and short forehead with a deep scar on the upper part, deep-set eyes, large and thick nostrils, the head high and narrow at the top."[1] Good Lamarckians, French psychiatrists conceived criminals as inadequately adapted organisms who transmitted their defects from generation to generation.[2] They labeled these so-called organisms "degenerates"—to use a term first employed in France by B. A. Morel in his *Traité des dégénérescences* (1857). Legislators exploited psychiatric language to justify harsh penalties, including capital punishment and the Relegation Act of 1885, which sent recidivists to New Caledonia for life.

[1] Emile Laurent, *Sadisme et masochisme* (Paris: Vigot Frères, 1903), pp. 183, 111. All translations herein are mine unless otherwise noted.

[2] As Robert Nye argues, in France the idea of degeneracy combined biological notions of criminality with sociological ones. Robert Nye, *Crime, Madness, and Politics in Modern France* (Princeton: Princeton University Press, 1984), p. 126.

But despite legislators' rhetoric, the origins of the Relegation Act were political rather than medical. It was passed during a period of labor unrest, and politicians, remembering the Paris Commune, conflated political and criminal deviance and took a hard line toward both.[3] And in spite of the denunciations of so-called degenerate populations and the harshness of the penal measures, French courts judged criminal responsibility according to a classical conception of free will. Though psychiatrists' relationship to the legal system was becoming increasingly complicated, their main task was to decide whether the delinquent was sane or insane, that is, whether the criminal could be held legally responsible for the crime.

In this context, psychiatrists began to promote a distinction between the incurable recidivist and curable criminals.[4] They relaxed what Nye identifies as the "presumption, initiated by Morel and underscored by Valentin Magnan, that degeneration was largely an irreversible process."[5] They advocated a positivist focus on the criminal body now in the interests of rehabilitation rather than repression. In the name of rehabilitation and hence for the "good" of the criminal, medical men sought to make punishment fit the criminal rather than the crime and hence challenged the primarily

[3] Nye, pp. 66–67. See also Patricia O'Brien, *The Promise of Punishment* (Princeton: Princeton University Press, 1982), p. 293.

[4] For a discussion of this shift, see See Lion Murard and Patrick Zylberman, "De l'hygiène comme introduction à la politique expérimentale, 1875–1925," *Revue de Synthèse* 55 (July–September 1984), 313–41. The idea of rehabilitation itself was not new. In the early years of the nineteenth century, the great French alienist Philippe Pinel advocated the most humane possible treatment of the mentally ill, and between 1810 and 1840 as well, the whole prison system in France was reformed on the basis of humane techniques of punishment whose purpose was to bring the individual back to reason. The inspiration for the reforms was rooted in the Enlightenment and in particular in Cesare de Beccaria's 1764 argument in favor of the abolition of torture and capital punishment. He based his analysis on the moral duty of society toward each of its members, whether the victim or the perpetrator of crime. On the nineteenth-century reforms, see O'Brien, *Promise of Punishment*, pp. 48–49. On the history of nineteenth-century French psychiatry, see Jan Goldstein, *Console and Classify: The French Psychiatric Profession in the Nineteenth Century* (Cambridge: Cambridge University Press, 1987), esp. pp. 64–119. For an overall analysis of the penal system and the meaning of "discipline" through rehabilitation, see Michel Foucault, *Discipline and Punish*, trans. Alan Sheridan (New York: Vintage, 1979). For an anti-Foucauldian assessment of prison reform in France, see also Gordon Wright, *Between the Guillotine and Liberty: Two Centuries of the Crime Problem in France* (Oxford, Oxford University Press, 1983).

[5] Nye, p. 323.

moral considerations still used to evaluate criminal behavior. As the penologist Raymond Saleilles put it in his classic work on the individualization of punishment, the punishment should correspond to the "perversity of the agent" rather than to the nature of the crime.[6]

Psychiatrists delineated intermediate states between sanity and insanity to permit a more refined interpretation of criminal responsibility and thus allow for a more "humane," because more scientific and studied, treatment of criminals. They thus reasoned that if responsibility were to be determined by doctors as well as by lawyers, no one who could be judged by the trained medical eye as irresponsible would be wrongfully interned, and by the same token, no responsible criminal would escape justice. As Jan Goldstein maintains, psychiatrists had their own professional interests at heart rather than those of the criminal. They sought to make these intermediate zones the province of medical expertise, to assert that "insanity and the 'intermediary' nervous pathologies shared an essential nature, making it only logical that the latter be entrusted to the already proven experts on insanity—hence the importance of the new label—*demi-folie.*"[7] But because of what one historian has called a crisis in public and judicial confidence in medical expertise, psychiatrists chose to remain on the sidelines of legal decision making. The contradiction between the increasing demands being made on psychiatrists and the increasing lack of confidence in their expertise can be partially explained by the expanding categories of mental illness—those intermediate states between sanity and insanity or normality and pathology. By the early twentieth century, psychiatric nosology had become so complex that psychiatrists were required to clarify its categories for juries trying to decide the degree of criminal responsibility, even as the complexity was overwhelming the psychiatrists themselves. Psychiatrists could not run the risk of seeing madmen everywhere, nor could they risk presenting evidence to jurors which was not empirically convincing.[8]

[6] Raymond Saleilles, *L'Individualisation de la peine* (Paris: Felix Alcan, 1898), p. iv. In practice, psychiatrists were committed to a peculiarly French marriage of these positivist convictions and a moral concept of liberty, which most considered necessary for social coherence. See Wright, pp. 127–28, 174–77.

[7] Goldstein, p. 333.

[8] For a more general discussion of the ins and outs of this "crisis," see Nye, pp. 227–64.

It was not until after the Great War that an increasing number of psychiatrists supported reforms aimed at replacing legal with medical diagnoses of the criminal, that is, making legal definitions of responsibility correspond to advances in psychiatry and criminology. We can speculate about the reasons for this shift. Jacques Donzelot has argued that psychiatric power expanded along with the welfare state, which transformed the relationship between individuals and public authority.[9] Many psychiatrists saw themselves as leaders in the mission to regenerate French morals, especially by combating alcoholism, prostitution, and venereal disease—social problems that many believed the war had exacerbated.[10] Many thought France's psychic health was at stake. One observer wrote that "the frequency [of crime] had increased so much that it had become part of everyday life, almost . . . banal." The legal scholar Lucien Mialane declared that the influence of economic misery on adolescent criminality was insignificant; the real cause of rising juvenile crime rates was a new psychic restlessness, which "seem[ed] to be one of the most characteristic traits of contemporary psychology." Medical men perceived alcoholism and prostitution as the inevitable consequences of a society that rewarded egotism and the "fast life" and offered "restless youth" nothing to live for.[11] They sought to increase their moral and professional power by facilitating, wrote Yvonne Marie Swiller, a broad "social adaptation and moral reeducation" for a people "weakened and humiliated," as well as for "morally deficient women."[12]

The most zealous proponents of medical intervention were the members of the Ligue Nationale Française d'Hygiène Mentale, founded in 1920 by the eminent psychiatrists Edouard Toulouse and G. Genil-Perrin. One of its intellectual ancestors was the social hygiene movement, which was organized as early as 1902 to combat alcoholism, tuberculosis, and syphilis. It represented the exten-

[9] Jacques Donzelot, *The Policing of Families* (New York: Pantheon, 1979).
[10] For a discussion of these social problems and their link to female criminality, see Chapter 2.
[11] Frédéric Boutet, *Crime d'aujourd'hui, crime d'autrefois* (Paris: Librairie des Champs-Elysées, 1928), pp. 7–8; Lucien Mialane, *La Criminalité juvénile* (Paris: Les Presses Modernes, 1921), p. 61. For a broader discussion of the social context of these developments, see Chapter 2.
[12] Yvonne Marie Swiller, "Déficiences morales féminines," *EC* (June, July, August 1930), 188–93.

sion of public health into a more comprehensive program of social discipline through which doctors sought to improve the so-called quality of the species by eliminating impediments—poor natal care,'veneral disease, and so forth—to healthy procreation. Most important, doctors, Lamarckians that they were, hoped to obstruct what they presumed was hereditary transmission of diseases from generation to generation.[13]

Following a model of social hygiene, the league sought to regulate deviants through a general reform of social institutions according to "scientific" criteria—by adapting institutions to the biological and neurological needs of human beings. It called on citizens to abstain from alcohol and from sex outside of marriage, but such appeals had never been taken as seriously in France as in Anglo-Saxon countries. As one advocate noted, his "hygiene manual" was an effort to adapt prophylaxis, including celibacy and temperance, to French culture, to a "Latin" and, hence, according to him, "a more or less hostile public."[14] But after the Great War the league became increasingly popular, and it even had some influence on public health policy.

The league, taking its inspiration from Belgian and American models,[15] also promoted penal and asylum reform, proposing a system of rehabilitation centers as a better way to combat perceived social evils. The league capitalized on the postwar political and psychic climate to encourage these reforms and tried most of all to shift mental health care away from alienism to psychiatry, from the asylum to the psychiatric hospital, and hence from repression to rehabilitation, from the treatment of the dangerous criminal to detecting and helping those individuals who occupied intermediate zones between normality and pathology. In 1922 Edouard Toulouse was officially received at the Hôtel de Ville in

---

[13] Marcel Jaeger, Le Désordre psychiatrique: Des politiques de la santé mentale en France (Paris: Payot, 1981), p. 85. On the origins of social hygiene, see William H. Schneider, Quality and Quantity: The Quest for Biological Regeneration in Twentieth-Century France (Cambridge: Cambridge University Press, 1990), pp. 48–54.

[14] Dr. Paul Chavigny, Psychologie de l'hygiène (Paris: Flammarion, 1921), pp. 6–14.

[15] According to Marie-Thérèse Lacroix-Dupouy, a National Committee for Mental Hygiene was established in the United States in 1909 to endorse a more "humanistic" treatment of prisoners. After 1920, its influence spread to Europe and Latin America. "Les Services ouverts dans les asile" (Thèse, University of Paris, 1926), p. 16.

Paris after a conference at the Sorbonne on mental hygiene attended by eight thousand people attested to popular support for his cause.[16] That same year, he and another activist in the league, Roger Dupouy, founded the Institut de Prophylaxie Mentale located at Sainte Anne's Hospital in Paris. Converted into the Hôpital Henri Rouselle in 1926, it included a research laboratory, an outpatient clinic, and teaching rooms.

Many psychiatrists associated with the league thus insisted on the importance of replacing legal analyses with medical ones in order to ensure the success of rehabilitation, for the first step in a successful rehabilitation program was determining who could and who could not be cured. Along these lines, the criminologist Paul Schiff argued that the only means to reclaim criminals and psychopaths was through a "reeducative segregation based on a medical and psychiatric foundation instead of a punitive segregation based on a juridical one."[17] As Frédéric-Jean Desthieux remarked, the league was undertaking no less than a "vast sanitary and social reorganization necessary to the regeneration of the social body" when it insisted on the substitution of medical for legal intervention in social life:

Since the individual has not been appropriately educated, rare are those sick people who will turn themselves over to psychiatric care. How can they even know they are ill? Will their entourage even allow them to seek help? Psychiatrists can predict all accidents (Dr. Dupouy affirms it). When they are not predicted, it is because of a defect in social organization. Society accepts that 65 thousand of its curable citizens be interned each year—forever. Society does not demand that the doctor be the assistant of the sick and the defender of society.[18]

Paul Schiff perhaps put it most bluntly when he argued that psychiatrists could not continue to claim that a criminal was both abnormal and responsible for his or her crime when legal logic had always equated abnormality with nonculpability; instead, he insisted, legal concepts had to be reformed in accord with psychi-

16 "Chronique," HM 20 (May 1925), 110–12.
17 Paul Schiff, "Les Anormaux devant la refonte du code pénal," EP no. 4 (1934), 82.
18 Frédéric-Jean Desthieux, Scandales et crimes sociaux (Paris: La Pensée Française, 1924), pp. 171, 178–79.

atric knowledge, moral sentiment had to give way to science.[19] Whereas Raymond Saleilles had made the same argument about the inconsistency of medical attitudes toward the criminal at the turn of the century, he had insisted, as had most doctors, on a fundamental separation between medical and legal domains, a separation Schiff, Toulouse, and others during the interwar years firmly rejected.[20]

This insistence on replacing legal with medical diagnoses clearly manifests expanding psychiatric power. More important, it provides one window on how that power was expanded and why it took the theoretical forms it did. Of course, psychiatric expansion was linked to the relationship between psychiatry and the state. As William Schneider has argued, by the 1920s, social hygiene was indistinguishable from public health, and doctors became agents in the state's effort to use science to regenerate a presumably declining and defective population. Moreover, the National League for Mental Hygiene was closely linked to the French Eugenics Society and had broad connections to influential legislators concerned with health questions.[21] But in order to address how the medicalization of punishment shaped the reception of psychoanalysis, I want to focus instead on the efforts of psychiatrists to distinguish normal from abnormal criminals, curable from incurable ones, to define the intermediate classificatory space between normality and pathology and identify those who represented a social danger.

Identifying Criminals: Reform Proposals

The question of asylum reform was brought to the fore in 1924 when the trial of the psychiatrist and league member Roger Dupouy resuscitated the discussion of criminal responsibility which had begun at the end of the nineteenth century. Dupouy had been accused by the Tribunal of the Seine of violating the law of 1838 by admitting into his open-service clinic at Château de Fontenay a patient who should have been placed in an asylum. Dupouy was finally acquitted because the expert psychiatrists called in to judge

---

[19] Schiff, "Les Anormaux," p. 84.
[20] Saleilles put it this way: "People can give up bread for a short time . . . [but] they cannot give up justice" (pp. 146–47).
[21] Schneider, pp. 135–40, 181–86.

the patient's mental state could not agree on whether she required internment or not. The tribunal attempted to clarify earlier definitions by defining an *aliéné* as someone who could "compromise public order and who presents a danger to himself or to others," but this clarification made the psychiatrists' task no easier.[22] How, after all, were they to determine whether Madame H. was dangerous? It was becoming increasingly difficult to make such a judgment with any confidence. As Dupouy himself put it, "Clinically mental illness is impossible to define. It is not an autonomous illness, characterized by an ensemble of determinant causes, of objective symptoms that can be easily perceived and controlled by any observer. It is constituted by an infinite series of the most different, the most opposed, and the most contradictory psychopathic states."[23]

The accusation of Dupouy and one of the rationales behind his acquittal—the confusion among psychiatrists over whether his patient was mentally ill—were part of a political struggle within the psychiatric profession which it is not my intention to discuss.[24] More important for my purpose is that the rationale was in fact only a symptom of the more general dissolution within psychiatric discourse of a clearly recognizable boundary between the normal and the pathological. It was not that psychiatrists were confused about what constituted pathological behavior. The problem was that they could no longer seem to link behavior to a diagnosis of pathology in any coherent way, despite their efforts to discover a scientific basis for criminal responsibility with which to assess who could be rehabilitated and how.

In 1921 one E. Garçon commented that "the progress of experimental psychology and psychiatry had ruined the simple idea that all men who were normal could be held responsible for their crimes." He went on to note, as turn-of-the-century psychiatrists

[22] Edouard Toulouse, "A propos d'un procès récent," *L'Informateur des Aliénistes et des Neurologistes* (July–August 1924), 168–69. The imprecision of the term *aliéné* had been alluded to several times in the latter half of the nineteenth century. See Goldstein, p. 332.

[23] Roger Dupouy, "L'Internabilité des malades mentaux et l'internement des aliénés," *La Consultation* (December 1924), 234.

[24] Many psychiatrists judged Dupouy and Toulouse to be too extreme, too willing to infringe on the individual liberties of patients. See "Le Referendum sur les services ouverts et sur la situation du Dr. Toulouse," *L'Aliéniste Français* (March, 1933), 139–44.

had already argued, that there was no "precise limit between madness and reason." While the "judge feels powerless to penetrate the mystery of conscience and calls on the alienist, the most enlightened alienists refuse to respond to these questions, which they declare beyond scientific resolution." The solution had been sought in various theories of criminal responsibility, most of which had failed to shed much light on precisely how to detect real criminal intent, how to distinguish between normal criminals and pathological ones.[25] Henri Verger put it this way: "It is impossible to establish a direct relation between [pathological anomalies of character] and the criminal act."[26]

A criminal act could be explained as dementia (in which case the criminal was not responsible at all), as the product of the economic and corollary psychological situation of the subject, or as a moment of temporary insanity in an otherwise normal individual, provoked by a friend's treachery perhaps, or a lover's infidelity. In this way psychiatry attempted to envision all possible organic, social, and emotional causes behind a crime and to take these into consideration when asked to determine a criminal's juridical responsibility for his or her crime. Yet it remained baffled by crimes that offered no such rationally explicable motivation.

Paul Guiraud commented in a 1931 article in *L'Evolution Psychiatrique:*

Science is possible only if it admits, at least as a postulate, the rigorous determination of the phenomena that it studies. Psychiatrists must thus be convinced that all psychopathic acts, as extravagant and unexpected as they are, have causes as precise as the most normal kinds of behavior. However uncertain and hesitant, the study of apparently unmotivated murders can raise interesting problems. While conserving my entire independence from orthodox psychoanalysis, I think in cases of this type it is necessary to admit the possibility of unconscious motivating factors. . . . using the terminology of Freud, we must distinguish crimes of the ego and crimes of the id [*soi*]. In the first case, the individual acts of his own will and with the illusion of freedom; in the second, the organism directly

25 E. Garçon, "Le Code de l'école d'anthropologie criminelle," *Journal des Débats,* July 8, 1921, pp. 63–65.

26 Henri Verger, *L'Evolution des idées médicales sur la responsabilité des délinquents* (Paris: Flammarion, 1923), pp. 155–56.

obeys the id [*ça*], and the ego remains a surprised spectator, passive and sometimes resistant.[27]

Because of the insufficiency of psychiatric categories to explain "inexplicable" criminal behavior, Guiraud, obviously no proponent of psychoanalytic method, insisted on the necessity of considering unconscious motivation. He was not alone in his frustration. Psychiatrists realized that if science could not establish a correlation between a criminal act and a specific, appropriate cause, then the entire enterprise, as Guiraud had pointed out, was seriously threatened. Henri Claude, for example, wrote in 1932 that more and more psychiatrists were having trouble deciding who was lucid at the moment of a crime and who was not.[28] Without a relatively clear definition of what constituted normality, and hence of what kind of behavior could be expected in a given context, it was impossible to judge to what extent the criminal could be held responsible for the crime.

The psychiatrist M. G. Calbairac remarked that what was so problematic about postwar crime was that its perpetrators were often "insufficiently psychotic to intern."[29] In 1930 a psychiatrist named Truelle wrote an inconclusive case study about an apparently well-adjusted worker who had killed his boss for no appreciable reason. "B.," he claimed, "shows no signs of pathology," and his crime is "inexplicable."[30] Dr. Paul Chavigny acknowledged that criminals could no longer be identified by appearance alone, and he found it profoundly troubling that doctors, at least those with prolonged experience, "now know that anomalies frequently appear, even very frequently, in individuals whose family milieu, whose refined education, and whose professional, worldly status would, or so it would seem, guarantee against such accidents."[31]

Along these lines, another psychiatrist, Paul Courbon, sought to

[27] Paul Guiraud, "Les Meurtres immotivés," *EP* no. 2 (March 1931), 25–26.
[28] Henri Claude, *Psychiatrie médico-légale* (Paris: G. Doin, 1932), pp. 1–40.
[29] M. G. Calbairac, "Les Répercussions de la Grande Guerre sur la criminalité en France," *EC* (March–April 1928), 18.
[30] Truelle, "Un Cas curieux de psychologie criminelle," *EC* (July–August 1929), 228.
[31] Dr. Paul Chavigny, *Sexualité et médecine légale* (Paris: J. B. Baillière et Fils, 1939), p. 21.

redefine the concept of mental lucidity (with reference to the criminal act) as mental "validity" (*validité*) since, according to him, lucidity was only the appearance of validity (i.e., the ability to reason).[32] He noted a frequent discrepancy between a patient's words, which might show no sign of pathology, and that patient's quite pathological acts. Several other psychiatrists corroborated Courbon's observation. Marie-Thérèse Lacroix-Dupouy warned that one must never judge a patient on the basis of his or her speech alone, for there existed a great discrepancy between speech and action, as well as between speech and writing.[33] It was this discrepancy between speech and writing that fascinated the young Jacques Lacan.[34]

The penal and asylum reforms proposed during the early 1930s should consequently be understood in Foucauldian terms as an attempt to construct the criminal, to make the criminal "visible." Among the most far-reaching proposals were the replacement of the word *dementia* by *états mentaux pathologiques* in article 64 of the penal code—an old issue;[35] the creation of annexes in prisons for the psychiatric study of criminals to facilitate crime prevention and determine who could or could not be rehabilitated; and the establishment, as an alternative to asylums, of open-service clinics in hospitals, for mental patients not necessarily requiring internment.

In a plea for the reform of the penal code, René Charpentier, an eminent psychiatrist, claimed that given the multiplying nuances of psychopathology as understood by modern psychiatry, the definition of criminal responsibility in the code had become obsolete.[36] Furthermore, he argued, since the traditional concept of moral liberty had not proven demonstrable, science had to find a new criterion for judging criminal responsibility. New psychiatric discoveries had replaced the old notion of dementia, formerly used

[32] Paul Courbon, "La Lucidité et la validité mentales," *AMP* 82 (1924), 111–14.
[33] Lacroix-Dupouy, pp. 25, 88–100.
[34] Jacques Lacan, J. Levy-Valensi, Pierre Migault, "Ecrits inspirés: Schizographie," *AMP* 89 (1931), 508–22.
[35] The earliest reform of the code took place in 1832, when a measure allowing "extenuating circumstances" permitted a more nuanced conception of criminal responsibility. See Nye, p. 28.
[36] René Charpentier, "A propos de la réforme du code pénal," *AMP* 91 (1933), 354.

to excuse criminals, with a panoply of diverse mental states under whose influence individuals could be held at least partially responsible for their crimes. These discoveries motivated the requested word change in article 64, which represented an attempt to modernize the conception of criminal responsibility in keeping with the recognition that dementia had been erroneously used to characterize a whole range of pathologies that were not necessarily demential.

The construction of annexes was an old idea justified in both old and new terms. In 1907 the Dubief Bill proposed special quarters for the criminally insane, which psychiatrists vigorously supported by declaring that vast numbers of social misfits were roaming the streets. In reality, according to Nye, they believed the quarters would "ensure a new flow of public appropriations and the subsidizing of the latest technology for the treatment of the mentally ill."[37] After the war, M. Blacque-Belair and others deemed new annexes in prisons necessary to control the "vagabond children" orphaned during the war, as well as to hold prostitution in check.[38] But it was also hoped that long periods of individualized observation in special quarters could help clarify the relationship between motive and act, word and deed, and reality and appearance. Psychiatrists advocated "asylum-prisons" where criminals would remain for longer periods of time and yet be treated more humanely than in the past.[39]

The difficulty of making a clear determination of the degree of responsibility was further compounded by an apparently increasing number of "simulators"—criminals, that is, who pretended to be mentally ill in order to escape punishment. Simulation had always been a problem, but psychiatrists in the past had been able to detect it with relative ease. During the interwar years, however, increasing numbers of criminals seem to have mastered the art of deception, or more likely, simulation did not increase as much as

[37] Nye, p. 244.

[38] M. Blacque-Belair, "Proposition de résolution concernant l'examen des détenus et des condamnés, ainsi que la création d'annexes psychiatriques des prisons et de laboratoires d'anthropologie criminelle," HM 26 (1931), 44.

[39] Dr. André Ceillier, "Exposé d'un projet de loi concernant la création d'annexes psychiatriques dans les prisons, de laboratoire d'anthropologie criminelle, et de maisons d'observation pour enfants vagabonds," HM 26 (1931), 22.

psychiatrists' anxiety about detecting it. One man, condemned to twenty years of hard labor for theft and murder, managed to fool psychiatrists for two years. Another woman simulated madness so effectively that psychiatrists were convinced she had been instructed by another prisoner or by her lawyer.[40] Psychiatrists argued that simulation would be more difficult to pull off in annexes, where prolonged close observation would be possible. "It is relatively easy," wrote Blacque-Belair, "to act like a madman for half an hour a day, but it is almost impossible to keep it up for an entire week without . . . being unmasked."[41]

Finally, the rationale behind the proposal for open services was to permit the institutional differentiation of "real" *aliénés* from psychopaths and criminals who did not necessarily require internment. In an open letter to the minister of health, Dr. Henri Baruk envisioned open services as a multilevel reform whose main goal was medical prevention. Open services would consist of outpatient consultations, of observation within hospitals, and of "closed" services for patients who were temporarily "antisocial."[42] This effort to differentiate between curable and incurable patients would give psychiatrists a larger role to play outside the asylum, and it represented an attempt to work out on an institutional level all the confusion in psychiatry about how to define an *aliéné*. If they could study patients over long periods of time in a friendly, unthreatening atmosphere, psychiatrists hoped they could discover how to identify the psychopath.

Psychiatrists cited a number of reasons for the necessity of open services, the most frequent of which was to establish links between general practitioners and psychiatrists to avoid misdiagnosis. "Considering," one psychiatrist claimed, "that a certain number of *aliénés* and neurotics escape all medical expertise and that in certain cases only specialists can identify them," increased surveillance of all those detained during and after their release was absolutely necessary to ensure the liberty of all. In this way, the

[40] Drs. Lagriffe and N. Sengès, "Sur un cas de simulation de troubles mentaux ayant duré de novembre 1920 à janvier 1922," *AMP* 86 (1928), 237; E. Martimor, "Un Cas de simulation de délire systématisé," *AMP* 86 (1928), 68-75.

[41] Blaque-Belair, "Proposition de résolution," p. 37.

[42] Henri Baruk, "La Question des services ouverts et l'évolution de la psychiatrie médicale," *L'Aliéniste Français* (February 1933), 77.

system would effect the maximum amount of social control with a minimum violation of individual rights. *Aliénés* would be seen not as criminals but as patients, and open services would offer a more constructive alternative to the asylum than prison.[43]

This argument was even reiterated in Georges Inman's popular *Voyage au pays des déments*, which advocated open services and drew a portrait of the ideal hospital. It included a psychiatric ward, a ward in which all patients could be observed, and an asylum for the chronically ill, subdivided into wards for incurables, "idiots," and the demented. Inman described the aim of the reforms as essentially humanitarian: "In France we have for too long considered abnormality as a rare exception, so rare that we . . . marginalized the scientific study of deviance and conceived it simply as an aberration without importance . . . too easily conceiving the abnormal individual as a monster when, in more humane terms, he is . . . a sick person."[44] He only echoed Baruk's judgment that "the notion of the madman who should be isolated must make way for the notion of a nervous, ill person who should receive preventive treatment." And as we have seen, this shift from the madman to the sick person was part and parcel of another shift. Said Baruk, "Exclusively medico-legal and social psychiatry must make way for *medical psychiatry.*"[45]

Thus, when they advocated open services, psychiatrists justified the extension of medical power in the name of a progressive rehabilitation platform that included an apparatus of outpatient services, home visits, and a coherent organization of centers for mental prophylaxis under the umbrella of the Office Publique d'Hygiène Sociale. Open services were implemented by the Popular Front government in 1936 because Lucien Bonnafé and others on the Left believed that such a program would wrest medical service from the "closed hospitals of the bourgeoisie." The government treated medical care as a right, not a privilege, and thus turned it into a truly public function.[46]

[43] Anonymous discussion about construction of annexes in prisons, *AMP* 89 (1931), 312. See also Henri Claude, "Les Aliénés en liberté," *AML* (April 1933); and "Discussion du rapport de M. Henri Claude," *AML* (October 1933), 554–73.

[44] Georges Inman, *Voyage au pays des déments* (Paris: Editions des Portiques, 1934), pp. 210, 193.

[45] Baruk, "Question des services ouverts," p. 76.

[46] Jaeger, p. 85. It is also worth noting that the league's emphasis on the malleability of the organism dovetailed well with the socialists' belief that the environ-

The reforms were thus part of a process through which, in the interests of social order, psychiatrists took over the right to define who was and who was not a criminal. This new emphasis on rehabilitation—on regulating rather than exiling deviant minds and bodies—marked one more phase in a long-term transition Jacques Donzelot identifies, from "restricted psychiatric expertise to general psychiatric expertise," in which medical men conceived themselves no longer as technicians of the body but, in the words of Lion Murard and Patrick Zylberman, as "scientists of the human."[47] But after the war, when the criminal body and the criminal act came to be seen as insufficient to determine criminal responsibility, when it became the preeminent task of the psychiatrist to determine the perversity of the agent, the agent (and hence his or her perversity) proved impenetrable. Just when psychiatrists won the right to draw a line between reason and madness according to the looser criteria permitted by the various *demi-fou* diagnoses, the line proved impossible to draw.

But how to reconcile the dissolution of an easily identifiable criminal character with the expansion of psychiatric power? I believe that the impenetrability of the criminal character did not challenge psychiatrists' power so much as it effected shifts in the deployment of that power (from prison to psychiatric hospitals, from asylums to outpatient clinics, from an overt hostility to psychoanalysis to an increasing tolerance of it). That is, psychiatrists' efforts to replace legal with medical diagnoses were not simply the product of an expanding disciplinary apparatus in which power is, as Michel Foucault put it, exercised rather than possessed."[48] Rather, they were the product of a historically specific dialectic. The medical discussion and elaboration of *demi-folie* during the interwar years in fact provides a good example of the dialectic through which the refinement of a diagnostic category meant to

---

ment shaped human nature. It is worth remembering that Enrico Ferri, a follower of Cesare Lombroso, was a Socialist. This relationship between Socialists and scientific determinism, for better or worse, dates back to the mid–nineteenth century. See Daniel Pick, *Faces of Degeneration: A European Disorder, c. 1848–c. 1918* (Cambridge: Cambridge University Press, 1989), pp. 72–73.

[47] Donzelot, p. 127; Murard and Zylberman, pp. 322–23. Thus, as Michel Foucault has argued, "health" became indistinct from a normative construction of "ideal man." Foucault, *The Birth of the Clinic: An Archaeology of Medical Perception*, trans. A. M. Sheridan Smith (New York: Vintage, 1975), pp. 22–37.

[48] Foucault, *Discipline and Punish*, p. 26.

consolidate psychiatric power led to the reconstruction of the theoretical foundations of psychiatry (or at least opened the way for a consideration of psychoanalysis). In fact, the increasing medicalization of deviance brought about a greater reliance on psychiatric expertise and yet also revealed its fallibility. This paradox becomes clear when we examine the role French psychoanalysts played in the reevaluation of crime and the criminal.

Autopunition

Psychoanalysts supported the gradual transformation of juridical verdicts into vehicles permitting more thorough scientific study of criminals. Yet for them, such reforms offered less a resolution to the problem raised by the discovery of new kinds of deviants than a recognition that the problem did indeed exist. The psychoanalyst René Allendy argued that a medicalized form of punishment might reduce the crime rate but that only a psychoanalytic study of criminal behavior could resolve the problem criminals had raised. Referring to a criminal who risked the death penalty by murdering a man from whom he had stolen only two hundred francs, Allendy remarked:

> In this case the problem remains without a real response until these last few years, since physical or [conscious] mental motives were sought to explain the crime. That is why criminological theories offer no real solution. We have seen that even when theft is involved, murder cannot be entirely explained by material gain. More often than not, material gain is not an issue at all. . . . The number of murders committed for their own sake remain the majority.

Allendy went on to cite the crimes of Sylvestre Matuschka and the Papin sisters, celebrated criminal cases of 1931 in which the murderers seemed to have no motives for their crimes.[49] Matuschka was a Hungarian who derailed trains for pleasure. Though prone to religious ravings, he was an ideal husband and father whom the tribunal declared normal and hence responsible for his crime. The

---

[49] René Allendy, "Le Crime et les perversions instinctives," *Crapouillot* (May 1938), 11–12, 27.

Papin sisters brutally murdered their employer and her daughter for no apparent reason. The scientific inexplicability of these crimes, as well as other less dramatic examples, became the point of departure for a psychoanalytic reinterpretation of psychiatric discourse that made inroads into French criminology even when psychoanalysis was neglected or theoretically repudiated in virtually every other area of study.[50]

The study of madness and crime led psychoanalysts to question the epistemological foundations of positivist analysis. Psychoanalysts claimed that the study of unconscious processes was the only means by which to relate the symptoms to the causes of pathological behavior. They believed the notion of criminal responsibility should be redefined according to the mode and degree of the ego's participation in the criminal act. Crime could therefore be seen as symptomatic of a particular structural relationship among the id, the ego, and the superego.[51]

As Paul Guiraud's statement about the necessity of considering unconscious forms of motivation indicates, such an explanation

[50] In France psychoanalysis was so marginalized that, as Jean-Pierre Mordier claims, a psychoanalytic perspective was not even considered in the postwar discussion of neurosis. In England, however, it was a war issue, shell shock, that opened the medical profession to psychoanalysis. It is difficult to explain why the French reacted differently. Perhaps the refusal to use psychoanalysis to understand shell shock may simply testify to the strength of the resistance to Freud among medical professionals. On the other hand, it is worthwhile to recall that it was André Breton's encounter with victims of shell shock that inspired his interest in psychoanalysis. During the First World War, Breton worked as an intern at the psychiatric center of the French Second Division. Mordier, p. 132; Roudinesco, *Lacan and Co.*, p. 21.

[51] See René Allendy, *La Justice intérieure* (Paris: Denoël and Steele, 1931); Henri Codet et René Laforgue, "Echecs sociaux et besoin inconscient de l'autopunition," *RFP* 3 (1929), 448–63; Angelo Hesnard and Laforgue, "Les Processus d'autopunition en psychologie des névroses et psychoses, en psychologie criminelle, et en pathologie générale," *RFP* 4 (1930–31), 3–84; Laforgue, "Les Mécanismes d'autopunition et leur influence sur le caractère de l'enfant," *RFP* 3 (1929), 735–45; Laforgue, "De l'angoisse à l'orgasme," *RFP* 4 (1930–31), 245–58; Laforgue, "Remarques sur l'érotisation des relations sociales de l'homme," *RFP* 4 (1930–31), 565-88; Laforgue, "Sur la psychologie de l'angoisse," *Le Médecin d'Alsace et Lorraine* no. 7 (April 1930); Paul Schiff, "Les paranoïas et la psychanalyse," *RFP* 8 (1935), 43–105; Hugo Staub, "Psychanalyse et criminalité," *RFP* 7 (1934), 469–89; J. R. Beltran, "La Psychanalyse en criminologie," *RFP* 4 (1930–31), 487–507. These are among the most relevant articles. Apart from Freud's work, one of the most influential psychoanalytic studies of crime was Theodor Reik's *Geständniszwang und Strafbedürfnis: Probleme der Psychoanalyse und der Kriminologie*, published in 1926.

had a great deal of power in view of the relative failure of positivist methodology to decipher criminal motivation. Nevertheless, psychoanalytic studies of crime were vigorously attacked. When psychoanalysts proposed basing criminology on psychological categories, psychiatrists believed they planned to take over the entire judicial process and that they hoped to reorient it along psychoanalytic lines. Jules Romains, who had published an important introductory article about psychoanalysis in the *Nouvelle Revue Française* in 1922, remarked that the psychoanalytic "cure" was unacceptable from a legal point of view; its prescription that we liberate ourselves from repression by killing our fathers and marrying our mothers was simply unrealistic.[52]

G. Genil-Perrin, doctor in chief of the asylums of the Seine and cofounder of the Ligue Nationale Française d'Hygiène Mentale, spent a tremendous amount of energy combating the perceived threat of psychoanalytic intervention in criminology. He wrote an article (and later, a book) questioning the value of analysis in the aftermath of the seventeenth Congrès de Médecine Légale de Langue française, held in 1932 on the topic of psychoanalysis in legal medecine.[53] A psychiatrist identified only as Dide expressed the opinion that "psychoanalysis has a tendency to challenge social order." It was not an isolated opinion, but it is important that he felt he had to state it, for French psychiatrists had never before bothered to take psychoanalysis so seriously.[54]

Genil-Perrin was most concerned by what he considered the surreptitious infiltration of psychoanalysis into areas where, in his opinion, it really had no business being. One of the areas he identified was the legislature. He cited a report presented by a legislator to the Chamber of Deputies about the creation of psychiatric annexes in prisons which demonstrated a surprisingly sophisticated grasp of psychoanalysis and included a reference to a work by the Austrian analysts Franz Alexander and Hugo Staub, *Le Criminel et ses juges*. He also noted the use of psychoanalysis in at least two prominent legal cases. In one, which involved a woman who had shot her lover, the psychiatrist who testified noted that the woman was someone in whom "acts of reflex predominated over acts re-

[52]Jules Romains, *Problèmes d'aujourd'hui* (Paris: Editions Kra, 1931), p. 136.
[53]G. Genil-Perrin, "La Psychanalyse en médecine légale," *AML* (May 1932), 274–371. See also his *Psychanalyse et criminologie* (Paris, 1934).
[54]Dide, "Psychanalyse et criminalité," *Paris Médical* (July–August 1932), 41.

flected on, and psychoanalysis would no doubt reveal the complex ideas dormant in her subconscious."[55]

Genil-Perrin expressed surprise that psychoanalysis had been taken seriously enough to guide politicians in drafting legislation. Nevertheless, he and other psychiatrists recognized, however reluctantly, that Freud's work at least had the merit of drawing attention to the psychological aspect of criminality, a tendency already marked within French criminology. They recognized that Freud had dared to confront the conceptual problems from which psychiatrists had recoiled. According to the criminologist Paul Provent, the concept of the unconscious, if used judiciously, could help psychiatry to distinguish more accurately between the normal and the pathological and to systematize its knowledge of criminal behavior.[56]

But the most influential psychoanalytic study of any criminal, and the second legal case cited by Genil-Perrin, was Marie Bonaparte's analysis of the pseudonymous Mme Lefebvre, whose trial became a cause célèbre. It appeared in the first issue of the *Revue Française de Psychanalyse* in 1927.

Mme Lefebvre had killed her pregnant daughter-in-law for no apparent reason, and Bonaparte's attempt to make sense of her incomprehensible crime was seen as tantamount to excusing its gravity. Bonaparte claimed that "Mme Lefebvre belongs to that category of the insane whom the public refuses to consider mad because they have fully conserved their lucidity, their memory, and their reason."[57] From a psychoanalytic perspective, she maintained, the appearance of sanity is a poor indicator of a criminal's interior mental lucidity, and it was wrong to assume that the absence of symptoms could be taken as evidence of culpability. Bonaparte felt that the progress of science depended on doing away entirely with the "archaic" notion of criminal responsibility by replacing verdicts with psychoanalytic (i.e., medical) diagnoses,

[55] Genil-Perrin, "Psychanalyse en médecine légale," pp. 274–76, 276. See Franz Alexander and Hugo Staub, *Le Criminel et ses juges* (Paris: Nouvelle Revue Française, 1934), originally published as *Der Verbrecher und seine Richter: Ein Psychoanalytischer Einblick in die Welt der Paragraphen* (Vienna: Internat. Psycho-analytischer Verlag, 1929).

[56] Paul Provent, "Le Freudisme et criminologie," *EC* (May–June 1927), 71. See also Provent, "La Psychoanalyse et le droit français," *AML* (January 1933), 9–14.

[57] Marie Bonaparte, "Le Cas de Mme Lefebvre," *RFP* 1 (1927), 193.

and in stating this view, she articulated an affinity between the orthodox Freudians in the Société Psychanalytique de Paris and the hygiene movement. She went on to claim that the important question concerned not the criminal's responsibility but whether he or she was internable. Yet even Bonaparte conceded that this type of legal innovation presented an unresolvable problem from a practical point of view. Mme Lefebvre, she argued, should be treated in an asylum, not imprisoned, and yet she could not justifiably be retained in an asylum when she manifested no chronic symptoms of mental illness. While the penal system had to be reformed to eliminate the outmoded conception of criminal responsibility and to replace punishment with medical treatment, such a reform could not accommodate the paradox that, according to Bonaparte, Mme Lefebvre had killed her daughter-in-law precisely *in order to be punished.* Such a diagnosis in fact precluded any conceivable legal resolution.[58]

By shifting the object of study away from clinical symptoms to unconscious processes, psychoanalysts reversed the psychiatric conception of penal reform. Crime was no longer the problem that needed to be explained but was itself the resolution of a deeper, usually unconscious problem—the need for self-punishment. In the concept of what the French called *autopunition* psychoanalysts thought they had found a way to establish a scientifically grounded relationship between psychic motivation and clinical (or lack of clinical) symptoms. In so doing, they believed they had resolved the mystery of criminal behavior.

In an article published in the *Revue Française de Psychanalyse* in 1930–1931, Angelo Hesnard and René Laforgue wrote:

Among the recent acquisitions of psychoanalysis, it is the incontestable importance of . . . autopunition in human life that has been most seriously echoed in our psychological comprehension in general and

[58] Ibid., pp. 194–98. For a different point of view from Bonaparte's, see Paul Voivenel, *Les Belles-Mères tragiques* (Paris: La Renaissance du Livre, 1927). In his book, Voivenel discusses the disagreements among psychiatrists over Mme Lefebvre's responsibility for her crime. As late as 1935, a doctor writing in *L'Esprit Médical* remarked that psychiatrists should not be permitted to testify in criminal cases and cited Mme Lefebvre's case as an example of why their testimony was unadvisable: three psychiatrists claimed she was responsible and two claimed she was not. M. Coulon, "Psychologie et psychiatrie," *EM* (January 1935).

in our therapeutic attitude in particular. The study [of autopunition] has even appeared so capital to some of us that we expect of it . . . a veritable transformation . . . of our young science, of a nature that will profoundly modify the teachings of the psychology of neuroses, of psychiatry, of criminology, and of pathology in general.[59]

While they warned against the overuse of autopunition as a catchall diagnosis, their enthusiasm was widespread among French analysts. Hesnard and Laforgue's article was expanded into a book in 1931 titled *Les Mécanismes de l'autopunition,* and many other articles helped diffuse the concept.[60] An entire issue of the *Revue Française de Psychanalyse* was devoted to explaining human society in terms of the psychic paradoxes of autopunition (in the context of explaining the origins of artistic and religious inspiration, termed "magic thought"), and Sophie Morgenstern claimed: "At present, analysts are giving birth to new ideas that suggest that the pervert commits criminal acts because of an exaggerated sentiment of culpability; he seeks in this way to punish himself and thereby seeks the moral satisfaction that comes with his own guilt."[61]

In *La Justice intérieure,* René Allendy argued that "from one end of pathology to the other, from organic illnesses to psychic troubles, we find, hidden insidiously behind all suffering, the guilt complex that implies an unconscious consent to suffering . . . and it seems finally that this paradoxical masochism is the most prevalent, the most constant of all human tendencies."[62] It is no coincidence that Marie Bonaparte diagnosed Mme Lefebvre's crime as motivated by a need to punish herself, and Lacan, inspired by Freud's writings on paranoia, explained the inexplicable murder committed by the Papin sisters in 1931 as a form of autopunition linked to their repressed homosexuality.[63]

Freud had developed the concept of autopunition in order to explain various obsessional neuroses. He used it to evaluate the

[59] Hesnard and Laforgue, "Les Processus d'autopunition," p. 4.

[60] See note 51.

[61] *RFP* 7 (1934), including articles by René Laforgue, Adrien Borel, and others; Sophie Morgenstern, "La Prophylaxie infantile et son rôle dans l'hygiène mentale," *RFP* 4 (1930–31), 140.

[62] Allendy, *La Justice intérieure,* pp. 240–41. See also René Allendy, "Les Représentations et l'instinct de la mort," *EP,* ser. 2, no. 1 (1929), 11–26.

[63] Jacques Lacan, "Motifs du crime paranoïaque. Le Crime des soeurs Papin," *Minotaure* 3–4 (1933), 25–28.

"moral masochism" of the supremely "sensitive conscience" as well as to explain the desire to fall ill, to fail, or to commit crime. The origin of self-punishment (Freud called it a "need for punishment") was the introjection of a sadistic impulse:

> It might be said that the death-instinct active in the organism—the primal sadism—is identical with masochism. After the chief part of it has been directed outward towards objects, there remains as a residuum within the organism the true erotogenic masochism, which on the one hand becomes a component of the libido and on the other still has the subject itself for an object. . . . under certain conditions the sadism or destruction instinct which has been directed outward can be introjected, turned inward again. . . . It then provides that secondary masochism which supplements the original one.

Freud went on to distinguish between the normal moral conscience and moral masochism:

> In the first, the accent falls on the heightened sadism of the super-ego to which the ego subjects itself; in the last, it falls instead on the masochism in the ego itself, which seeks punishment, whether from the super-ego within or from parental authorities without: . . . the sadism of the super-ego is for the most part acutely perceived consciously, while the masochistic impulse of the ego as a rule remains hidden from the person and must be inferred from his behavior.

Furthermore, moral masochism eroticizes guilt, makes it a source of libidinal pleasure: "Conscience and morality arose through overcoming, desexualizing, the Oedipus-complex; in moral masochism morality becomes sexualized afresh. The Oedipus-complex is reactivated, a regression from morality back to the Oedipus-complex is under way."[64]

The subject thus unconsciously desires to be guilty, "craves" an unconscious and eroticized "punishment and suffering," and this desire manifests itself in various ways and in various neuroses. For example, referring to obsessional neuroses, Freud remarked:

> If it is asked why the ego does not also attempt to withdraw from the tormenting criticism of the super-ego, the answer is that it does man-

[64] Sigmund Freud, "The Economic Problem of Masochism" (1924), in *General Psychological Theory* (New York: Macmillan, 1963), pp. 195, 199, 199–200.

age to do so in a great number of instances. There are obsessional neuroses in which no sense of guilt whatever is present. In them, as far as can be seen, the ego has avoided becoming aware of it by instituting a fresh set of symptoms, penances, or restrictions of a self-punishing kind.[65]

Here, self-punishment suspends the ego's fear of the superego and manifests an unconscious desire to be guilty which is at once fulfilled (through masochistic pleasure) and repressed (because the pangs that accompany a conscious sense of guilt are absent).

Marie Bonaparte introduced Freud's concept in France in her study of Mme Lefebvre, but it was not until Henri Codet and René Laforgue published an article on autopunition in 1929 that it became the topic of much theoretical debate in France.[66] Hesnard and Laforgue's 1931 book summarized the positions of Ernest Jones, Freud, Sandor Ferenczi, and Wilhelm Stekel on autopunition and its relation to the formation of the superego. All these positions represented variations on or elaborations of Freud's original idea that the self-punitive impulse was the socialized form of an unconscious, introjected sadistic or aggressive drive.

What was most important for French psychoanalysts such as Hesnard, Laforgue, Allendy, and Schiff was that autopunition answered all the questions raised by the psychiatric study of crime which framed the conceptual context of their investigation. It often manifested itself without clinical symptoms and was sometimes recognizable only in expressions of remorse, in strong resistance to clinical treatment, in sexual or nonsexual masochistic fantasies, or in slightly exaggerated quirks of behavior that could not be clearly designated as pathological.[67]

Paul Schiff noted that autopunition was especially valuable in the study of paranoia and claimed that Alexander and Staub's and Paul Guiraud's psychoanalytically oriented studies of criminals had permitted him to analyze a perpetrator of "these incomprehensible crimes" with fruitful results.[68] Hesnard and Laforgue boldly claimed that the psychological diagnosis was more useful than the psychiatric diagnosis, which was helpful only when doctors had to

---

[65] Sigmund Freud, *Inhibitions, Symptoms, and Anxiety* (New York: Norton, 1959), pp. 43–44.
[66] Codet and Laforgue, "Echecs sociaux."
[67] Hesnard and Laforgue, "Les Processus d'autopunition," pp. 14, 37n.
[68] Schiff, "Les paranoïas et la psychanalyse," pp. 89, 93.

deal with real psychopaths. They argued that psychoanalysis could substitute a "judgment of self-punishment for vague and uncertain notions of attenuated responsibility" and that hereafter judges and juries would see the benefit of sending criminals to "special establishments" and emphasizing social defense through prevention, "la prophylaxie du crime."[69]

At the same time, in a debate reviewing Alexander and Staub's psychoanalytic study of criminal behavior all the analysts present agreed that the main problem with the book was the incompatibility of its theoretical proposals with its practical propositions. How could its insistence on psychoanalytic cure be reconciled with the necessity of punishing criminals? The important contribution of the book was to offer an original explanation of the unconscious motives behind criminal behavior. But because those motives were sought in unconscious forces over which the criminal had little control, he or she could not be held responsible in traditional legal terms for the crime. The criminal, in other words, was normal and yet not responsible. Charles Odier noted that Alexander and Staub claimed that penal justice was necessary to assure "social equilibrium" and yet insisted that the punishment of criminals was "irrational" because it in fact encouraged crime. The analyst Edouard Pichon declared that as much as psychoanalysts wanted to do away with the concept of free will in the context of criminal justice, their insistence that a criminal could be held responsible after being psychoanalyzed only reinforced the idea of free will in new terms. After all, on what grounds could one argue that the criminal exercised free will after he or she had been cured? If psychiatrists were committed to the concept of unconscious motivation, they could not claim that only criminals were subject to its tyranny.[70] The question here was thus not, as Jules Romains and others surmised, whether the criminal should or should not be held responsible for the specific crime committed. The question was how to distinguish between responsible and irresponsible criminals.

Crime, furthermore, represented what analysts called a nonsymbolic attempt to resolve an internal conflict. The *passage à l'acte*,

[69] Hesnard and Laforgue, "Les Processus d'autopunition," p. 81.
[70] Review of the debate by Charles Odier, "Comptes Rendus," *RFP* 3 (1929), 550, 552.

as they called it, was a symptom of a self-punitive drive that could not be represented in symbolic form like other obsessions. In the latter, unconscious guilt could be "seen" (as an image literally perceived by the patient in some forms of obsessional neurosis) or was symbolized in some way by the patient's behavior. Franz Alexander, Hesnard and Laforgue noted, "has demonstrated that a large number of criminals execute the crime with the unconscious purpose of resolving some serious internal conflict, because their mental constitution does not permit them to achieve this aim imaginatively or symbolically, as does that of [other] neurotics."[71]

According to Freud, neuroses, unlike psychoses, transpose repressed desire into symbols or behavior symbolic of the original desire. For example, Alexander and Staub diagnosed a young man who took taxis without being able to pay the fare as fleeing symbolically from unconscious desire for his mother. They argued that he unconsciously sought legal retribution (not to mention the taxi driver's wrath) and that his obsession with aimless taxi rides was a form of autopunition linked to an unresolved Oedipus complex.[72]

Crime, however, was nonsymbolic. In the self-punitive drive, as Marie Bonaparte discovered in reference to Mme Lefebvre, and as all the analysts recognized in their debates about the efficacy of traditional forms of criminal justice, pleasure and punishment cannot be differentiated from each other, so that pleasure always refers only to the punishment that makes it possible. That is, because autopunition fulfills desire by punishing it, because the crime frees the perpetrator from guilt by sustaining the desire to be guilty, its motive or origin has no referent. The desire to be guilty—the motive behind the crime—becomes transparent only at the moment the guillotine blade falls; its "reason" could be understood only when the patient, paradoxically, lost his or her head.

If the motive behind apparently unmotivated crime was self-punishment, then the conceptual problem confronting both psychiatrists and psychoanalysts who tried to make punishment more efficacious could not be resolved on a practical (i.e., legal) or— though this was not an issue until Lacan redefined the problem— theoretical (i.e., epistemological) level. How could society effectively punish criminals who unconsciously wanted to be

---

[71] Hesnard and Laforgue, "Les Processus de l'autopunition," pp. 72–73.
[72] Alexander and Staub, p. 209.

punished? How could society "cure" criminals without encouraging their pathology? Crime, like Mme Lefebvre's act of murder, could not be accommodated by any medico-legal discourse or legal solutions.

Lacan's Interpretation

In a 1950 lecture, "Theoretical Introduction to the Functions of Psychoanalysis in Criminology," Jacques Lacan claimed that "the calamities of the First World War having marked the end of [its] pretensions, Lombrosian theory was obsolete [*rendue aux vieilles lunes*] and the simplest respect for the proper conditions of any human science, those which we believe to have invoked in our exordium, were applied to the study of the criminal." He remarked that criminology throughout the nineteenth century could not accommodate crimes whose nature "escaped a utilitarian register," whereas psychoanalysis could explore such crimes—apparently unmotivated ones—without dehumanizing the criminal.[73] This lecture about the insights with which psychoanalysis had provided criminology had roots in Lacan's long-standing interest in criminal behavior, which he had explored in depth in his medical thesis, *De la psychose paranoïaque dans ses rapports avec la personnalité* (1932).

At that time Lacan was at the beginning of his medical career, which he had initiated in 1926 in Paris at Sainte Anne's Hospital under the direction of Gaston de Clérembault and Henri Claude. Lacan was from a traditional, Catholic, well-to-do background, though, unlike most of his colleagues, he had nontraditional interests: He began frequenting avant-garde circles in 1931 and had contributed to the surrealist periodical *Minotaure*, founded in 1933 by Georges Bataille and André Masson.[74] His connections to sur-

---

[73] Jacques Lacan, *Ecrits* (Paris: Seuil, 1966), pp. 135, 134.

[74] Bataille and Masson were dissident surrealists who hoped *Minotaure* might become a forum for those disillusioned with Breton and his followers. Bataille's biographer Michel Surya notes, however, that from the first issue its direction was taken out of their hands by Breton and others, including Picasso. Bataille and Masson did, however, remain occasional contributors. Lacan was also a participant in Bataille's group Acéphale and married Bataille's ex-wife Sylvie. Michel Surya, *Georges Bataille: La Mort à l'oeuvre* (Paris: Librarie Séguier, 1987), pp. 238–39, 347–

realists such as Salvador Dali and to more shadowy avant-garde figures such as Bataille shaped his interest in madness, particularly in mad women, and rendered him sympathetic to Freud's ideas; his thesis represented the first sophisticated use of Freud in any major French study of mental illness.[75]

Lacan's thesis was an effort to understand what motivated a young woman in full possession of her intellectual faculties and with no explicable reason to try to murder an actress with whom she had never had any personal contact. His 1933 article titled "Motifs du crime paranoïaque" similarly concerned the incomprehensible crime of the celebrated Papin sisters, who had mutilated and murdered their *patronne* and her daughter: "To the judge, they gave no comprehensive motive to explain their act: they expressed no hatred, no grief toward their victims; their only concern was to share entirely the responsibility for the crime. To three medical experts, they manifested no signs of psychic or physical disturbance."[76] By analyzing the questions posed by apparently unmotivated crime in *De la psychose*, Lacan approached the more general epistemological problem in psychiatric study created by the absence of a necessary correlation between what he called a specific "characterology" (i.e., clinical symptoms) and the subject's "personality" (i.e., broader psychological makeup). He argued that all psychiatric discourse concerning paranoia had been primarily descriptive, classifying paranoid delirium according to clinical symptoms and explaining its causes in terms of a particular "morbid constitution" that marked an individual's organic predisposition to paranoia.[77]

While the notion of a constitution corresponded to clinical reality, it described only the symptoms of the delirium without explaining how its content was organized. For example, Aimée, the subject of Lacan's case study in *De la psychose*, had no clinically observable memory problems, and yet memory loss was an impor-

49. For additional biographical details on Lacan, see Roudinesco, *Lacan and Co.*, pp. 101–47.

[75]Dali used Lacan's *thèse* to develop his own theory of "paranoid-critical" art. For a discussion of the larger context within which Lacan wrote his *thèse* and its significance, see Roudinesco, *Lacan and Co.*, pp. 110–16.

[76]Lacan, "Motifs du crime paranoïaque," p. 25.

[77]Jacques Lacan, *De la psychose paranoïaque dans ses rapports avec la personnalité* (Paris: Seuil, 1980), p. 53.

tant component of her delirium. As long as proponents of "constitutionalist" theories could not explain the actual structure of the delirium, it would be impossible to define a specific set of symptoms as paranoid except on a superficial, descriptive basis lacking empirical rigor and explanatory power. Constitutionalists, in short, could not explain what motivated the apparently fortuitous crimes of paranoids because they conceived those crimes as secondary, as the consequences of organic factors that provoked psychological "errors."[78]

Lacan claimed that while constitutional factors had to be taken into account in understanding the origin of any psychopathology, only psychoanalysis, which understood delirium as a complicated projection of the subject's personality (instead of as an impoverished form of normality), could demonstrate the relationship between the causes and symptoms of paranoia. Only psychoanalysis could further the psychiatric study of paranoia because it explored the delirium as a structure, as a complex of psychic resistances to a specific psychological context, and hence conceived the paranoid as a person rather than as an ideal "type."

Lacan thus merged a phenomenological interest in lived experience with a psychoanalytic emphasis on unconscious structures. He argued that Aimée's crime was caused by her relation to a particular familial context and explained both her and the Papin sisters' crimes in terms of a "self-punishment paranoia."

In keeping with his theoretical convictions, his analysis recounted Aimée's personal life in detail. She had already manifested erratic or disturbed behavior in the early months of her marriage. She was pathologically jealous of her husband and was herself apparently "frigid." Her delusions began to be systematic when her first child was stillborn and were increasingly pronounced after the birth of her second infant, a boy. Aimée's elder sister, a recent widow who had no children, came to live with the couple not long after they had been married and eventually took over the household tasks as well as the care of Aimée's son. After her sister's arrival, Aimée's delusions worsened. She imagined her coworkers whispering behind her back, believed she could identify veiled slanderous references to herself in newspaper articles, and insisted that all her persecutors were engaged in a conspiracy to end her

[78] Ibid., pp. 74–75.

son's life. Most of Aimée's persecutors were individuals who had successfully achieved goals Aimée had set for herself but not attained. Her female persecutors were successful society women, often actresses, and Aimée imagined herself as having the requisite if as yet unrealized talent.

Lacan argued that Aimée in fact both hated and loved her persecutors because they represented the woman Aimée wanted to be but knew unconsciously she would never become. Such feelings of inadequacy, furthermore, were rooted—as Freud had argued in his own analysis of paranoia—in Aimée's unconscious, unacceptable homosexual desire, which she transposed into hatred of her real love objects. As in Freud's schema, homosexual desire also implied the narcissistic inability to distinguish between self and other. Her delusions were the product of identification with a projected other—Aimée's sister, who represented Aimée's mother—for whom her persecutors were symbolic substitutes:

The image that represents her ideal is also the object of her hatred. Aimée strikes in her victim her externalized ideal, just as the *passionnelle* strikes the sole object of her hatred and her love. But the object attacked by Aimée had no more than a purely symbolic value, and her deed brought her no sense of relief. And yet with the same blow which had made her guilty before the law, Aimée had struck herself, and when she understood as much, she experienced the satisfaction of a wish fulfilled. The delusion no longer serving any purpose, disappeared. The nature of her cure demonstrates, we believe, the nature of her illness.[79]

Aimée's crime therefore represented an unconscious desire for self-punishment. In trying to kill the actress, she both expressed and punished her intolerable love for her sister, for the persecuting other in whom Aimée also saw her ideal self.

The concept of autopunition explained Aimée's cure as well as Lea and Christine von Papin's tranquillity after committing their crimes, cures that expressed a form of psychic relief inexplicable in constitutionalist terms. Furthermore, such crimes did not fall into the category of crimes passionnels because neither Aimée nor the

[79] Lacan, *De la psychose*, p. 253. I have used Jeffrey Mehlman's translation of most of this passage as it appears in Roudinesco, *Lacan and Co.*, p. 114.

von Papin sisters were plagued by the remorse that usually weighed so heavily on the perpetrator of a single crime of passion. By showing how the crime functioned as a form of self-punishment, as the "arrested development of the personality at the genetic stage of the superego," Lacan noted, psychoanalysis could resolve the cause-and-effect problem raised by supposedly inexplicable crimes: "What is original and precious in such a theory [autopunition] is that it has permitted us to establish the determinants in certain psychological phenomena of social origin and meaning, those we define as phenomena of the personality. . . . such a hypothesis . . . explains the meaning of the delirium." Using the psychoanalytic concept of self-punishment, Lacan reconceived the relationship between cause and effect in psychiatry and in fact supported the penal and asylum reforms proposed at the time to remedy overzealous and often misapplied punishment.[80]

But Lacan did not just use autopunition to introduce a more sophisticated version of Freud into France, nor did he resolve the medico-legal problem created by the psychoanalytic study of unmotivated crime. Instead, he used autopunition to recast Freud's concept of ego formation in a new light. Aimée's self-punitive drive not only described the "hidden" or "other" (repressed)[81] self that explained her otherwise inexplicable behavior but also structured Lacan's innovative concept of "self" development—of ego formation and hence of what he later termed the imaginary structure of the self. In short, Lacan did not seek to cure the pathology but used the pathology as a sort of cure, as a means of redefining the structure of human (and hence criminal) motivation *tout court*. Thus, on one level, he used autopunition to structure human behavior in a new way, but on another level, he replicated its paradoxical structure (using pathology as a cure) in his own method. I will take each of these levels in turn.

In his thesis, Lacan reiterated Freud's concepts of ego and superego formation in order to demonstrate that Freud's theory made possible a structural and relational rather than functionalist analysis of psychic development. He linked Aimée's apparently unmoti-

[80]Ibid., pp. 349, 252, 303.
[81]Lacan's concept of repression is not Freudian. In his work *repression* usually means "alienation," as I will point out when it is important. The idea of alienation does not develop, however, until the mirror-stage period, and is not really elaborated in full until much later. Thus, for consistency, I use *repression*.

vated crime in particular to her early, narcissistic (and hence imaginary) identification with others. According to Freud, narcissistic identification is characterized by a lack of differentiation between ego and id, and secondary narcissism describes the process by which the ego (which is a mental projection of the body's surface) differentiates itself from the id through identification with others whom the ego wants "to be" (the subject's ego-ideals, such as Aimée's sister).

In "Mourning and Melancholia" (1916) and "Group Psychology and the Analysis of the Ego" (1921), Freud began to link identification with introjection, and in *The Ego and the Id* (1923) he defined the superego in terms of "a setting up of the object inside the ego."[82] The ego and superego are formed through a process of identifying with and introjecting love objects, the superego, through introjecting authority figures (the incest interdiction represented by the father) in particular. Ego formation is congruent with and organized by a "reality principle," and the ego's function is to mediate between the id and the external world, to avoid unpleasure by defending the id from external interference. The reality principle thus develops to promote pleasure but resorts to delayed gratification and other tactics in order to achieve it. The ego for Freud was thus, above all, an agency of adaptation centered on consciousness and perception, on "reality."

Lacan, however, claimed the "reality principle is in no way separable from the pleasure principle."[83] Freud's 1923 topography, in which the ego appeared as an agent of synthesis and adaptation—of reality—was abstract, he said, and did not account for the concrete terms of ego development. The genesis of autopunition, however,

clearly reveals the concrete structure, imitative in nature, of one of the vital foundations of cognition. . . . the question arises of knowing if all knowledge is not originally knowledge of a person before it is knowledge of an object, if the notion of an object may be, for humanity, a secondary acquisition. . . . this exposé of Freudian doctrines of the ego and the superego brings out the scientific accessibility of all research into a concrete tendency . . . in opposing it to the confusion

[82] Freud, *The Ego and the Id,* excerpted in *The Freud Reader,* ed. Peter Gay (New York: Norton, 1989), p. 638.
[83] Lacan, *De la psychose,* p. 324.

born of all efforts to resolve in genetic terms a problem of a gnosological [gnoséologique] order such as that of the ego, if it is considered as a locus of conscious perception, that is, as the subject of knowledge.[84]

Thus, to the extent that Lacan elaborated precisely how his analysis of Aimée's self-punishment paranoia helped explain ego formation, he suggested that the narcissistic identification structuring the autopunitive tendency is best characterized as an imbrication of ego and id. That is, in Aimée's case, reality and pleasure could not be easily distinguished. Her reality as it was constituted through identification was always an illusion about reality, a projection of narcissistic desire onto an other. In ego formation, he suggested, the ego is not clearly differentiated from the id; instead, as in autopunition, identification involves a misrecognition (Aimée's imposition of her own distorted reality on the world) of reality which constitutes what is real, a repression of the truth about the self (that it is inadequate, guilty, homosexual, etc.) which fulfills its narcissistic desire. But Lacan has not yet distinguished himself from Freud. He simply suspects that the master may have begged the question of ego formation, and he developed and sharpened this suspicion in his work with Aimée.

The Mirror Stage

Lacan developed his insights into ego formation most fully in his innovative and unpublished paper on the mirror stage, delivered at a conference in Marienbad in 1936 and in revised form in 1949 at the Psychoanalytic Congress in Zurich.[85] Lacan argued, as had

[84] Ibid., p. 326. Borch-Jacobsen has also pointed out to what extent Lacan's analysis of Aimée was indebted to Hegel, though he expressed that indebtedness only in veiled terms. I am, however, more interested in how Aimée's crime simply cannot be accommodated by a Hegelian schema (the *Aufhebung* of self and other) and, further, how the context for Lacan's analysis is broader than his reading of German philosophy. Borch-Jacobsen, pp. 26-29.

[85] The 1936 paper was delivered at the International Psychoanalytic Congress at Marienbad. Its contents were reiterated in Lacan's 1938 article on the family (see Chapter 2) and Lacan delivered another, definitive version in 1949 at the Zurich International Psychoanalytic Congress. The paper was published in *Ecrits* in 1966 as "Le Stade du miroir comme formateur de la fonction du je," *Ecrits*, pp. 93–100. The

Freud, that the ego was formed through identification, but he gave a different account of the process by which that formation occurred. As some critics have noted, the paper was influenced by Lacan's early interest in Aimée's *méconnaissance* (misrecognition) and also by psychologist Henri Wallon's work on child development.[86] In 1931, three years before publishing his celebrated work *Les Origines du caractère chez l'enfant,* Wallon had published an article in the *Journal de Psychologie* titled "Comment se développe chez l'enfant la notion du corps propre," in which he argued that infants take their mirror images for themselves.

Lacan's originality, however, derives from his use of Kojèvian terms to revise Freudian concepts. We may recall that Kojève gave a series of celebrated lectures at the Ecole des Hautes Etudes between 1933 and 1939, attended by prominent intellectuals, Lacan among them. As Elisabeth Roudinesco and Martin Jay note, he looked to Kojève's stress on man's primordial lack in order to turn Wallon's emphasis on specular self-identification into a negative dialectic in which human consciousness is formed through interaction with the desire of the other.[87]

After Marx, Kojève transformed Hegel's analysis of the master-slave relationship into a metaphor for class struggle, but he defined the struggle for freedom in existentialist rather than Marxist

---

English version is "The Mirror Stage as Formative of the Function of the I," in *Ecrits: A Selection,* trans. Alan Sheridan (London: Tavistock, 1977), pp. 1–7. For an interesting discussion of the history of its publication, see Gallop, *Reading Lacan,* pp. 74–92.

[86] Benvenuto and Kennedy, p. 44; Roudinesco, *Lacan and Co.,* p. 158; and Macey, p. 111 indicate the link with Aimée's case history but do not explain it. For a discussion of Wallon, see Roudinesco, *Lacan and Co.,* pp. 66–71. Lacan was also influenced by Elsa Köhler and Charlotte Bühler's work on transitivism, in which children's identities were thought to be shaped through empathizing with others. Lacan refers to them in *Ecrits: A Selection,* pp. 1, 5.

[87] See Martin Jay, untitled, unpublished manuscript; Roudinesco, *Lacan and Co.,* pp. 137–42. For other discussions of Lacan's relation to Kojève, see Macey, pp. 95–99; Edward Casey and J. Melvin Woody, "Hegel, Heidegger, Lacan: The Dialectic of Desire," in Joseph Smith and William Kerrigan, eds., *Interpreting Lacan* (New Haven: Yale University Press, 1983), pp. 75–88; Wilden, pp. 179–82, 284–93. For the most extensive discussion of Lacan's Hegelianism and "Kojèvianism," see Borch-Jacobsen, esp. pp. 1–96. Influences other than Kojève include Roger Caillois's article on mimesis, which appeared in *Minotaure* in 1935 and which Lacan cites in the mirror-stage essay, and Jean-Paul Sartre, who himself contributed to the demolition of the transcendental ego. For a discussion of Sartre and Lacan, see Macey, pp. 103–5; Jameson, p. 379; Wilden, in Lacan, *Language of the Self,* p. 160.

terms, as a struggle for recognition by the other (for the desire of the other) in which the slave is willing to risk his life for an essentially imaginary gain. Kojève maintained that class struggle would pass only when the desire for the desire of the other was satisfied. At the same time, he also implied that history was propelled by an ever-unsatisfied desire for recognition by the other, and thus in fact he refused Hegel's emphasis on the ultimate *Aufhebung* of the difference between self and other, subject and object. As Elisabeth Roudinesco has so aptly put it, "Kojève was thus condemned to read Marx into Hegel and Hegel with Heidegger."[88]

But why did Lacan read Kojève the way he did? How can we explain the relationship between his early criticism of Freud and his later use of Kojève? In his article on the mirror stage, Lacan (quite characteristically) mentioned everyone from whose ideas he borrowed except Kojève and Wallon. Instead, he returned to his own early discussion of Freud. We should not, he claimed, "regard the ego as centered on the perception-consciousness system, or as organized by the 'reality-principle'—a principle that is the expression of a scientific prejudice most hostile to the dialectic of knowledge. Our experience shows us that we should start instead from the *function of méconnaissance* that characterizes the ego in all its structures."[89] According to Lacan, the mirror stage occurs when the infant is between six and eighteen months old and constitutes one of the formative events in human development. During this period, the infant begins to recognize and to identify with its image in the mirror and to derive from it an imaginary sense of wholeness, totality, which it experiences with jubilation. At the same time, this identification with its own body as an other constitutes the subject as his own rival, so that its very unity is permeated with distress, fragmentation, and aggressiveness that the subject later projects onto other, usually sibling, rivals.

The infant's "self," or ego, is thus not innate but constructed, as Kojève had asserted about human consciousness, through its identification with an other, in this case, through the reified gaze in whose reflection it (like Aimée) misrecognizes its self. It is this misrecognition (the taking of itself for a unified entity) that constitutes identity, this fantasy of wholeness that constitutes the

[88] Roudinesco, *Lacan and Co.*, p. 140.
[89] Lacan, *Ecrits: A Selection*, p. 6.

reality of selfhood, this self-alienation that, paradoxically, constitutes the self. The self is not, as Freud had contended, constituted by an increasing adaptation to reality facilitated by the ego's mediating, repressive function; instead, as in the structure of autopunition, the self is constructed through a misrecognition of reality which is always repressed, a misrecognition of truth (the truth about the real fragmentation, helplessness, and lack that defines human identity), whose repression constitutes pleasure (the infant's jubilation before its image). It was this moment, in which the self's truth was always already alienated, that Lacan later termed the imaginary.

Lacan's concept of the imaginary represented the subversion of conventional boundaries between normality and pathology implicit in autopunition, the subversion represented by the conflation of reality and pleasure. But Lacan reconceived those boundaries in terms of a repression that was always experienced as pleasure, in terms of a pathology (autopunition) always structured into the normal self. The imaginary structure of the self was thus both a reflection of and a response to the dissolution of any clear line of demarcation between the normal and the pathological effected by incomprehensible or "unmotivated" crime, albeit a response mediated by Lacan's absorption of other texts—of Wallon and Kojève in particular. He used Aimée's crime as a metaphor for an ego that is always an illusion trapped within the mirrors of its own making, and he used the logic of a "self-punishment paranoia" to structure the collapse of the id and ego into an imaginary *moi* conceived as the site of a repression that is always already pleasurable.[90]

---

[90] Lacan thus placed object relations at the center of ego formation itself: "This form [imaginary identifications] would have to be called the Ideal-I, if we wished to incorporate it into our usual register, in the sense that it will also be the source of secondary identifications, under which term I would place the functions of libidinal normalization. But the important point is that the form situates the agency of the ego, before its social determination, in a fictional direction, which will always remain irreducible for the individual alone" (*Ecrits: A Selection*, p. 2). Ellie Ragland-Sullivan notes along these lines that "the pre-mirror, fantasmatic merging with images is what Lacan has called primary identification; his secondary identification is the mirror-stage fusion with others as objects (Freud's secondary narcissism). Lacan therefore views Freud's secondary narcissism, with its attributes of permanence as manifest in ego-ideals (others), as the basic process of humanization, as well as the cornerstone of human interrelations." Ragland-Sullivan, p. 35.

Or, going further, we could say that Lacan used Kojève's discourse about the constitution of human consciousness to transform what was *already* implicit in Aimée's crime into a theory of
human development in which the struggle for freedom, for autonomy and subjecthood, is inseparable from an ever-unsatisfied desire
for recognition. The crime propelled by the desire for the other's
desire reveals that the struggle will never cease, because no "other"
desire will ever compensate for the primordial lack at the heart of
human consciousness. Aimée's crime, in other words, dramatizes
the tragic human struggle to be free of others, whose recognition
human beings always desire: the struggle to be free of the mirrors
that are *at once* the source of human slavery and human pleasure.

Aimée Revisited

When Lacan returned to Aimée in a 1946 lecture later reprinted
in *Ecrits*, he sought to illustrate the relationship of the imaginary
to paranoid psychoses in new terms that reflected his increasing
interest in language (though not yet linguistics). He also made the
"desire of the other" more explicit. Lacan returned to the problem
of "psychical causality" and criticized the inadequacies of behav-
iorist and functionalist theories of psychic development. He
stressed the importance of phenomenological insights and the contribution of Maurice Merleau-Ponty in particular.[91] Lacan brought
up Aimée's case again in order to develop his earlier argument that
madness was not evidence of an impoverished mind, of a falling
away from reality, but of an irreparable self: "Madness, far from
being an accident befalling an organism because of its frailties, is
the permanent virtuality of a rift opened in its very essence").[92]
Paranoids are mad not because their selves are irreparable but because they seek to mend the inevitable rift between the real, irreparable and the ideal or imaginary self. Their effort to blur the essentially permanent discord between who they are and the ideal to
which they aspire constitutes the motive behind unmotivated or
inexplicable crime, its "cause." The crime may liberate Aimée

---

[91] Lacan, "Propos sur la causalité psychique," *Ecrits*, p. 179. The reference is to
Merleau-Ponty's *Phenomenology of Perception*, published in 1945.
[92] Ibid., p. 176.

from her guilt, may "cure" her, but at the same time it reinforces the discrepancy between who she is and who she wants to be which is at the origin of her paranoia (it sustains the desire to be guilty).

As Lacan put it, crime describes a paradoxical movement toward liberty which, because it is itself a form of madness, is always a prison. Madness is a form of liberty and yet also marks its limits.[93] The megalomania symptomatic of paranoid behavior, we recall, is actually part of a dialectic of self-glorification and self-punishment, a form of compensation for feelings of inadequacy vis-à-vis expected social roles: Aimée felt inadequate as a wife and mother. The paranoid thus tries to resolve the discrepancy between her real and ideal selves by constructing an illusory ideal that is a symbolic inversion of real feelings of guilt and inadequacy in a psychic operation that liberates her from those feelings (functions as a defense against them) at the same time as it drives her to crime in order to sustain her illusion.

Yet we know that the criminal act necessarily fails to reconcile the paranoid with her ideal, though within the psychological structure of paranoia that reconciliation is its "purpose". While the crime liberates the paranoid from the unconscious guilt at the origin of her delirium, while it "cures" her, it reveals the absence at the heart of the ego which constitutes her selfhood, since selfhood can be defined only in terms of an imaginary self, in terms of a series of failed attempts to identify with an ideal. Her self, then, is a hollow, empty structure, an absence perpetually replenished by the delirium, by an illusion that disguises the painful lack that is really there.[94] Hence Aimée felt unburdened after her crime but remained trapped in a world of mirrors in which she would misrecognize herself again and again.

Crime thus designates what Lacan called the "limits of signification" (or, in Aimée's case, what he calls the limits of "resistance")[95]—the limits, that is, of the various representational structures that constitute the self. The cause of crime is an attempted cure that is always a form of pathology, always a slippage of the subject into the open rift of madness, which, in her endless attempts to reconcile reality and ideal, endlessly re-presents the

[93] Ibid., p. 176.
[94] Ibid., pp. 187–88.
[95] Ibid., p. 168.

self. This desire to create a self when in fact no original self exists forms the crux of an epistemology that questions the very possibility of epistemology; an incurable madness paradoxically constitutes the rationale behind criminal action. The criminal act marks the limits of knowledge, of signification; it reveals that the self is an illusion (or, better yet, only a reflection in the mirror) and yet convinces its perpetrator that something is really there.

For Lacan, then, the criminal act was not just symbolic of our "deeper being." It did not suggest an unconscious underneath consciousness, a hidden self to be discovered by perspicacious analysts. Instead, the criminal act symbolized a self whose truth could not be represented because it was perpetually displaced, because the criminal act was a form of pathology that was always also a cure, a liberation from guilt that sustained the desire to be guilty. The ego was now an imaginary structure whose function was to resist at all costs the absence at its origins, and it was the criminal act that marked that absence.

Lacan thus argued in his 1950 article on criminology that the quest for the objective, comprehensible motives of crime was but a pathological attempt to construct a coherent individual, a self, when no such entity existed. He condemned the penal reforms he had tacitly approved in 1932 as part of a "sanitary penology" aimed at "affirming the individualistic ideal." In fact, he claimed, all of human history (particularly the history of the human sciences) was but a repetition of Aimée's tragic, pathological gesture (analogous to the one that "drove the old revolutionary of 1917 to the bench of the accused in the Moscow trials").[96] History thus repeated Aimée's gesture because

> it might be said that at every moment [man] constitutes his world by his suicide, the psychological experience of which Freud had the audacity to formulate, however paradoxical its expression in biological terms, as the "death instinct."
>
> In the "emancipated" man of modern society, this splitting reveals, right down to the depths of his being, a neurosis of self-punish-

[96] Ibid., pp. 138–39, 145, 175. Lacan's account of the shift from the theological subject to the bourgeois subject is remarkably similar to the one Michel Foucault developed later. Lacan also argued that positivist reforms aimed at humanizing the criminal in fact represented a new deployment of bourgeois power through a new representation of the self from the eighteenth century on.

ment . . . with the psychasthenic forms of its derealizations of others and of the world, with its social consequences in failure and crime. It is this pitiful victim, this escaped, irresponsible outlaw, who is condemning modern man to the most formidable social hell . . . ; it is our daily task to open up to this being of nothingness the way of his meaning . . . a task for which we are always too inadequate.[97]

Psychoanalysis promises a devastating critique of this "social hell," which the criminal symbolizes but which all human beings live; it can demonstrate to what extent this splitting exposes the construction of the social order as illusory or imaginary. But because the basic process of humanization is not just symbolized but *structured* by self-punishment (the conflation of pleasure and repression), human beings will necessarily keep plunging themselves into a hell from which psychoanalysis will never be adequate to rescue them. In 1975 Lacan explained his reluctance to publish his thesis after so many years by claiming that there was no *relationship* between paranoid psychosis and the self: They are the same thing. The self is always a figment of the imagination; "the core of our being," Lacan said, "does not coincide with the ego."[98] That core is always someplace else.

This perpetually displaced self, as I have argued, represented Lacan's reconstruction of the self's boundaries in terms of a repression that is always a pleasure and, hence, represented a new and compromised subject: one whose actions are necessarily driven by illusions, generated by an other within. His "solution" to the theoretical problems raised by unmotivated crime thus made its motives explicable (and hence, presumably, curable) and at the same time conceived them as a permanent dimension of the human psyche, as motives, then, for which there was no cure. That is, he insisted that criminal behavior had to be explained—that it was indeed other—at the same time as he defined the self in terms of an other. While Lacan thus hopelessly compromised the concept of rehabilitation (how can one cure a pathology that structures human development?), while the analyst lost his or her position as expert, one could by no means dispense with analysts, pursuing tasks for which they will always be inadequate.

[97] Lacan, *Ecrits: A Selection*, pp. 28–29.
[98] Lacan, quoted in Macey, p. 212.

But how to have it both ways? That is, how to envision crime as pathological and at the same time identify psychosis with the self and hence obliterate the crime, which becomes but another attempt to escape from or acknowledge the social hell into which we are all plunged? And how then to legitimate expertise—the need for and privileged position of the analyst—while eroding its foundations, while refusing a normative concept of psychic health?

This paradox is rooted in the history of the imaginary. As I have argued, autopunition was the structure Lacan used to organize other intellectual influences—Kojève, Wallon—and the aporia to which it leads was already implicit in psychoanalysts' attempts to solve the epistemological problem posed by unmotivated crime. Autopunition served to legitimate psychoanalysis. It proved the novelty and worthiness of psychoanalytic insights into an issue that psychiatrists were finding increasingly difficult to resolve in positivist terms. Lacan, however, spelled out its full implications, which Marie Bonaparte and those present at the colloquium reported by Charles Odier had explored only tentatively. Lacan's concept of ego formation served at once to define, to "recognize" the self's structure in new terms (and hence privilege psychoanalysis as an instrument of recognition, if not of knowledge in the sense of truth), and to insist on the fundamental *méconnaissance* of all attempts at recognition. Or to use Paul Bercherie's terminology, the imaginary is "Lacanianism's blind-spot."[99] The imaginary both describes a blind spot, a lacuna that is the core of the self, and is itself the blind spot of Lacan's theory; it describes on two levels a recognition that must always also be a misrecognition.

Lacan's imaginary thus must be seen as the culmination of psychiatrists' and psychoanalysts' attempts to deal with the dissolving boundaries between the normal and the pathological symbolized by the criminal, as the culmination of an effort to assert the power of science, which comes, dialectically, to restructure the foundations of science, of psychoanalysis. The blind spot (the lack of a dialectical resolution) implicit in the structure of autopunition became Lacan's primary insight and the point past which his theory of knowledge could not "see." As I have argued thus far, the dialectic of self-punishment which structures self-formation describes a truth that is at once revealed and lost. To repeat the

[99] Bercherie, p. 58.

argument more precisely: the *passage à l'acte* is the moment when an unconscious drive to self-punishment paradoxically gives the self its form, when the desire to be an other whom one cannot be is satisfied because unsatisfied, repressed. The dialectic of self-punishment thus suggests that the self can be known only when it is repressed, the self's truth (its pleasure) is accessible only when it is lost.

But Lacan, good doctor and psychoanalyst, did not so much want structures in ruin as he wanted to ruin certain cherished structures. Lacan was no celebrant of the imaginary—and hence no celebrant of criminals—even though he believed that Aimée's pathological gesture was the structuring metaphor of the self. He viewed the imaginary as a trap. And it is perhaps not surprising that it was through a devaluation of mothers—after all, Aimée's psychosis entailed an overidentification with a strong mother, transferred to her sister—and a reevaluation of fathers that Lacan began to theorize a way out.

Many critics have suggested that Lacan's fascination with Aimée's psychosis went hand in hand with a more general fascination with the female as well as the criminal other.[100] It is not clear, however, precisely how *female* otherness was structured into his concept of the self in historical and cultural terms—how, that is, criminality, and hence otherness, was gendered feminine (apart from the fact that Aimée is a woman)—until he began working on the social role of fathers. In the next chapter, I turn to female deviants, to fathers, and to another dimension of self-formation for which fathers prove to be indispensable. How successful, then, was Lacan's own effort to see beyond the blind spot he found at the heart of the self, and why would fathers necessarily be a privileged locus of sight?

[100] Roudinesco makes this observation in *Lacan and Co.*, pp. 20–21; so does Catherine Clément, *The Lives and Legends of Jacques Lacan* (New York: Columbia University Press, 1983), pp. 53–101; and Grosz, p. 6. For a critique of woman as other in Lacan, see Alice Jardine, *Gynesis: Configurations of Woman and Modernity* (Ithaca: Cornell University Press, 1985), pp. 159–77.

Chapter Two

Gender Complexes

If the theoretical problem of unmotivated crime challenged psychiatric expertise and rendered many, though not by any means all, medical men sympathetic to the insights afforded by psychoanalysis, most doctors represented the immediate criminal threat to social order in terms of gender—in terms, above all, of nonconformist, "deviant" women. This chapter examines the relationship between the psychiatric and psychoanalytic constructions of female criminals and the young Lacan's effort to save men and women from the trap of the imaginary. In order to address that relationship, we must turn once again to the perceived dissolution of the boundaries between the normal and the pathological after the Great War. This time we are concerned with the boundaries between normal and pathological women. I focus on how female deviance came to symbolize a crisis of male authority which began in the late nineteenth century and crystallized after 1918. Second, I examine how these representations of female deviance both symbolized and shaped a new representation of the (male) self as other in the work of psychiatrists, psychoanalysts, and Lacan. Of what did Lacan construct the (male) self? Of what did Lacan construct his resolution of the conflation of self and other represented by the imaginary?

The New Woman

French cultural critics had long linked national decline and moral decadence to female deviance. When the French lost the Franco-

Prussian War in 1870, the defeat was attributed to a peculiarly French malaise manifested in a declining birth rate. As the historian Angus McLaren has demonstrated, after 1870 the social control of women's bodies was deemed essential to the health of a nation threatened by a sluggish birth rate, and women's "unnatural" efforts to control family size—through abortion, infanticide, or any other means—became the focus of a campaign that culminated in the 1920 law forbidding the sale and distribution of contraceptives and literature about how to use them.[1] Countless satires and political tracts linked France's so-called loss of virility to depopulation and depopulation to feminism, to women's refusal of their designated social roles.

The "New Woman"—as journalists dubbed the sexually independent woman—had, one reported, "ranged herself perversely with the forces of cultural anarchism and decay."[2] The misogyny of much fin-de-siècle art and literature—the portrayal of women as monsters, vampires, or abominable criminals and of men as their victims—was in many ways a male fantasy of female potency (and of male impotence) which linked cultural dissolution and decay to female power.[3]

Prewar medical texts conceived women as repositories of sexuality that had to be contained and controlled. Female sexuality defined female nature and was perceived as the source of both women's power and their weakness. Women were considered both nymphomaniacal and passive, sadistic and masochistic, and men were thereby conceived as both their innocent prey and their inevitable masters. This contradictory logic suggested that all women were potentially deviant: Normal women contained and hence repressed their sexuality, whereas deviant women made it discern-

[1] Angus McLaren, *Sexuality and Social Order: The Debate over the Fertility of Women and Workers in France, 1770–1920* (New York: Holmes and Meier, 1983), pp. 169–70. See especially chap. 9, "Abortion as Birth Control," pp. 136–153. The 1920 law forbade the mere advocacy of abortion or birth control. The penalties were fixed at a fine of one hundred to three thousand francs plus imprisonment for six months to three years.

[2] Linda Dowling, quoted in Elaine Showalter, *Sexual Anarchy: Gender and Culture at the Fin-de-Siècle* (New York: Viking, 1990), pp. 38–39.

[3] On the connection between "modernism and masculinism," see Sandra Gilbert and Susan Gubar, *No Man's Land: The Place of the Woman Writer in the Twentieth Century* (New Haven: Yale University Press, 1988), esp. pp. 125–62. See also Showalter, pp. 144–87.

ible and identifiable, symbolized it. Medical men equated female sexuality with female power and used the pseudoscientific construction of sexual difference as a pretext for both identifying and controlling it.

Female sterility, embodied by the lesbian, was frequently used in fin-de-siècle literature as a metaphor for all that was *contre-nature* (against nature), juxtaposing a specific social concern about female sexuality with a medical discourse about deviance.[4] Female sexuality freed of its procreative functions operated as the metaphor par excellence for a contaminated, because excessive, sexuality that served as a conceptual link among the standard nineteenth-century deviants: the prostitute, the homosexual, and the criminal-madman. All were believed to be tainted by a degenerate, because excessive, sexuality, and all were seen as metaphorically sterile and hence unproductive. Many famous characters of fin-de-siècle literature—Zola's Nana, Wedekind's Lulu—exemplify the medical definition of deviance, which represented disease as sexual insatiability, often linked with working-class status: They are all compelled to sell or offer their bodies for pleasure; they cannot help but want more, and they drive themselves to sickness and death in order to get it.

Before the Great War, deviance was increasingly linked to a degenerate sexuality. In considering perversion, nineteenth-century medical men often did not distinguish between biological dysfunction and the moral character of the sufferer and thus used the biological defect as a metaphor for the pervert's soul.[5] Sexual and other deviants were assimilated into a larger category of degenerates, individuals who were physiologically defective and hence diseased, perverts whose aberration was quite literally written on their bodies. As Sander Gilman has written, "The identity of the Other, whether social outcast, marginal member of society, or sexual degenerate, is carried in his or her appearance. The Other looks different."[6]

---

[4] Nicole Albert, "Lesbos et la décadence: Images du sapphisme dans la littérature décadente," *Diplôme d'Etudes Approfondies, Université de Paris* 4 (1988).

[5] For a general discussion of this development, see Michel Foucault, *The History of Sexuality* (New York: Vintage, 1980). See also Arnold I. Davidson, "Sex and the Emergence of Sexuality," *Critical Inquiry* (Autumn 1987), 17–48.

[6] Sander Gilman, *Difference and Pathology: Stereotypes of Sexuality, Race, and Madness* (Ithaca: Cornell University Press, 1985), p. 70.

Although this medicalization of deviance survived the war and the biologically "natural" remained an important reference for writers and doctors who sought to justify their vision of morally appropriate behavior, the distinction between normal and abnormal individuals and hence between natural and unnatural practices had become increasingly tenuous by the turn of the century. Many physiological theories of character disorder had been discredited, and the development of dynamic psychiatry suggested, as one psychiatrist concluded rather dramatically in 1899, that "only 3 percent of the population is normal as we have defined it."[7]

Already in the early 1900s, the external signs of deviance—the degenerate appearance associated with abnormality (and almost always with a particular race, class, and gender)—were increasingly acknowledged to be unreliable indicators. Instead, all individuals, regardless of appearance (or race or class), became potentially suspect, potentially guilty of concealing a pathological character. Medical men conceived female deviance and prostitution in particular as a universal tendency, a potential implicit in female nature to which various kinds of crimes (prostitution above all) were visible clues.[8] When the clues themselves were absent or concealed, medical (or state) intervention became more imperative. Dr. Eugène Prévost argued that abortion, in contrast to infanticide, was a specifically modern crime because both the crime and the women who perpetrated it were or could be made invisible. Abortion, he insisted, was a crime of sophisticated urbanites who had perfected the art of deception.[9] On another note, Dr. G. St. Paul claimed that homosexuals could not necessarily be recognized by their appearance, that, contrary to common assumptions, they were an invisible population.[10]

[7] Dr. Joanny Roux, quoted in Chavigny, p. 51.
[8] See Gilman, p. 55.
[9] Dr. Balthazard and Eugène Prevost, *Une Plaie sociale* (Paris: A. Maloine, 1912), pp. 27–29. Angus McLaren (p. 140) has noted that after 1880 all working-class women regardless of martial status began to be suspected of performing abortions: instead of the seduced and betrayed (and desperate) domestic, the suspect was a married woman seeking to control the size of her family. The shift was part of the hysteria concerning the demographic crisis and the need to control all women.
[10] Dr. G. St. Paul, *Thèmes psychologiques: Invertis et homosexuels* (Paris: Vigot Frères, 1930), p. 11. This edition is a reprint of a version published in 1896, but the preface is revised. For a problematic, because homophobic, discussion of the debates about male homosexuality and the (primarily German and Austrian) challenges to

But in spite of this new emphasis on concealment, the portrait of the deviant remained that of a working-class individual who was somehow marked and could be identified and controlled. Even so-called clandestine prostitutes in the late nineteenth century were conceived as threatening, paradoxically, because of their increasing *visibility*. One observer remarked that clandestine prostitution "advertises itself and has become arrogant; if it was hidden before, it shows itself today."[11] In spite of some alarm about the demimondaines (mostly kept prostitutes), who moved easily and often undetected between different levels of society, it was not until after the war that the absence of a clearly definable or identifiable deviant nature correlated with a new image of the deviant. Doctors and writers effected a broader cultural shift in the image of the deviant away from a visible, discernible, and hence controllable threat.

By the 1920s deviants were conceived more generally as uncontrollable, characterized by their invisibility and ability to evade justice.[12] Both adolescent and female criminals were described less in terms of their brutality or their degenerate appearance than in terms of their stealthiness and their cunning. Whereas the prewar discourse referred to both male and female criminals in hordes and bands and evoked the physical marks of deviance—the depraved milieu, the sinister gaze, the jaundiced skin—after 1918 criminals were characterized as "reptiles,"[13] as slippery and obscure figures whose actions were impossible to interpret or predict. Clearly, the shift originated in the late nineteenth century (as did almost all social and cultural developments that culminated after the war), and the female images of interwar modernism were heirs of the fin de siècle, but the war helped mobilize old images in new ways and in so doing created a new kind of female deviant symbolic of widespread moral anarchy. And the strategies of social control designed to meet the threat of this modern deviant were new as well.

---

the idea that homosexual men bore corporeal signs of their perversion, see Antony Copley, *Sexual Moralities in France, 1780–1980: New Ideas on the Family, Divorce, and Homosexuality* (New York: Routledge, 1989), pp. 135–54.

[11] Félix Carlier, quoted in Jill Harsin, *Policing Prostitution in Nineteenth-Century Paris* (Princeton: Princeton University Press, 1985), p. 242.

[12] I use invisibility not in its literal sense (though it is often applicable) but rather as a metaphor to describe a new experience of the threat posed by deviance.

[13] Mialane, pp. 8–9.

The perceived shift from visibility to invisibility in conceptions of criminal deviance was part of a changing perception of social order itself and, in particular, of the relationship between the sexes. Female cunning was frequently invoked as a literal cause of post-war anarchy and more often as a metaphor for a world in which no one could be trusted, in which things were frequently not what they seemed, and in which fathers had lost their authority. Medical men in particular represented political threats in terms of gender. Women's repudiation of traditional gender roles and the new relationships between men and women were the presumed causes of social disorder, and the New Woman—now dubbed *la garçonne* (the bachelor-girl)—once again became the symbolic center of moral crisis. Her deviance was the metaphor for the new utilitarianism, frivolity, and selfishness contemporaries viewed as characteristic of the postwar years.[14]

The loosening of morals to which crime was to be attributed had begun before 1918 and had been held partly responsible for the demographic crisis that became an issue after the French defeat in the Franco-Prussian conflict. Nevertheless, the First World War was perceived to have encouraged this new morality at the same time as it turned the demographic crisis into catastrophe: Thousands of young men had lost their lives. As many historians have argued, particularly in trying to understand the appeal of fascism, the war was generally conceived to have eroded the spiritual values it was originally supposed to foster. Crude utilitarianism, especially a lust for money, was only one significant reflection of the "new" egotism of young men and women. Their elders accused them of refusing the kind of deep emotional commitment that their parents had made to each other and of consequently shirking the responsibility of marriage and family.[15]

[14] The prolific French writer Victor Margueritte coined the term *la garçonne* in 1922.

[15] On the general issue of sexuality and social order after the war—an enormous topic with many dimensions that I cannot cover here except as they relate to the debate about criminality—see Yvonne Delatour, "Le Travail des femmes pendant la première guerre mondiale et ses conséquences sur l'évolution de leur rôle dans la société," *Francia* 2 (1974), 482–501; James F. MacMillan, *Housewife or Harlot: The Place of Women in French Society, 1870–1940* (Sussex: Harvester Press, 1981). MacMillan has demonstrated that despite the perception of moral crisis due to women's repudiation of normal gender roles after the war, in reality marriage increased as the stigma of remaining single became more difficult to bear (p. 126). Interestingly

As panicked male leaders saw it, just when national security required that women devote themselves more exclusively than ever to reproduction, the war had freed them from traditional social roles because it allowed them to work outside the home and in jobs traditionally reserved for men and it gave new life to feminist demands for the vote. It liberated both women and men from the social and sexual obligations imposed on them by marriage as men left home for extended periods of time. The increased liberty of both women and young men and the newfound social and economic independence of many women—or rather, their demands that that independence be institutionalized to prevent its loss—thus coincided with an imagined crisis of the race, which women's autonomy was perceived to exacerbate.

Between the late 1920s and 1930s, Dr. Robert Teutsch compiled the opinions of journalists, doctors, and other social commentators on the "woman question," and published them in a collection purporting to analyze the impact of feminism on French social and moral life. The collection appeared in 1934, the year of the fascist riots at the Place de la Concorde and twelve years after Victor Margueritte published *La Garçonne*. Teutsch believed feminists threatened social order. "Females who do not want to live as real women," he said, "conscious of the duties their dignity requires, must sooner or later be corrected . . . or sent back to the unworthy ranks from whence they came. It is one of the only ways to save our society from certain sources of moral putrefaction."[16] Dr. M. de Hell expressed the same sentiment with as much conviction but less venom:

> The man, the foundation of the home, the family, of class, of peoples, and of nations, the man can play his predestined role only if he can root himself in it with dignity and permanence, sentimentally and materially. Woman is created and born into this world above all in

---

enough, the idea of a moral crisis expressed in these terms was also said to plague the medical profession—the eventual focus of our interest. In a survey conducted in 1930 in *L'Esprit Médical*, most doctors concluded that medicine itself was in moral crisis because young doctors trained after the war had committed themselves to the profession for material gain rather than emotional satisfaction. *EM* (September 1931), 6.

[16]Dr. Robert Teutsch, *Le Féminisme* (Paris: Société Française d'Editions Littéraires et Techniques, 1934), p. 261.

order to make it possible for him to do so. If she refuses to remain in her natural place, she will contribute to social danger. Such is the ABC of all societies.[17]

Such remarks expressed the general attitude toward what was perceived as women's selfishness as well as a fantasy about its consequences which was mirrored in the perception of youth. The journalist Claude Barjas noted what he called the "arrogance of youth today." "Young generations, those that came of age just after the war, are full of dryness and cynicism; they glorify vices which were not always considered so refined, and manifest a real contempt for all that has to do with love or sentiment."[18] Another writer, Lucien Descaves, described a young boy who hated any kind of criticism and claimed that he was a typical specimen of the new generation, whose "arrogance is extreme. . . . The adolescent, regardless of the milieu from which he comes . . . is conscious of only one thing: his superiority."[19] Adolescents shared the attitudes and the behavior of women in a world in which men and the noble values associated with paternal discipline had disappeared. "Men no longer exist," wrote André Lichtenberger. "The child is disappearing. When women do not exploit men they challenge their authority. The number of divorces increases incessantly. Our women are like those spoiled children who ask for the moon but don't know what to do with it once you give it to them."[20]

The threat posed by women's independence and the new cynicism of youth was perhaps most literally represented by the rising number of female and minor criminals after the war, as well as by a perceived acceleration in the spread of venereal disease, attributed to a lax attitude toward prostitution and to the new and reckless sexual mores.[21] Most commentators on crime statistics

[17] Quoted ibid., p. 260.
[18] Quoted ibid., p. 242.
[19] Quoted ibid., p. 79. See also Henri d'Alméras, *La France dévorée par les poux* (Paris: Collections des Frondeurs, 1933), pp. 20–22.
[20] Quoted in ibid., p. 200.
[21] The historian Gordon Wright has argued that since 1789 every war in France except the Great War has produced "bursts of reform talk, and even some action in the realm of crime control" (pp. 175–76), but it would be incorrect to assume the French were indifferent to criminal issues after the war. Instead, we need to understand what they defined as criminal and note how that definition was connected to perceived social threats and fantasies about their origins.

commended the diminution of violent crime after the war, and shifted the focus of their concern to the alarming increase of female and juvenile criminality and to the threat to the race presumably posed by prostitution.

Most writers admitted that crime statistics were in many instances unreliable because the war had interrupted official record taking and criminal prosecution. The dramatic diminution of violent crime during and immediately after the war was exaggerated by the highly irregular context created by mobilization. The contingent of the population from which most criminals emerged— young, working-class men—had been mobilized; many crimes were not recorded because they were tried in military instead of civilian courts; and there were no statistics at all in the northern departments that had been invaded by the Germans. Thus the crime increase that statistics recorded after 1920 represented less a real augmentation of deviance than a stabilizing of crime patterns at a prewar level.[22]

Yet contemporaries interpreted the dramatic rise in female and juvenile criminality as evidence that the war had effected important cultural changes whose traces marked all of France's most cherished institutions, the patriarchal family in particular. If writers were reassured by a diminution in violent crime, they were alarmed by the increase in new kinds of crimes against property, marriage, and family morality. One lawyer claimed that crimes against morality (*attentats à la pudeur*)—including rape, indecent exposure, and abuse of minors (conceived as male crimes)—had decreased, but cases of abortion, adultery, and infanticide (conceived as female crimes) nearly doubled after 1920.[23] It is significant that these "crimes" all represent a repudiation of women's traditional roles as wives and mothers (as well as a distinction between sex and reproduction) and that their increase coincided

[22] Panagiote Yocas, *L'Influence de la guerre européenne sur la criminalité* (Paris: Jouve, 1926), p. 10. M. G. Calbairac, "Les Répercussions de la Grande Guerre sur la criminalité en France," *EC* 2 (March–April 1928), 63–70.

[23] Figures are from Yocas, pp. 18, 20–21. His statistics are confirmed by other sources. See E. Garçon, "La Criminalité pendant la guerre," *Journal des Débats*, May 27, 1921, p. 860; Paul Provent, "Informations," *EC* (January 1930), 28; René Allendy, "Le Crime et les perversions instinctives," *Crapouillot* (May 1938), 8–11. I am less concerned, however, with the exactitude of the statistics than with the common perception that female and juvenile crime increased dramatically.

with the perception of the threat "emancipated" women posed to the traditional family.

In 1913, according to Panagiote Yocas, 92 women had been condemned for infanticide; in 1920, 178 had been found guilty. The numbers he reported for abortion were similar: In 1913, 89 men (those doctors assisting the woman) and women were condemned, and by 1920 the number had risen to 126.[24] Furthermore, these numbers represented only a very small proportion of the abortions actually performed since most, to the dismay of many commentators, went undetected and hence unquantified. At a meeting of the Association for Sexual Reform in 1933, one participant estimated the number of abortions at about one million a year.[25] In a separate text, another doctor reiterated this figure.[26]

Prostitution was used as a metaphor for the luxury and laziness of postwar society, in which it was more frequent to "honeymoon than to do housekeeping or factory work," wrote Maurice Prax, even though "women could easily find other positions than horizontal ones . . . . [since] maids are needed by all the employment offices."[27] Prostitution was perceived to have increased and was linked, as it had always been, to the spread of venereal disease. The increase in cases of venereal disease after the war was attributed to the increasing reliance of soldiers on prostitutes, and by the end of the war prostitution was addressed as part of the larger problem of female criminality. During the war, legislation was passed with the aim of repressing the practice. In December 1916 penalties for procuring increased; in October 1917 prostitutes could no longer be employed by bars.[28] Reform-minded groups calling for the abolition of the *maisons de tolérance* (state-regulated brothels) resur-

[24] Yocas, p. 20.

[25] Jean Kun, *Les Principales Imperfections du code pénal* (Paris: Editions Domat-Monchrestein, 1933), p. 102. This figure is probably exaggerated since the author was in favor of legalizing abortion and wished to identify the number of women who would seek abortions even when it was illegal to do so. But most of these figures are unreliable anyway, since conservative writers also inflated numbers, trying to shock their own constituencies by describing a situation that was presumably out of control. William Schneider gives the figure of 500,000 (p. 177).

[26] H. Mondor, *Les Avortements mortels* (Paris: Masson, 1936), p. 7.

[27] Quoted in Maurice Hamel and Charles Tournier, *La Prostitution: Enquête* (Nice: Palais Marie-Christine, 1927), pp. 103, 62.

[28] Corbin, p. 335.

faced during the 1920s, and in 1928 the minister Justin Godart in Grenoble proposed legislation to recriminalize prostitution and begin programs of moral and sexual preventive education.[29] Other cities in Alsace, including Strasbourg, Mulhouse, and Hagenau, followed suit. In fact, by 1920 there were only thirty *maisons* left in all of Paris.[30]

But most important, as crime was literally feminized, its threat was reconceived as invisible. As Lucien Mialane noted, "brutal criminality since the war has ceded its terrain to delinquency," to crimes at which women and minors, as Yocas put it, excel.[31] They were crimes that, if not literally committed by women, were gendered feminine because they were characterized by cowardice, cunning, and manipulation. This type of "expertise" was attributed to the *garçonne,* whose motives and behaviors differed from those of her nineteenth-century sisters. Her crimes were not brutal, driven by hunger and marked by the sordid trappings of poverty (as prostitution was often conceived in the nineteenth century). They were characterized above all by a rejection of "honest" work and by sloth; they were motivated less by greed or necessity than by pleasure. This argument also indicated a shift in the perceived class basis of crime. "When hungry prostitutes disappear," wrote Urbain Gohier, "lazy and vain prostitutes take their place."[32]

Thus, whereas less-than-generous commentators had long accused women of enjoying prostitution, though they were often forced into it by circumstance, in the interwar years moralistic

---

[29] See *L'Expérience de Grenoble* (Grenoble: Association Dauphinoise d'Hygiène Morale, 1933); and Jacques Siau, *La Prostitution devant la loi, la morale, et l'hygiène* (Lyon: BOSC Frères, 1931), p. 66.

[30] Corbin, pp. 336–37.

[31] Mialane, pp. 8–9; Yocas, pp. 42–43.

[32] Gohier quoted in Hamel and Tournier, p. 116. Victor Margueritte's *Prostitutée* (Paris: Bibliothèque Charpentier, 1907) offers (as Margueritte's novels always do) a good characterization of attitudes toward prostitution in the late nineteenth and early twentieth centuries. The prostitutes are all poor, working-class women, victimized by evil, irresponsible men, who are usually rich and in good social standing. Hardworking, orphaned Annette becomes a prostitute because she is arrested by accident in one of the indiscriminate roundups frequent at the turn of the century; Rose's employer makes her pregnant and throws her out of the house, having infected her with syphillis to boot. Rose dies at the end and Annette becomes a high-class hooker in order to take "vengeance" on men. Margueritte sought to expose the hypocrisy of attitudes toward prostitutes, even if his appeal was conventional and kitsch.

rhetoric claimed over and over that pleasure constituted prostitutes' central motivation in choosing their trade. Paul Bureau
insisted that "all women who sell their bodies are not constrained
to do so by violence, trickery, or misery."[33] He also claimed that
abortion was increasing because married women now wanted to
avoid the consequences of indulgence with their *poilu* (soldier).[34]
Dr. Léon Bizard argued that "misery is no longer an excuse" for
prostitution and claimed that prostitution "is no longer confined
to the bottom end of society and . . . has little by little infiltrated
those milieus where before it was exceptional to find bad morals
among young women and especially young girls."[35]

Prostitution had been the metaphor par excellence for social con-
tamination in the nineteenth century; it had represented an identifiable symbol of danger that had to be swept away by indiscriminate roundups and incarceration. Now Bizard's location of deviants
in all milieus paradoxically linked it to the dissolution of clear
marks of criminality. In fact, as Alain Corbin has noted, as the
maison close declined, new, more open, and yet hidden forms of
prostitution were made possible, in part because women could now
go out alone without risking scandal.[36] The representation of danger thus shifted because the prostitute was fast becoming Every-
woman. Max and Alex Fischer predicted that "in fifty years time,
professional prostitution will have completely disappeared, sub-
merged by amateurism, by the elegant woman, the pretty woman,
the woman who does it for nothing."[37] This conflation Atina
Grossman identifies, of the "honest woman and the whore,"[38] this
shift in the perceived class basis of prostitution, expressed most
clearly the idea that all criteria normally used to place women
morally as well as socially had dissolved.

In an investigation of postwar prostitution, Jean-José Frappa remarked that one of the most urgent questions confronting social
analysts was how to tell whether a woman was a prostitute and

[33] Paul Bureau, *L'Indiscipline des moeurs* (Paris: Blond and Gay, 1921), p. 289.
[34] Literally, the word means "hairy."
[35] Léon Bizard, *La Vie des filles* (Paris: Grasset, 1934), pp. 95, 47.
[36] Corbin, p. 337.
[37] Fischers, quoted in Hamel and Tournier, p. 82.
[38] Atina Grossman, "The New Woman and the Rationalization of Sexuality in
Weimar Germany," in Ann Snitow, Christine Stansell, and Sharon Thompson, eds.,
Powers of Desire: The Politics of Sexuality (New York: Monthly Review Press, 1983),
p. 156.

how to prove it beyond a doubt.[39] In a book about prostitutes' lives, Léon Bizard wrote:

> It has become very difficult to differentiate at first sight an honest woman or a pure young girl from a whore. . . . All women, from the adolescent to the grandmother are molded according to the same model: they wear lipstick and powder their faces, have pearly eyelids, long black lashes, painted nails, platinum or red hair . . . ; they all smoke, drink cocktails, loiter at dancing halls, drive cars. . . .
>
> Given the promiscuity of these bodies that are not always comparable to Venus, how can we place them? Which is the marquise, the wife of the wealthy industrialist? or simply the woman of easy virtue? What an embarrassing question and what a difficult problem to solve![40]

In the same vein, Dr. Teutsch claimed that "we are drowning in the immense legion of prostitutes and pimps; it is becoming more and more difficult to distinguish them at first sight, [because all women] dress indecently and provocatively." And Joë Bridge summed up this sentiment most forcefully: "Do you feel capable of registering all women . . . the music-hall performers, typists, saleswomen, honest women, petty-bourgeois women whose duped husbands earn six hundred francs at this or that government office? . . . Don't you see prostitution everywhere around us? It is a rising torrent in the process of submerging us all!"[41]

At the same time, this drowning of conventional distinctions between honest women and whores (and hence between normal and deviant women) blurred the boundaries between masculinity and femininity. Bizard linked the fading of the demarcation between honest women and whores to an "increase" in prostitution, and that increase to the emancipation of women, to their desire to compete in a male world. Several other writers echoed his opinion, correlating emancipated women with prostitutes. Because the garçonne chose several partners when and where she wanted, she inverted gender roles, and therefore many men conflated what they

[39] Jean-José Frappa, *Enquête sur la prostitution* (Paris: Flammarion, 1937), p. 29.
[40] Bizard, p. 45.
[41] Teutsch, pp. 124; Joë Bridge, quoted in Hamel and Tournier, p. 131.

perceived as her desire to sleep with every man with a desire to be a man. As Teutsch saw it, most prostitutes and most women who had abortions sought pleasure in the autonomy afforded by aborting their infants or selling their bodies; prostitutes were attracted to the profession by a "spirit of luxury" and the "taste for vice."[42] The moralistic Paul Bureau noted that prostitution, abortion, and infanticide were being practiced by married and unmarried women alike in order to avoid the obligations imposed on them by their sex.[43]

As we have seen, in the nineteenth century, many doctors and others believed prostitution merely externalized an intrinsically deviant female nature. But after the war prostitution became a metaphor for the uncertain status of female gender identity, for the *dissolution* of a distinctive female nature. The deviant woman no longer affirmed sexual difference, she metaphorized sexual *sameness*, for in the words of one commentator, she was at once a "superman" and a "superwoman." When she acted as an autonomous individual, when she chose her partners when and where she wanted, she usurped male prerogatives and, in so doing, acted out the insatiable longing and lack of self-control which purportedly characterized female nature.[44] When she acted as a man she did not transgress or invert her so-called nature but expressed it. In other words, the deviant or criminal woman no longer transgressed or inverted gender roles but marked their fluidity, marked the reification of gender itself.

Like the image Armand Villette used in 1907 to describe prostitutes' overcrowded living quarters—"Human forms are effaced in a flesh without individuality"[45]—men's fantasized inability to differentiate between the marquise and the street girl symbolized a world without a stable center of power, in which the patriarchal norms necessary to define sexual difference had dissolved, and in which sexual identity, like bodies, could be bought and sold. This shift from sexual difference to sameness mirrored the perceived

[42] Teutsch, p. 124.

[43] Bureau, pp. 39–40, 113.

[44] Anonymous review of André Gybal, *Ma Femme et son amant,* in *Le Grand Guignol,* no. 33 (December 1926), 178–79.

[45] Armand Villette, *Du trottoir à St. Lazare* (Paris: Editions Henry-Parville, 1925), p. 181. This is a reissue of the 1907 work.

dissolution of gender boundaries and at the same time represented an effort to redefine them. It did not, therefore, just reflect male power, but generated shifts in its form and content.

The Medical Response

The medical establishment divided into two camps in response to this "crisis" of male power: conservatives—natalists—on one hand, and progressives—neo-Malthusians and members of the Ligue Nationale Française d'Hygiène Mentale—on the other. Yet, as we shall see, they shared the same fundamental attitude toward the deviant woman even if they proposed different solutions to the problem she embodied.[46] Conservative natalist doctors diagnosed the problem as one of male impotence and sought to restore the traditional model of paternal authority to remedy postwar anarchy. Yocas, a conservative, gave two causes for the rise in female criminality: the participation of women in social life, which had exposed them to new temptations, and the general loosening of matrimonial ties. He attributed the overall rise in crime to the difficult conditions of wartime existence and, most significantly, to the absence of men: "The husband and father, the two guardians of family morality, had left for the front [and] moral order was not able to be maintained in their absence. Familial anarchy has been the result of that absence and this is perhaps the most serious reason [for the increase in female and juvenile criminality]."[47]

Most conservative commentators shared Yocas's opinion. Dr. M. G. Calbairac insisted that after the war crime, though related to anatomical lesions or social milieu, was above all the product of a general moral vacuum created by the absence of paternal authority. In his view, single women were more prone to suicide, infanticide,

---

[46] In his study of French eugenics, William Schneider has noted to what extent that movement was part of broader reform movements aimed at biological regeneration since the late nineteenth century. Both natalists and neo-Malthusians were interested in controlling the population, and in France they united behind this common goal. After the Great War, however, their strategies for control clashed increasingly, as eugenicists became more extreme (the league, as I noted earlier, was loosely allied with the French eugenics movement). Both groups shared the goal of controlling women's bodies, but Schneider gives gender only a cursory treatment. See Schneider, pp. 32–33, 181.

[47] Yocas, pp. 44–45.

and prostitution than those who were married, and the numerical disparity between men and women gave free reign to casual sexual relationships and adulterous liaisons instead of marriage.[48] And the criminologist J. A. Roux attributed the rise in juvenile criminality to the absence of fathers.[49]

These opinions were widespread among critics of the new morality, as well as critics of feminist demands for equality. The writer E. Garçon claimed that it was "necessary to seek the cause of this recrudescence [of female criminality] in the absence of the husband and the loosening of family discipline. Is the moral direction of the spouse," he asked, "thus not entirely useless to women?" The criminologist Evangèle Kyrkos attributed juvenile criminality to the absence of fathers and the "bad behavior" of mothers during the war. Dr. K. A. Wieth-Knudsen, a foreigner and a favorite of antifeminists, claimed that "modern legislation related to marriage has . . . [stripped] all veritable authority from the father, thus compromising the education of his children and leaving the field open to the asocial and amoral instincts of women." Finally, the prominent lawyer Charles Lefebvre declared that it was not in the "law but in our morals that paternal authority has lost its vigor."[50]

But the National League for Mental Hygiene and the psychoanalysts who shared its concerns conceived the problem differently. As the prominent psychiatrist Edouard Toulouse saw it, traditional male authority had been rendered dysfunctional by women, who could no longer be bound, identified, or defined in old ways. Most women refused to tolerate arbitrary male authority because the war had made them aware of a double standard that restricted their freedom, and in the postwar sexual marketplace it had become difficult to distinguish "women who are not for sale" from those who were seeking "sexual recreation"—that is, from those who were presumably prostitutes. Toulouse declared that the war had acted as a "school of sexual liberty," in which women had

[48]Calbairac, "Les Répercussions," pp. 69–70.
[49]J. A. Roux, "Ce que sera la criminalité après la guerre," *Revue Politique et Parlementaire*, April 10, 1917, p. 42.
[50]Garçon, "La Criminalité pendant la guerre," p. 860; Evangèle Kyrkos, "Les Causes de la criminalité juvénile" (Thèse, University of Rennes, 1931), p. 35; Dr. K. A. Wieth-Knudsen, *Le Conflit des sexes dans l'évolution sociale et la question sexuelle* (Paris: Marcel Rivière, 1931), p. 177; Charles Lefebvre, *La Famille en France* (Paris: Marcel Giard, 1920), p. 144.

been encouraged to try to eradicate the "irreducible and natural differences between the sexes," and that conservative demands that men and women return to outmoded social roles were therefore unrealistic.[51]

Psychiatrists' perception that the New Woman had forever blurred gender distinctions effected a shift in their focus away from female deviance per se to male authority and to the relationship between men and women, to shaping, says Atina Grossman, "the heterosexual couple in a way that also disciplined women."[52] As Dr. J. Laumonier noted with alarm, "The trouble stirring in feminine souls is the result of the universal anarchy of which man first made himself the champion."[53] The new focus on disciplining women by attempting to regulate male sexuality represented a methodological shift away from a morally based definition of sexual difference to a rationally based one, the same shift from morality (e.g., free will) to "science" which I identified in my discussion of asylum and penal reform, which was theoretically indebted to proponents of social hygiene, the biologically based movement for social reform. That shift also implied that sex and gender—one's biological sex and one's sex role—were related functionally rather than naturally, although doctors confounded what was deemed functional with what was deemed natural. This shift was perhaps best represented in France in the agenda developed by the Ligue Nationale Française d'Hygiène Mentale.

The league's agenda was primarily one of moral regeneration through greater state control of sexuality. It thus encouraged what could be termed "sex reform."[54] "During this epoch of reconstruction," Dr. Robert Chable remarked, "it is important that sexual life be subject to reform, not to return it to another age . . . but to place it in its true hygienic and social role as a procreative function and

---

[51] Edouard Toulouse, *La Question sexuelle et la femme* (Paris: Charpentier, 1918), pp. 57, 16.

[52] Grossman, p. 154.

[53] Laumonier, quoted in Teutsch, p. 263.

[54] Grossman, p. 154. The term was used in Weimar Germany to describe a broad movement of socialist doctors and writers seeking to "rationalize" sexual life. In France it was not used in any official manner. The French movement was not nearly as widespread as in Germany because its neo-Malthusian undertones were highly unpopular. In the medical world, however, it represented an important postwar development. On France, see Schneider, pp. 116–256. On the German case, see Grossman, pp. 154-71.

not as an instrument of debauch."[55] Most of the proponents of sex reform sought to avoid the debauchery symbolized by the New Woman by rendering men and women sexually functional according to the objective needs of the state through a vast sexual education program that would eliminate the double standard. "Men and women" insisted the hygienist Paul Good, "should no longer be subject to two different moral and social laws."[56] He argued that they should be considered "equal but different," using the old idea espoused by several Christian commentators and now by women's groups and so lending it scientific or functional legitimacy.[57] Such demands for equality nevertheless worried medical men. In reference to sex reform, Dr. René Bion asked, "How can the biologist not be worried by a society that tends to conflate men and women more and more? How can he not be frightened by the assertions of certain reformers who believe they have found a remedy to current problems by making uniform the social activity of two beings that nature has so profoundly differentiated?"[58]

In spite of what some medical men interpreted as its radical implications, the league's endorsement of women's equality was contradictory. Doctors sought, for example, to domesticate women by emancipating them. Hence they advocated equal rights and education for women, but with the goal of making reproduction more efficient. They wanted to use education to socialize girls more effectively into their "natural" social roles and to give women a

[55] Dr. Robert Chable, *Education sexuelle et maladies vénériennes* (Neuchâtel: Editions Forum, 1921), p. 6.

[56] Paul Good, *Hygiène et morale* (Paris: Editions Je Sers, 1931), p. 8.

[57] The Catholic Emmanuel Gounot suggested that the family be structured like a government in which the father is the president and the mother minister of the interior. He went on to argue that the absolute authority of the father should be limited but that the wife should necessarily obey the husband: "To obey is not a humiliation; obeying and commanding are two duties, two complementary functions; to obey and to command equally serve the common good." Emmanuel Gounot, *L'Epouse et la mère en droit français* (Lyon: Chronique Sociale, 1927), pp. 10–12. A popular women's magazine took a startlingly similar line, declaring that the husband must rule like a "constitutional monarch"; he would not rule arbitrarily, for the wife would act as parliament: "The husband of the modern wife must be considered by her as the representative of a will that is common to both of them." ("Ce que toute jeune femme doit savoir," *La Vie et le Coeur*, March 25, 1932, pp. 4–5).

[58] Dr. René Bion, *La Nature féminine et le féminisme* (Lyon: Chronique Sociale de France, 1927), p. 28.

political stake in the nation so they would feel obliged by patriotic duty to become mothers. Toulouse, for example, claimed that separate agrégations for boys and girls were not unjust but irrational. Because the female agrégation required a superficial knowledge of several subjects rather than a profound knowledge of one, the preparation was in fact more exhaustive than that required of the boys: "We could not have found a better way to harden young girls, to desexualize them, to render them unfit for childbirth."[59]

Consistent with this attempt to reconstitute sexual difference in functional terms, the league also repudiated conservative nostalgia about a golden age of noble fatherhood and based its reform proposals on the functional requirements of the state rather than on an appeal to the father's natural authority. It joined others in supporting the transfer of paternal authority to the state when the father was judged incapable of effectively raising his children and so advocated legislation that punished men who had not provided their families with basic subsidies for over three months. They praised the reform of the Napoleonic code which gave the mother power over the fate of her children at all times rather than only in the father's absence.[60]

The historian Jacques Donzelot has equated this kind of legislation with the emasculation of the father, linking the erosion of men's power within the family to the erosion (which he mourns) of masculinity itself.[61] And in fact, as the league sought to resexualize women in an appropriate fashion, it also sought to desexualize men or, as some horrified onlookers warned, to castrate them. For the new man constructed by sex reformers was above all a chaste one.

Bureau and other conservatives considered this new emphasis on male chastity (from which other virtues "logically" followed) an emasculating response to social crisis.[62] The hygiene movement,

[59] Edouard Toulouse, *La Question sociale* (Paris: Editions du Progrès Civique, 1921), p. 198.

[60] Mothers were given the right to exercise the prerogatives of paternal authority after July 3, 1915, and the Senate gave women the right to become legal guardians in March 1917.

[61] Donzelot, *Policing of Families*.

[62] Bureau, pp. 549–50. Bureau is referring to an article by Toulouse on male chastity. Teutsch, another conservative, claimed (pp. 111–12) that male virginity led to impotence and depression. One of the commonest responses to the endorsement of male chastity was that it would lead to homosexuality. In fact, much conservative

however, embraced it, and it received an important popular reso-
nance in the work of the novelist Marcel Prévost. The sociologist
Gaston Richard celebrated male chastity as a transcendent spiritual quality that expressed men's true nature, whereas female
chastity was merely a functional necessity to which women were
obliged as "generators of the race."[63] Most doctors linked their
endorsement of male chastity to the "scientific" recognition that
sexual desire was not an uncontrollable, savage force but a "spiritual phenomenon," as Chable put it, which could be controlled
and channeled without harming the body.[64] New scientific information proving that male continence would not atrophy the re-
productive organs made possible what Dr. Frank Escande identified
as "a perfect correlation between a moral ideal and scientific
laws."[65] Male chastity was, in his opinion, a rational response to
moral crisis which would oblige women to follow men's moral
example and resume the femininity they had repudiated.

Chastity was thus envisioned as a scientifically sound method of
ensuring the healthy propagation of the race because it would limit
the number of unwanted births and prevent the spread of venereal
disease while promoting a spiritual ideal. Male chastity outside of
marriage would ensure that unmarried women would once again
feel the comforting mantle of male protection without fear for
their safety and that married women could expect responsible,
faithful husbands. Doctors in the league argued that old ideas
about the father's absolute rights over his wife and children, as well
as all notions of male superiority, had to be discarded in favor of
treating women as equal but different if the social and sexual order
was to foster happiness and guarantee national security. In other

commentary expressed anxiety about the "elitism" of male homosexuals, in response to André Gide's defense and celebration of it in *Corydon* (1924).

[63] Gaston Richard, *L'Evolution des moeurs* (Paris: Gaston Doin, 1925), p. 252.

[64] Chable, p. 46.

[65] Dr. Frank Escande, *Le Problème de la chasteté masculine au point de vue
scientifique* (Paris: Librarie J. B. Baillière et Fils, 1919), p. 193. See also Louis Fiaux,
Enseignement populaire de la moralité sexuelle (Paris: F. Alcan, 1908), p. 41. The
notion of endorsing chastity through sexual education had been advocated by the
social hygiene movement in 1906 and 1910 as a remedy for veneral disease, but had
run into obstacles both because of the controversial nature of sexual education and
because a majority of doctors believed that the sexual instinct was an untamable
force that could not be tampered with. See Escande, pp. 56–69. Escande also notes
that the issue of male chastity did not become important until after the war, pp. 46–
47.

words, men would have to repudiate the double standard that allowed them sexual license without threatening their respectability. Paul Chavigny cited America's "chaste" and yet "great" men—the presidents of Harvard and the University of Chicago—to demonstrate that the two qualities were not mutually incompatible.[66] Paul Good quoted an unidentified "great poet," on the virtues of male chastity.[67] Frank Escande cited Tolstoy's *Kreutzer Sonata*, and almost everyone considered Marcel Prévost's novel *L'Homme vierge*, which celebrated male chastity as a noble response to women's treachery, an exemplary moral tract.

The League for Mental Hygiene thus sought to resolve the crisis of male authority by representing this old aristocratic image of paternal authority in new, functional terms. Doctors attempted a return to chivalry when they made chaste virility the scientific rather than natural foundation of masculinity. The league's ends were thus traditional, although their means and terms of debate were not. Though it represented a reformist current allied in some respects to the political Left, its efforts are best seen as an adaptation of patriarchal values to new, more technocratic forms of social organization (including a belief in eugenics and euthanasia and hence in the "scientific" regulation of culture)—a strategy not incompatible, for example, with the objectives of the Vichy government.

It is difficult to judge the leagues' real impact on family policy. It does not seem to have had an important practical influence except in the realm of public health reform. Nevertheless, its celebration of a chaste and noble virility cut across and contained political differences, and its blend of traditionalism and functionalism was attractive, for different reasons, to both Left and Right alike. Therefore, the league's apparent privileging of the state's over the father's rights did not, as Jacques Donzelot has argued, bring about the "neutralizing" or "effacing" of paternal power.[68] Nor did its emphasis on functionalism over ethics institute sexual equality.

[66]Chavigny, *Sexualité et médecine légale*, pp. 85–86.
[67]Good, p. 63.
[68]Donzelot considers women the agents of the father's entrapment and thus always complicitous with the state as it attempts to efface paternal power. He claims that "family patriarchalism" was destroyed in favor of a "patriarchy of the State." (p. 103), but he divorces in a confusing way the patriarchal state from the power of men. In fact, in his account the state destroys their power. Even more

If the image of the new man—the new, functionalist construction of men's and women's equality—represented men's anxieties
about the dissolution of gender boundaries, it also represented a
means of reinforcing them in new terms. Paradoxically, male power
now derived from its own discretion, its refusal to pronounce its
power as powerful. To describe men and women as equal but different was to articulate equality as gender difference. But how exactly
can equality be so articulated? How could the solution to the problem of dissolving gender boundaries (equality) be the same as the
cause of it (equality)? Where, in other words, was the difference?

Psychoanalysis

Psychoanalysts also sought to reestablish sexual difference in
functionalist terms that would reinstate the harmony between the
sexes which the New Woman was said to have shattered. As Marie
Bonaparte suggested, they wanted to help the female deviant adapt
nonneurotically to the reality principle by building sexual difference on rational rather than repressive foundations. In so doing,
they used psychoanalysis not to repudiate but to provide a more
convincing justification of the league's remedies for what most
analysts defined as postwar neurosis. French psychoanalysts did
not challenge a functionalist model of psychic operations; instead,
they assimilated psychoanalysis into a functionalist framework in
which deviance could be scientifically controlled through a more
sophisticated analysis and regulation of the mind, an analysis that
conceived pathology, in Angelo Hesnard's words, as "an absence of
virility [in the case of men] and of femininity [in the case of wom-
en]."[69] René Laforgue put it this way: "We must take medical and
social action at once. Medical for the sick, social in order to form

---

confusingly, Donzelot views women as agents of the state and also its victims. He
argues that the work offered to women was designed to be but an extension of
female domestic activity *in order to give men the illusion of patriarchal power.*
First, it is not clear why male power in this context is illusory. After all, men had
real legal and economic power over women, who could not even vote. Second, it is
also unclear who is neutralizing patriarchy, who is effacing male power. The state,
which clearly limits women's professional activity for the benefit of men, to use
Donzelot's image, "floats." Its power base is genderless. Donzelot, pp. 103, 40.

[69] Angelo Hesnard, "Culture psychanalytique et clientèle psychiatrique cour-
ante," *HM* 25 (1930), 52.

the teachers and pedagogues whom society trusts with the future of youth, the generation of tomorrow. I even think that the greatest effort of psychoanalysis should be directed toward social order, to organize mental hygiene . . . and to create a favorable environment for normal development."[70]

In 1930 René Laforgue and Sacha Nacht published an article in the league's journal, *L'Hygiène Mentale*, concerning the insights psychoanalysis could offer within a framework of mental prophylaxy. They declared that the main goal of analysis was to "render reality as palatable as possible by replacing each instinctively derived pleasure with fulfilling experiences that are both realizable and rational."[71]

The orthodox Freudian Marie Bonaparte declared that analysis facilitated the progressive evolution of humanity. It could help men learn to be "stronger, more virile, and more adult" because, in contrast to religious exhortations to be kind and good and strong, psychoanalysis was "intimately adapted to the reality principle." Because sexual education directed sexual instinct in a rational and hence healthy manner, she argued, it would eliminate both male and female neuroses: It would restore virility to men and hence their capacity for work; it would permit women to develop their "maternal instinct" fully without being exploited by the patriarchal double standard that took advantage of women's sensuous nature as well as their natural passivity.[72] Essentially, she maintained that psychoanalysis would render men and women once again "equal but different," though she did not use these words.

Other analysts shared Bonaparte's diagnosis of modern neurosis as rooted in a diminution of male virility which sexual education could remedy by restoring male and female complementarity. John Leuba stigmatized the social rejection of sexual difference not because it was unnatural but because it was dysfunctional:

The modern woman, obliged by the economic changes that followed the war to work like a man, to challenge him in all the professions, has made herself virile. Living as man's equal, she has destroyed her

[70] René Laforgue, "La Névrose familiale," *RFP* 9 (1936), 354.
[71] René Laforgue and Sacha Nacht, "Considérations psychanalytiques sur l'hygiène mentale," *HM* 25 (1930), 48.
[72] Marie Bonaparte, "La Prophylaxie infantile des névroses," *RFP* 4 (1930–31), 132, 104.

charm. Spouses, each working on his own, return to each other in the evening like two business associates, and in this respect form homosexual couples.

The collective neurosis of the postwar years is characterized . . . by a rising amount of impotence of both sexes but especially of men. Abolish the sexual attraction of women and you abolish the possibility of sublimation.[73]

Elsewhere, giving an "objective" rather than ethical analysis of social crisis, he declares: "It is the refusal of femininity that has, I believe, . . . the most serious social consequences. This refusal affects all kinds of things since the rebellious woman [*la femme révoltée*] who calls herself a feminist . . . who seeks to supplant men in all domains and inculcates other women to have only contempt for them, and the masochistic woman who . . . castrates her infants through her excessive tenderness . . . tend to create household environments disastrous for children."[74]

René Laforgue described the "typical bourgeois family" after the war as comprising a weak man, a tyrannical woman, a passive son, and a frigid or lesbian daughter. The woman's contempt for men gives her the desire, he claimed, "to study, to be a lawyer, a doctor, an engineer," and her husband will most likely be a "passive intellectual." The woman thus tries to "reverse the roles of the spouses," or she manifests other deviant symptoms—frigidity, homosexuality, or nymphomania. She is motivated by an unconscious refusal to accept her femininity and seeks out weak men likely to accept her dominance, men who are themselves neurotic postwar products. Finally, her children mirror the parental relationship: "The boys will have a tendency to become girls, the girls to become boys, even though [this tendency] does not always manifest itself in the same manner."[75]

The analysts Ilse and Charles Odier's portrait of the neurotic family is strikingly similar. In their subtle attempt to outline the specifics of female superego development, they demonized female authority as contributing to a diminution of paternal virility and

---

[73] John Leuba, "Notions élémentaires de biologie psycho-sexuelle," *RFP* 7 (1934), 536–37.

[74] John Leuba, "La Famille névrotique et les névroses familiales," *RFP* 9 (1936), 397.

[75] Laforgue, "La Névrose familiale," p. 344.

the consequent masculinization of the daughter, whose superego is developed in accordance with a maternal rather than paternal interdiction. The image they paint in their case history is nearly identical to Laforgue's: the mother "is evidently herself neurotic . . . the victim of an extraordinary masculinity complex. She reigns in the family circle and even outside of it in her activity as feminist and suffragette. Her husband . . . is weak, an intellectual, an artist who bends before his formidable spouse in order to have some peace."[76] The Odiers conclude that the young victims of maternal despotism are not fundamentally homosexual, as a preliminary diagnosis would indicate, but perfectly normal women driven to lesbianism by a strong mother.

Psychoanalysts thus shared the general consensus that the root of social problems was women's "irrational" refusal of femininity and sought to make women accept their "natural" role by proposing that fathers take a new initiative. In the postwar years, they insisted, fathers had become pathologically weak, indifferent, or severe. Laforgue and Hesnard declared that "a weak father does not allow his sons to become men or his daughters to become women."[77] Laforgue argued elsewhere that men who threw themselves into their work at the expense of their families and lovers betrayed an inability to "give [themselves] to another" and in fact an unconscious wish "not to want to give oneself." While this withdrawal was sometimes blamed on women's new assertiveness, women's assertiveness was also blamed on male passivity—hence Laforgue's and Ilse and Charles Odier's passive intellectual. Weak men's wives took on a masculine persona and were encouraged by their husband's indifference to frequent questionable milieus, or they were normal and hence turned, with predictably disastrous results, to their children for comfort.[78]

But from a functional point of view harsh fathers were most undesirable. Tyrannical fathers, like weak ones, also feminized boys and made girls virile. The tough disciplinarian, Leuba claimed, inevitably inspired fantasies of vengeance in his wife and

[76] Ilse and Charles Odier, "Contribution à l'étude du surmoi féminin," *RFP* 4 (1930–31), 664.

[77] Angelo Hesnard and René Laforgue, "Les Processus d'autopunition en psychologie des névroses et psychoses, en psychologie criminelle, et en pathologie générale," *RFP* 4 (1930–31), 81.

[78] Laforgue, "La Névrose familiale," p. 346.

daughter. Moreover, his daughter's hostile attitude toward men would drive her to take female lovers, and his son would develop a strong erotic attachment to his mother, overidentifying with maternal tenderness in flight from paternal terror. Leuba also maintained that male overidentification with the mother was one of the dangers inherent in families run by strong women.[79]

The ideal father was thus authoritative but gentle. Like the league, psychoanalysts took an old image of paternity and represented it in functional terms. More realistic perhaps than their brethren or more conscious of the power of repressed sexual impulses, the psychoanalysts did not recommend chastity but, like the league, supported a range of sexual reforms—sexual education, medical intervention in the family—designed to strengthen the father and hence social order in general by rendering him more gentle, more giving, more powerful through his willingness to give up power. The father had to be nurturing but strong, gentle but virile.

The aristocratic image of the gentle father was most forcefully expressed by Edouard Pichon, who, along with Laforgue and the analyst Henri Codet, sought to adapt psychoanalysis to a French cultural and intellectual tradition in a more sophisticated fashion than that used by orthodox French Freudians such as Bonaparte.[80] Pichon in particular rejected all functional and biological theories of the libido, the family, and neurosis, claiming that "there was absolutely no proof" to support such interpretations.[81] Even so, he used the psychoanalytic model of the neurotic family and the *garçonne*'s role in it as his starting point. He repudiated psychoanalysts' recourse to a medical model of culture and argued instead that paternal authority, if it was to be rendered functional and hence to be effectively restored, had to be grounded in the civilizing force of morality. But Pichon sought only to do explicitly what other psychoanalysts had done implicitly: to ground the concept of "equal but different" in science and in this case, in a revision, neither quite functionalist nor Freudian (though drawing on both), of psychoanalytic theory.

[79] Leuba, "La Famille névrotique," p. 391.
[80] See Chapter 3.
[81] Edouard Pichon, "La Famille devant M. Lacan," *RFP* 11 (1939), 110–111. See also Elisabeth Roudinesco's reading of this piece: "M. Pichon devant la famille," *Confrontations* no. 3 (Spring 1980), 209–26.

Pichon claimed that neurosis was best explained in terms of the absence or presence of moral self-control and in particular what he called the acceptance or refusal of sexual difference: "In sum, clinical psychopathology teaches us clearly that in the West every human being who does not possess enough self-control [*maîtrise de soi*] to accept sexual difference and all that results from it . . . will become neurotic." He went on to identify "two aberrant types" of women who "stubbornly resist normal sexual order": the feminist and the "easy woman" (*la cocotte*). Both represent a fundamental loss of self-control typical of women without male guidance. Feminists in particular have "genital problems, are avowed or latent homosexuals, or are frigid." To prevent the "effacing of feminine characteristics and a unification of the social roles of both sexes" and to promote sexual difference while preserving men's and women's spiritual equality, Pichon sought to restore paternal authority by justifying it in innovative psychoanalytic terms that represented an extension of an antiformalist linguistic argument.[82]

A trained linguist, Pichon rejected the Saussurian insistence upon the distinction between language and thought and argued that ideas about reality and reality itself were indistinguishable. This monism, as Roudinesco has noted, was implicit in the title of the multi-volume grammar he had written with his uncle, *Des mots à la pensée*.[83] It also characterized his antifunctionalist explanation of why paternal authority should be obeyed and hence of why male authority best ensured the maintenance and perpetuation of an ideal social order.

Pichon, whose political allegiance was with the proto-fascist Action Française, believed that patriarchy was the ideal form of social order because it was the basis of language. He noted that in Indo-European languages the male represents the generic and the female is inscribed as other and different. To this observation he coupled an anthropological one: patriarchal language took the normal, biological differences between men and women and transmuted them into the "cultural differentiation of humanity into two blocs," depriving instinctive passions not of their power but of their brutality.[84] Patriarchal culture was thus a transparent expression of

[82] Edouard Pichon, "A l'aise dans la civilisation," *RFP* 10 (1939), 29, 27, 28.
[83] Roudinesco, "M. Pichon devant la famille," p. 212.
[84] Edouard Pichon, *Evolution divergente de la génitalité et la sexualité dans la civilisation occidentale* (Paris: Denoël, 1939), pp. 5–6. I cite the pamphlet, a copy of

patriarchal language, and it expressed and facilitated the progressive evolution of humanity toward ever higher levels of civilization, in which men became increasingly gentle toward and respectful of women.

This equation of patriarchy with civlization drew upon Freud but at the same time rejected the fundamental dynamics of the Oedipus complex. Pichon and Laforgue defined the mechanism of normal maturation not as a normative regulation of the sexual drive and the sexual object (i.e., the Oedipus complex) but instead in terms of an assumption that normality could be empirically determined. Pichon, along with Laforgue, argued that maturation was dependent on the child's capacity to separate from his or her mother. They explained normative development in terms of the child's moral capacity to repress its infantile desires and confront the world as an adult. This process was described as a passage from *captativité*, or dependence on the mother, to *oblativité*, or the sacrifice of the mother in exchange for the maturity represented by paternal law. As in Freud's schema, the mother functioned as temptation, the father as interdiction. Yet in contrast to Freud's theory, maturation depended on an *innate* moral capacity to sacrifice the mother and accept the father's law. Pichon denounced any refusal to obey male authority; yet he was unable to explain precisely how the capacity for sacrifice was constituted.

Patriarchy was thus both the producer and product of this mature individual. Pichon's entire theory was, after all, an attempt to justify in theoretical terms his belief that patriarchy was the only means of guaranteeing the health, survival, and evolution of cherished cultural institutions—indeed, the survival of civilization itself. But if it was tautological to argue that one did or should obey the father's law simply because one did or should, it was equally tautological to claim that patriarchy guaranteed the survival of civilization because it had thus far done so. To argue that thought mirrored language did not explain how it did or why it should do so. If women and men were equal but different, it was unclear precisely how and why the father was different even as he was equal, how his authority could be theoretically justified. Instead of grounding the functionalist insistence on patriarchal supremacy in

which can be found in the Bibliothèque Nationale. The article originally appeared in *RFP* 10 (1939), 461–70.

a more rigorous argument, Pichon's effort to make "equal but different" an empirical truth exposed the fragility of its premises. It was thus still unclear how equality could be conceived in terms of a gender difference, how an effort to ground that difference in science or language rather than nature explained and justified male difference and hence, in this context, male superiority.

Remaking the Patriarchal Family

Jacques Lacan addressed Pichon's theory and what it owed to Freudian analysis in his article on the family, written as a contribution to the *Encyclopédie Française* in 1938 and later published as *Les Complexes familiaux*. The article was commissioned by the psychiatrist Henri Wallon, whose theory about the child's gaze in the mirror Lacan used as the basis of his own innovative conception of the mirror stage, worked out around 1936 and developed in the article on the family. Lacan attacked Pichon and his followers' conception of psychic development, but he also rejected the functionalist analysis of Bonaparte, Leuba, and others and, in so doing, cut across both trends to forge an original reading of Freud.

Drawing on his knowledge of phenomenology and Freud and influenced by the communist theoretician Georges Politzer's rigorous critique of empirical psychology in *Les Fondements de la psychologie*, Lacan argued in *Les Complexes familiaux* that those psychoanalysts who tried to explain psychological development in terms of the passage from an inferior to a superior moral will, from *captativité* to *oblativité*, had developed an erroneous understanding of psychic activity.[85] Their conception of normal development, he said, begged the question of how that development took place:

This role of Oedipus correlates with sexual maturation. The attitude inaugurated by genital tendencies crystallizes the vital relation to reality according to its normal type. This attitude has been characterized by the terms gift and sacrifice, grandiose terms whose meaning remains ambiguous and hesitates between defense and renunciation.

[85] On Politzer's influence on Lacan, see Borch-Jacobsen, p. 22; Macey, pp. 101–2; Bercherie, pp. 55–56. Bercherie makes a case for the more general importance of Politzer's work for French psychoanalysis.

Through them [Freud's] audacious conception rediscovers the secret comfort of a moralizing theme: in the passage from *captativité* to *oblativité* the vital trial and the moral trial are . . . confounded.[86]

Lacan provided an alternative to this theoretical schema. He organized psychic development according to a three-tiered structure: the severance complex, the intrusion complex, and the Oedipus complex. At each stage he proposed a revision of Freud. His argument was original because he explained and organized psychic material not in terms of instinct or energy but in terms of its relationship to cultural representation. In contrast to Freud, who maintained that an analysis of the instinctive drives would clarify the complex, Lacan argued that the complex itself, the structural organization of the drive, explained the instinct. The complex, he said, was determined in relation to an object. Since all psychic relations are embedded in and organized by symbolic systems, they are constructed by, in, and through culture.[87]

Lacan declared that severance is characterized by "cannibalism," which is "fusional and ineffable," because prefigurative. Freud's own term, *autoeroticism,* was unacceptable because at this developmental stage, the ego (as we have seen in Chapter 1) is not yet constituted. Intrusion, the process of identification and constitution of the ego, was similarly conceived in terms of an initiation into representation symbolized by the specular image and the other, the rival "brother" with whom one identifies, whom one loves and hates (the mirror stage). Finally and most significantly for our purposes, the Oedipus complex defuses the aggressiveness implicit in the mirror stage (effects the "repression of sexuality" and "sublimation") and makes it possible for the individual to live peaceably in the world of others. In Lacan's words, it contributes to the "constitution of reality."[88]

According to Lacan, Pichon and his colleagues failed to explain the relationship between repression and normative sexual identity. They participated in "the most marked failure of analytic doctrine: neglecting the structure in favor of dynamism."[89] The normative

---

[86] Jacques Lacan, *Les Complexes familiaux dans la formation de l'individu: Essai d'analyse d'une fonction en psychologie* (Paris: Navrin, 1984), p. 58.

[87] Ibid., pp. 22–23.

[88] Ibid., pp. 55, 57.

[89] Ibid., pp. 58–59.

regulation of the relationship between desire and its object could be explained only in terms that would clarify the relationship between desire and its structure, the complex. In articulating these terms, Lacan both drew on and reinterpreted Freud's theory of superego formation. As Freud conceived it, normative demands are imposed on the ego through the child's identification with and introjection of the father, through which he at once compensates for and renounces the desire for the mother prohibited by paternal interdiction. This secondary identification, effected through the oedipal drama, supplants the primary fusion with the mother and serves as the child's vehicle into reality. Lacan agreed with Freud that the subject's narcissistic defense against desire allows for sublimation and that through this process normative (hetero)sexual identity was constituted.[90] But unlike Freud, Lacan argued that the father's function is itself determined by a cultural form of social organization, the patriarchal family. Like most psychoanalysts, Lacan recognized that the father's authority could no longer be justified by recourse to nature. He returned to Pichon's idea that patriarchal authority is rooted in cultural forms (e.g., language) rather than in "real" fathers but also repudiated Pichon's belief that the patriarchal family in its modern form is the natural basis of social and psychic organization. He maintained that analytic concepts such as imago and complexes had made the family the object not just of "moralizing paraphrases" but of "concrete analysis," that "the human family is an institution."[91]

For Lacan, thus, paternal authority is not derived from nature but is the product of social relations that have invested the father with it.[92] To support his argument about the cultural foundations of the modern family, Lacan pointed out how its form has changed in response to various social and cultural needs. He cited examples

[90] Ibid., p. 60. Since Lacan refers to girls but uses boys' experiences as normative I use the pronoun.

[91] Ibid., pp. 24, 13.

[92] Michael Roth contends that Freud did not necessarily conceive of paternal authority as natural, but Lacan clearly thought that he did, or he was at least responding to French psychoanalysts' uncritical assumption that he did, as well as to their belief that paternal authority was natural, even if they tried to justify it in functionalist rather than moral terms. I thank Michael Roth for pointing out the nuances in Freud's argument to me. See his *Psycho-Analysis as History: Negation and Freedom in Freud* (Ithaca: Cornell University Press, 1987).

from primitive tribal customs and from Roman society and noted the existence of matriarchal cultures in which authority was vested in the maternal uncle. He claimed that even Freud's own concept of Oedipus was the product of a very specific historical and cultural context characterized by a "social decline of the paternal imago," as Lacan called it. "Perhaps the sublime accident of genius is not enough to explain why it was in Vienna—then the center of a state that was the melting pot of the most diverse forms of family, from the most archaic to the most evolved . . . that the son of the Jewish patriarchy imagined the Oedipus complex."[93] That is, Freud's Oedipus was the product of a decline of traditional paternal forms of social organization and hence itself what one critic has called a "neurotic" Oedipus.[94] But what did it mean to claim that the Oedipus complex had a neurotic structure? What were the consequences of such a claim for its future? In other words, how did culture actually determine family forms and hence psychic development itself?

Now we have seen that Lacan was not averse to a decline of paternal authority. Yet he was alarmed by what he saw as the contemporary *form* of that decline. He argued that the weakness of the paternal imago once manifested in Freud's Vienna also characterized "the great contemporary neurosis," and at the end of his essay he linked the decline of traditional patriarchal culture to male homosexuality, and male homosexuality to the blurring of sexual boundaries between men and women. The whole problem, Lacan noted, can be traced, on the one hand, to an "excessive superego" (an overly authoritarian father) and, on the other, to excessively tender or excessively virile mothers. "In male homosexuality, he noted, "the essential role of the relationship between the parents has established itself clearly; analysts have emphasized to

[93] Lacan, *Les Complexes familiaux*, pp. 11–17, 72, 73.
[94] See Borch-Jacobsen's brilliant discussion, pp. 35–41. My analysis follows his closely, though I emphasize the relation between Lacan's text and a much broader sociocultural context, whereas he explores Lacan's struggle with the paradox inherent in the Oedipus complex itself. That is, as Borch-Jacobsen puts it, how can the boy learn to be a father he is also prohibited from being? How can secondary identification be a resolution to primary identification? How can identification be a resolution to the problems posed by identification? He argues, as I will, that Lacan finally cannot distinguish between the two types of identification in a theoretically convincing fashion.

what extent the mother is a domestic tyrant in the marriage, and the subtle or overt manifestations of this tyranny . . . reveal themselves to be a virile protest."[95]

But Lacan does not link male homosexuality (or any other symptom of paternal decline) to immorality; he ties it implicitly to what he called a "rupture of dialectical tension" between fathers and sons.[96] As Freud argued in *Totem and Taboo*, the father's "murder" is the basis of a powerful dialectic through which patriarchy was founded (the one Lacan claimed had been ruptured): the sublimation of the son's original crime against the father marks the founding moment of culture. The paternal imago, says Lacan, is "invested with repression . . . [and] projects repression's original force into the very sublimations that must overcome it."[97] But when dialectical tension is ruptured, all the repression with which the paternal imago is invested is no longer sublimated. That is, if "oedipal identification . . . [revives] the aggressive ambivalence immanent in the primal relationship to the object of identification [the *semblable*],"[98] then the rupture of tension effected by paternal decline renders it impossible to pass from this primary identification to a secondary or healthy one. It leads instead to a homosexual, sadomasochistic eroticization of the persecuting other whom one would like to be.

What Lacan meant by the "decline of the paternal imago" was therefore that oedipal identification had been arrested at an imaginary stage, when the son wants to be and is a rival of the father. Thus, Lacan warned of the dangerous *ambiguity* of the paternal imago, in which the father is the center both of prohibition, of "sexual revelation," and of sublimation, and he noted that the most common consequence of paternal decline was the neurosis "we call autopunition,"[99] which we know describes an arrested stage of

[95] Lacan, *Les Complexes familiaux*, pp. 73, 110.
[96] Ibid., p. 103.
[97] Lacan, quoted in Borch-Jacobsen, p. 39.
[98] Lacan, *Les Complexes familiaux*, p. 96. See also pp. 62–63, where Lacan speaks of the difficulty he has trying to differentiate primary from secondary identification.
[99] Ibid., pp. 103, 105. As he put it, "We have especially insisted on the dual role played by the father, insofar as he represents authority and yet is also the center of sexual revelation; it is the ambiguity of this imago, the incarnation of repression and the catalyst of an essential access to reality, to which we have ascribed the double progress, typical of a culture, of a certain temperament of the superego and of a progressive development of the personality."

development in which the self continues to confuse itself with the ideal other it wants to be.

I would thus argue that when Lacan referred to the "excess of paternal domination" characteristic of the modern nuclear family, he had in mind the narcissistic, sadomasochistic, *imaginary* identification with the father which he believed to be characteristic of modern cultures and especially of fascist movements. For in fact, Lacan contended that the appeal to tradition made in order to correct paternal decline actually reinforced it: "Religious ideals and their social equivalents easily play the role of vehicles of this psychological oppression, so much so that they are utilized to exclusionary ends . . . to signify requirements of a name or of the race."[100] That is—and here Lacan got back to his right-wing target, Pichon—the commitment to the triad of family, work, and country which culminated in the Fascists' celebration of the race was not the solution to but the *product* of the "social decline of the paternal imago." What better way to criticize Pichon than by insisting that the cultural ideals he so cherished were responsible for the "social progress" of "psychic inversion?" As Lacan put it, it is "under the forms of moral sublimity that the mother of the invert exercises her most categorically emasculating action."[101]

In modern culture and now in modern political movements, the difference between the secondary identification with the father's law and the primary identification with the father as rival has thus been absolutely blurred. The problem really amounts to a sophisticated rearticulation of the problem concerning the foundation of paternal authority and hence gender difference with which we are now familiar: How to distinguish between the dialectic of imaginary desire I defined in Chapter 1 and the dialectic of oedipal identification, between a neurotic father and a stable, strong one? How to distinguish the pleasurable and pathological (because self-punitive) repression that characterizes imaginary relations from the pleasurable (because purportedly compensatory) repression that characterizes resolved oedipal relations? And implicitly then,

---

[100] Ibid., p. 105.

[101] Ibid., p. 111. To imply, as Roudinesco does, that this passage represents a tribute to feminists and "pederasts" seems to me to be much too generous. Roudinesco, "M. Pichon devant la famille," p. 211. In a 1947 article Lacan described the psychic breakdown effected by the war in terms of a triumph of the imaginary. "La Psychiatrie anglaise," *EP* (January–March, 1947), 298–318.

what prevents contractual, democratic orders from dissolving into fascist tyrannies? How, in other words, could Lacan restore the father's difference?

It could not be done by restoring the father's so-called natural authority. As we have seen, Lacan believed that paternal authority was not a natural force but a cultural product, and he rejected right-wing solutions because he was convinced that they in fact contributed to the father's decline. At the same time, Lacan did believe that the function of sublimation had to be embodied by the imago of the father. Thus, while he claimed not to be "one of those who mourned the putative loosening of family ties," he also declared that "the ideologues who . . . countered the paternalist family with the most subversive critiques are not those who least bear its imprint." Or as he put it most pointedly: "Our experience has led us to designate the principal determinant of neurosis in the personality of the father, which is always deficient in some way, absent, humiliated, divided. . . . It is this deficiency that, in accordance with our conception of the Oedipus complex, exhausts the instinctive élan as it perverts the dialectic of sublimation."[102] Cultural decline cannot have a positive, dialectical function if it manifests itself as an erosion of the father's difference, his privileged role as agent of sublimation and hence culture maker. But how can the father save the world from imaginary aggression if his role as savior is nothing more than a fragile cultural invention liable to shifts in form and content at specific historical periods? How can the father be at once a privileged agent of sublimation and the (albeit unwitting) perpetrator of the sadomasochistic violence implicit in imaginary identification? Doesn't oedipal identification always necessarily revive "the aggressive ambivalence immanent in the primal relationship to the object of identification?"[103]

In fact, Lacan's essay on the family implicitly proposed to restore the father's difference, so fundamental to normative identification and cultural production, even as it eroded the concept of difference as it had heretofore been defined—in terms of the father's natural or scientifically grounded authority. Because he conceived the father's difference in symbolic (as a social imago) rather than natural

102 Ibid., pp. 72, 73.
103 Ibid., p. 96.

terms, Lacan no longer considered repression a moral adjustment to a reality principle manifested in the father's authority, as Pichon had insisted, nor did he believe, as Freud had argued, that repression produces the final, genital stage of a complex and progressive maturation process. Instead, Lacan suggested that the natural and, in modern cultures, the neurotic father had to be distinguished from the paternal imago. In cultures afflicted by paternal decline, he said, children identify with the (neurotic, overburdened, excessively authoritarian) "parental person" rather than with "that in his comportment which can be objectified," with a "symbolic" (Lacan does not yet use this term) authority rather than a real (and rival) one.[104]

Along these lines, Mikkel Borch-Jacobsen has argued that in this essay Lacan celebrated primitive societies precisely because they separated the real father (the father of prohibition) from what Lacan was later to call a symbolic one (the totem that effects sublimation).[105] Therefore the social imago of the father could not be confused with real fathers. The father remains the fundamental condition of normative identification regardless of the foibles of real men, regardless of the lack of natural or scientific basis for his authority. *This* father can thus function as an agent of sublimation to the extent that his revelatory function is always sublimated, "split" off from him or, to allude to one of Lacan's famous later "algorithms," "barred." That is, because the father is the fundamental condition of normative identification, of knowledge, there is no way of knowing that his own authority is not natural, no way of knowing, on another level, that he is the center not just of sublimation but also of prohibition, and hence no way, to repeat Lacan's words yet again, of reviving "the aggressive ambivalence immanent" in the relation to the "primary object of identification." The imaginary father can be "known," as it were, only when sublimated. Thus, as Lacan was later to make clear, sublimation invariably constitutes the instinct. That is why in this essay Lacan already privileged the structure of the complex over the instinct. It was (in this case the patriarchal) structure that, in his view, constructed the instinct and hence psychic reality itself.

104 Ibid., pp. 103–5.
105 Borch-Jacobsen, pp. 39–40.

I think already in 1938, the gendered self (what Lacan called "sexe psychique")[106] was born at the join of instinct (desire) and culture (patriarchy). Lacan insisted on the necessity of paternal authority; he thus used the father not as truth but as a symbol of a truth (that desire is a cultural product) always already repressed, and in so doing, he retained the patriarchal structure of sexual difference while insisting that male and female natures were not real but constructed, cultural symbols. He addressed the problematic status of the father after the war by making the father the anchor of reality while insisting that his status was illusory, rooted not in nature or instinct but in cultural norms. Although he referred to the New Woman only in veiled terms once or twice in his essay, Lacan made central to psychoanalytic theory what anxious perceptions of the New Woman had made all too clear: Male primacy was no longer as certain as it had once been. At the same time, he insisted on the "primacy of the male principle."[107]

Lacan's concept of the father represented the blurring of gender boundaries already implicit in psychoanalysts' construction of the relationship between equality and difference. He too reconstructed those boundaries in terms of an equality (the father loses his natural privilege and predominance) that was always experienced as a gender difference, in terms of "sexual indifference"[108] always already experienced as masculinity, and hence of an imaginary other already structured into the self. In so doing, he put French psychoanalysts' attempts to restore male power at the heart of analysis, he reiterated a patriarchal structure of sexual difference. But he effected that restoration only by redefining the foundations of patriarchy in new terms.

Lacan thus took psychoanalysts' problematic efforts to ground paternal authority in science to a striking, though perhaps not entirely unexpected conclusion: Didn't Lacan also use the preva-

---

106 Lacan, *Les Complexes familiaux*, p. 52.

107 Ibid., p. 111.

108 The term appears in Luce Irigaray, *Speculum of the Other Woman*, trans. Gillian Gill (Ithaca: Cornell University Press, 1985), p. 28. Teresa de Lauretis uses it in "Sexual Indifference and Lesbian Representation," in Sue-Ellen Case, ed., *Performing Feminisms: Feminist Critical Theory and Theatre* (Baltimore: Johns Hopkins University Press, 1990), p. 18. They use it to describe how masculinity itself becomes a term of sexual indifference, of gender neutrality. This idea is already implicit in this essay but is not developed until Lacan begins work on female sexuality much later.

lent notion of a father who was absent, humiliated, divided, and in decline as a metaphor for the dissolution of gender boundaries manifested by the specter of homosexuality and of the dominant, tyrannical woman? And didn't he too use the logic of "equal but different" to structure a collapse of gender boundaries into what he later called a symbolic father who is the site of an imaginary other (and hence of a potential homosexuality or femininity) always already sublimated?

Thus Lacan is a critic of patriarchy, but he really only quibbled with its forms rather than its necessity. He thus looked to patriarchy to stabilize patriarchy. To repeat, Lacan did not draw a new line between men and women but argued that the masculine self is an always repressed other. The oedipal "solution" proposed by Lacan thus suggested that the true self is accessible only when repressed, lost, given form *as a sexe psychique*. But what is this solution to the conflation of gender boundaries but a failure of (an unusually imaginative) imagination to envision alternatives to patriarchy? What does it mean but that Lacan, with the best of intentions to liberate the world from the ghosts of fathers—of French psychoanalysts, Pichon, maybe even Freud—could not finally imagine a world without some kind of father figure? And how, then, can we distinguish between the oedipal and the imaginary dialectic (how do we restore the father's difference—the normative function of Oedipus) except, finally, by accepting the psychoanalysts' word that he is indeed different?

The Symbolic

Lacan worked out the implications of this construction of sexual difference much later, when he developed the concept of the symbolic.[109] Here I want to offer only a brief summary of this difficult concept in order to describe how he developed the paradoxical notion of paternal authority implicit in *Les Complexes familiaux*. How, first of all, did this reconstruction of the father after 1953 "resolve" in new terms the discord between self and other which

[109] He also drew out some of those implications in his late discussion of female sexuality. In *Les Complexes familiaux*, Lacan was primarily interested in the construction of (male) gender identity and the restoration of the father.

the imaginary self cannot tolerate? As Lacan claimed, "the function of psychic development" is to "resolve [this primordial discordance between the ego and reality] by developing it."[110] In order to emerge from social hell, then, the subject must accept the alterity of the other, must accept the fact that his or her desire for the other will remain ever unsatisfied. Entry into the symbolic facilitates the acceptance of the otherness of the other: It splits the ego, resolves discord by developing it.

The symbolic is an entry into language effected by the "name of the father," which organizes, guides, and structures imaginary perceptions. This linguistic reinterpretation of the father's difference maintained the structures I have outlined thus far while redefining them in terms of language. Hence, Lacan argued that the father's "no" (the paternal interdiction), homophonic in French with the "name" of the father (nom du père), represents an initiation into the world of language through the introjection of the father's phallus conceived as signifier (hence conceived not as the penis but as the culturally privileged signifier of sexual difference, much like the father's symbolic role in Les Complexes familiaux). In Lacan's later work, this introjection is conceived as overcoming castration anxiety and hence as overcoming the desire to "be" the phallus which compensates for the mother's presumed castration. Through identification with the father's name, men move from being the phallus to having the phallus, and hence from a projection of themselves onto the mother to an assumption of a split identity.

In the late Lacan too, this belief in having the phallus is an illusion that is at the same time the fundamental basis of reality. That is, the phallus signifies the principle of sexual difference. It anchors reality because it represents the capacity to name and hence to differentiate from and compensate for the loss of (replace the desire for fusion with) the mother. The introjection of the father's incest prohibition enables us to pass from the narcissism of the mirror stage to social relations: from primary identification with the mother or the mirror image to a secondary identification with the father. At the same time, because the phallus is a signifier, that is, because it is part of a relational linguistic (i.e., Saussurian) system, it is not the "truth" about sexual difference. Instead, it

[110]Lacan, Ecrits, p. 187.

represents a truth about the constructedness of sexual difference that is always, in Lacan's word, "veiled."[111] For Lacan, patriarchy no longer functioned as the foundation of truth but became instead an anchor of cultural fictions.[112] That is, the father is both authentic and a charlatan, a man who doesn't know he is also always other.

[111] Lacan, *Feminine Sexuality*, p. 82. For a critique of Lacan's concept of the phallus, see Jacques Derrida, *The Post Card: From Socrates to Freud and Beyond*, trans. Alan Bass (Chicago: University of Chicago Press, 1987), pp. 411-96. For an interesting discussion of the relationship between Lacan and Derrida which tries to move outside both of them, see John Forrester, *The Seductions of Psychoanalysis: Freud, Lacan, and Derrida* (Cambridge: Cambridge University Press, 1990), esp. pp. 221–42.

[112] Many feminists believe that this argument, at least in its more recent version, constitutes a radical critique of patriarchy because, while it reinforces normative gender roles, it also theorizes to what extent they are constructed. See Jardine, pp. 159–77; Jane Gallop, *The Daughter's Seduction: Feminism and Psychoanalysis* (Ithaca: Cornell University Press, 1982); Mitchell and Rose, Introduction to Lacan, *Feminine Sexuality*, pp. 2–57; Ragland-Sullivan, pp. 267–308. There are also many articles pertaining to Lacan's understanding of feminine sexuality. For a lucid anti-Lacanian account, see Dorothy Leland, "Lacanian Psychoanalysis and French Feminism: Toward an Adequate Political Psychology," *Hypatia* no. 3 (Winter 1989), 81–103.

Chapter Three

Sight Unseen
(Reading the Unconscious)

Pleasure and reality, instinct and culture, madness and reason, self and other—the dichotomies that had structured debates about criminals and about deviance in general before the Great War—were being redefined in new terms. The debate about schizophrenia in interwar France offers yet another window on the dissolution of the boundaries between the normal and the pathological, and helps us better to understand precisely where Lacan located the other self and why he located it where he did. I first discuss the way in which the kinds of questions articulated in the previous two chapters were replicated in the theoretical terms used to redefine schizophrenia: Where and how to draw boundaries between full-fledged schizophrenics and functional ones? How to determine who was a schizophrenic and on what grounds? Second, I analyze how those terms became the basis for what one critic has termed the most original product of French psychoanalysis: the concept of scotomization.[1] And finally, I address how scotomization structured a new concept of the unconscious as an absolute other in French psychoanalysis and in Lacan's work specifically.

Schizophrenia

In the first years of the twentieth century the founding of two journals in France signaled the beginning of what could easily be

[1] Bercherie, pp. 55, 67n.

called a new era in French psychiatry. In 1904 the psychiatrist Pierre Janet launched the *Journal de Psychologie* with Georges Dumas. Both had propounded a fundamental identity of normal and pathological psychic mechanisms and posited a quantitative (functional) difference between them. In 1906 G. Ballet, J. Dejérine, A. Antheaume, and Henri Claude began publishing *L'Encéphale*, whose purpose was to end the isolation of mental pathology and thus to link it more intimately with neurology and psychology. They emphasized a "return to the clinic" to reinforce the image of the alienist as a scientist rather than a medical administrator, the role most psychiatrists played throughout the nineteenth century.[2]

The founding of these journals thus marked an important theoretical and professional transition in French psychiatry which culminated in the interwar years. In an open letter to the minister of public health in 1924, the psychiatrist Henri Baruk remarked approvingly that within the last few years French psychiatry had attempted to resurrect its own great clinical tradition. He claimed that psychiatrists were motivated by the desire to find stable ground between a "sterile" nosological system, which degeneracy theory had made of the study of heredity, and "philosophical" psychiatry, in which psychiatric analyses had come to resemble those of ethics or of sociology.[3] Baruk spoke on behalf of the psychiatric reform movement, pleading for the establishment of open services and stressing the importance of long-term observation of psychopathic behavior in facilitating the development of preventive medicine. In keeping with the league's language, he suggested that such strategies would remedicalize the psychogenesis of mental illness while moving away from the problematic nosological classification systems characteristic of nineteenth-century medicine.

This turn back to the clinic represented an attempt to clarify definitions of mental illness. For example, whereas psychiatrists had long questioned any simple dichotomy between the demented

[2] The term *alienist* was coined to describe the role of the doctor who directed asylums until the early twentieth century. The term reflects the increasing professionalization of psychiatry during the nineteenth century. The alienist was not simply a consultant to the lay administrator (as had been the case through the early nineteenth century) but the director of the establishment. This situation did not change until psychiatrists extended their sphere of influence beyond the asylum.

[3] Henri Baruk, "La Question des services ouverts et l'évolution de la psychiatrie médicale," *L'Aliéniste Français* (February 1932), 74.

and the sane, it was not until 1923 that dementia became obsolete as an acceptable psychiatric diagnosis; J. Rogues de Fursac made long-standing medical opinion official when he eliminated it from his *Manuel de psychiatrie*.[4] After 1923 other terms were developed for patients who appeared demented but were not—Chaslin's *folie discordante*, for example. No one, however, had persuasively accounted for the apparent discrepancy between a patient's intellect and his or her assumed mental deficiency.[5]

Dementia had long been conceived as a constitutional predisposition inherent in highly intelligent individuals, but Bénédict-Auguste Morel's insistence in 1860 that dementia praecox was rooted in a hereditary predisposition had proven far too general. He had not really explained the reasons why mental functions diminished and why that diminution was not always progressive. German-speaking psychiatrists were responsible for addressing the theoretical problems inherent in the model of degeneration. In 1893 Emil Kraeplin used the term *dementia* again but conceived it as one part of a degenerative process whose subcategories (dementia praecox, catatonia, and dementia paranoides) replaced the separate diagnostic categories of hebephrenia, catatonia, and paranoia. Sander Gilman describes how Kraeplin shifted the focus of his analysis away from "deterioration . . . to the phenomenology of the disease," to a study of the patient's language and artistic products.[6] Nevertheless, not until the early twentieth century did a new emphasis on the psychogenetic roots of mental illness lead to a definitive move away from nineteenth-century categories. The Swiss psychiatrist Eugen Bleuler's work, with its emphasis on psychopathology and its attempt to differentiate between different forms of dementia within a broad clinical framework, provided the most fruitful, if problematic, means of dealing with the issue at hand.

Bleuler had coined the term *schizophrenia* in 1911 as an alternative to Kraeplin's categories of dementia.[7] According to Bleuler,

[4] J. Rogues de Fursac, *Manuel de psychiatrie* (Paris: Felix Alcan, 1923), pp. 305–7. He replaced *démence précoce* with *hébéphréno-catatonie* (*schizophrénie*).

[5] J. Lautier, "Le Démembrement de la démence précoce," *AMP* 82 (1924), 299–300.

[6] Sander Gilman, *Disease and Representation: Images of Illness from Madness to AIDS* (Ithaca: Cornell University Press, 1988), p. 211. I have drawn on Gilman's discussion of schizophrenia, pp. 208–12.

[7] Bleuler's book was titled: *Dementia Praecox; or, The Group of Schizophrenias*.

schizophrenia defined different stages of mental illness depending on the degree to which a subject lost or maintained contact with reality. He noted that the causes of schizophrenia were unknown, though probably related to the physiology of the brain, but he focused primarily on symptoms rather than etiology. Bleuler claimed that the loss of contact with reality was the consequence of a fundamental dissociation that manifested itself in the patient's language. His attention to language marked Freud's influence, as did his definition of normality in experiential (i.e., as an attitude toward reality) rather than empirical terms.[8]

Bleuler provided a resolution to a difficult problem in nineteenth-century psychiatry, one that the concept of dementia illustrated. To accommodate the diversity of individual genealogies and symptoms, nosological categories had to be increasingly differentiated, making it difficult to establish any connection between individual symptoms and illnesses of a more general order. By introducing the notion of a psychopathological structure defined according to a broad criterion—the loss of contact with reality—Bleuler grouped apparently unrelated organic symptoms under a unified structure of which these symptoms were but various manifestations.

Although articles about Bleuler appeared in French as early as 1912, it was primarily through the devoted efforts of Eugène Minkowski that his work was diffused in France. Minkowski, a Polish refugee who had been Bleuler's student in Zurich, published a series of articles as well as a book about schizophrenia in 1927. Minkowski's most important article, "Impressions psychiatrique d'un séjour à Zürich," summarized Bleuler's revision of Kraeplin's categories and inspired a host of responses and criticisms.[9] Most French psychiatrists during the 1920s perceived a structural problem in Bleuler's conception of schizophrenia opposite to the one he had criticized in his predecessors. That is, the criterion he used was so extensive that virtually any form of behavior could be classified as schizophrenic regardless of its clinical symptoms.[10] Such was

[8] For a discussion of Bleuler, see Ellenberger, pp. 285–88.

[9] Eugène Minkowski, "Impressions psychiatrique d'un séjour à Zurich," *AMP* 81 (1923). Minkowski's book was titled *La Schizophrénie: Psychopathologie des schizoïdes et des schizophrènes.* (Paris: Payot, 1927).

[10] See, for example, P. R. Bize, "La Notion de contact avec la réalité: Le Contact ego-cosmos," *EP* no. 3 (1935) 3–21; Henri Claude, "A propos de la schizoïdie et la

the common ground of the various interpretations of Bleuler's work in France.

Bleuler's use of such an extensive criterion derived from his refusal to concern himself with the etiology of schizophrenia. Bleuler believed that its causes were probably organic and that psychic factors (e.g., personality structure) gave the symptoms their form. It was the symptoms he wanted to describe in a new way. Instead of trying to distinguish between endogenous and exogenous forms of schizophrenia, Bleuler discerned primary and secondary symptoms related to the dissonance between the patient and the world.

French psychiatrists were divided over how to interpret his work, and their discussion focused above all on the question Bleuler had avoided: the question of etiology. Henri Ey, an important representative of dynamic psychiatry, and Minkowski, who articulated a phenomenological version of psychopathology, both insisted in different ways that Bleuler believed in an organic etiology and that the loss of contact with reality was essentially the superstructure of a constitutional deficiency. Henri Claude, Adrien Borel, and Gilbert Robin argued that schizophrenic dissonance also had psychic causes that were frequently ignored. They maintained that those causes could be identified only through an analysis of the individual's constitution understood as a set of psychological as well as organic predispositions. Despite the importance of Ey's and Minkowski's ideas, Claude, Borel, and Robin's collective critique of Bleuler was the real point of departure for a *psychoanalytic* recasting of the psychiatric discussion about schizophrenia.

Claude's school was part of the *Evolution Psychiatrique* group, the first psychoanalytic current in France, whose journal of the same name appeared in 1925. In contrast to the group around the *Revue Française de Psychanalyse*, they were not Freudians (though there was some overlap between the two groups), but they sought, according to Paul Bercherie, "to use Bleuler's work in an attempt to reconcile Janet and Freud via a French reading of psychoanalysis

schizophrénie," *AMP* 84 (1926), 332–54; J. Dublineau, "Signification psychopathologique de la schizophrénie," *EP* no. 4 (1935), 33–81; Eugène Minkowski, "Démence précoce, schizophrénie, schizoïdie," *AMP* 84 (1926); G. Morsier and F. Morel, "Critique de la notion de la schizophrénie," *AMP* 87 (1929) 406–15; Gilbert Robin, "Les Frontières de la schizophrénie et de la démence précoce," *EP* no. 3 (1932), 91–103.

and by applying it to the field of psychiatry."[11] Claude, Borel, and Robin's collective critique of Bleuler was formulated in a series of articles published in various psychiatric journals between 1924 and 1926. They contended that Bleuler, by making schizophrenia the mental illness par excellence, had neglected the individual in the "totality of his elements." The biggest reproach one could make to the master was that "he had incorporated diverse illnesses into a vast synthesis, and in so doing sacrificed a precise delimitation of the mental disease in favor of the delineation of broad structures."[12] He had distinguished only four types: paranoia, catatonia, hebephrenia, and simple schizophrenia. This last category proved the most problematic, precisely because it represented cases in which the boundary between normality and pathology was blurry at best.

Kraeplin and Bleuler's designation of simple schizophrenia was, they believed, only a reformulation of Ulysse Trélat's *folie lucide*, a term he used to denote those individuals who were mentally ill but appeared normal. Within this category, Trélat had classified "erotomaniacs," kleptomaniacs, suicidal, jealous, and untrustworthy patients. Bleuler retained this classification, integrating it into the framework of schizophrenia itself. Claude, Borel, and Robin objected to this rounding up of every sort of social misfit into one category, and were especially critical of their subsumption under the even larger category of schizophrenia, where they were lumped with much more serious diseases. Equally problematic, in their view, was Bleuler's incorporation of illnesses diagnosed as demential under the rubric of schizophrenia. They argued that schizophrenia and dementia were not necessarily related.[13]

Claude, Borel, and Robin replaced the notion of simple schizophrenia with that of a schizoid constitution, a set of psychological tendencies that marked an inclination toward schizophrenic behavior, which could be divided into simple and latent forms.[14] According to Claude, schizophrenia was not an attitude toward reality, as Bleuler had claimed. Instead it was a habitual and clinically discernible psychological state, a constitution that had

[11] Bercherie, p. 67n.
[12] Henri Claude, Adrien Borel, Gilbert Robin, "La Constitution schizoïde," *L'Encéphale* 19 (1924), 209.
[13] Claude, "A propos de la schizoïdie," p. 334.
[14] Ibid., p. 343.

developed in relation to sociopsychological circumstances specific to a given individual but linked to a set of clinically verifiable symptoms common, in varying degrees, to all schizophrenics.[15]

To accommodate individual peculiarities, then, Claude, Borel, and Robin defined three successive stages of constitutional development: a schizoid constitution, schizomania, and schizophrenia. The schizoid constitution merely marked a tendency toward full-fledged schizophrenia but was in no way incompatible with normal life. Schizomania signaled a habitual tendency toward dissociation. Schizophrenia represented the final stage of a development that could be arrested permanently at any stage, a development, in other words, not fatally progressive.[16] This conception remained within the framework of Bleuler's thinking, in which schizophrenia was a matter of degrees of estrangement rather than of an absolute rupture with reality, but it specified more clearly the very different and complex forms of dissociation that actually existed.

Those forms of dissociation could be identified by different symptoms, which Claude, Borel, and Robin sought to systematize. Most of their work was devoted to articulating the symptomatology of the schizoid constitution, which manifested no diminished mental capacity, but a passive and indifferent attitude to the world, and a consciousness of the illness combined with a feeling of powerlessness before it. The three psychiatrists surmised that these symptoms originated in infancy and emerged gradually after some kind of emotional trauma.[17] They were thus primarily interested in evaluating the etiology of schizophrenia in patients who manifested no signs of intellectual deficiency but who were diagnosed as schizophrenic because of their difficulty in getting on

[15] It should be noted that "constitutionalism" usually referred to a physical rather than a mental predisposition to mental illness; so their use of the term in this way was confusing. Henri Ey tried to clarify the concept, which he claimed had become unclear because of the move away from degeneracy as an acceptable diagnosis and the "confused" efforts of Claude, Borel, and Robin to separate the psychic and organic components of schizophrenia in a more conceptually sophisticated way than had Bleuler. Ey argued that Claude et al. were not wrong but had misunderstood Bleuler's claim that schizophrenia was primarily a loss of contact with reality. See Henri Ey, "Position actuelles des problèmes de la démence précoce et des états schizophréniques," *EP* no. 3 (1934), 3–25; and Paul Guiraud and Henri Ey, "Remarques critiques sur la schizophrénie de Bleuler," *AMP* 84 (1926), 364.

[16] Claude, Borel, Robin, "Démence précoce, schizomanie, et schizophrénie," *Encéphale* 19 (1924), 148–50.

[17] Claude, Borel, Robin, "La Constitution schizoïde," p. 210.

in the world. Borel and Robin in particular gave priority to the psychological meaning of symptoms by explaining dissociation in terms of a psychological need to compensate for what the patient perceived as an empty, hopeless, existence. In so doing, they were influenced by the surrealist celebration of dreams and their relation to aesthetic creativity. Borel himself was the psychoanalyst of many writers and artists, including Georges Bataille, Michel Leiris, and Raymond Queneau.

Most of the patients they examined manifested identical symptoms. Borel and Robin called them dreamers of a particular order. They were to a pathological degree indifferent to their immediate surroundings but also gifted with extraordinary imaginative power and very high intelligence.[18] Their indifference distinguished them from other cases of psychotic delirium in which the subject's hallucinations became an objective reality externalized and interpreted. In contrast, dreamers such as "Marie B." were aware of their dissociation: "I said I was the Queen of Spain. Deep down I knew it wasn't really true. I was like a child who plays with her doll and who knows very well that her doll isn't alive, but who wants to persuade herself otherwise."[19]

Borel and Robin acknowledged the importance of Freud's theory of the unconscious, and they cited Freud along with the surrealists as one of their most important inspirations. Their interpretation of Freud was nevertheless filtered through French readings of his work. This filtering was especially evident in their reference to various forms of compensation, for example, Marie B.'s *rêveries morbides* (morbid daydreams), which they used to explain cases of schizophrenia with no apparent organic causes. Compensation described the way in which dreamers, who appeared normal but whose perceptions blurred the boundaries between reality and hallucination, filled up the empty places in their lives with either fantasies or creative work. Borel and Robin borrowed the term from Freud's French interpreters, who both reformulated and rejected the Freudian concept. Whereas Freud had defined compensation as sublimation, as a form of repression, the French psychiatrist M. Montassut argued that it was a voluntary evasion in which the patient created an imaginary world where his or her wishes could

[18] Adrien Borel and Gilbert Robin, *Les Rêveurs éveillés* (Paris, 1925).
[19] Adrien Borel and Gilbert Robin, "Les Rêveries morbides," *AMP* 82 (1924), 239.

be fulfilled. Montassut thus made no distinction between compensation and sublimation, and conceived the work of art as a "fecund form of compensation."[20] Along with the psychiatrist Maurice Mignard, he argued that his understanding of compensation, unlike Freud's, was nonsexual because many forms of neuroses and psychoses designated compensatory involved no sexual components.[21] His argument was thus based on a widespread and erroneous perception of Freudian theory as a form of pansexualism, and furthermore, it left ambiguous to what extent compensation described a conscious or unconscious process.

By reformulating schizophrenia as a specific set of constitutional tendencies, Claude and his fellow psychiatrists hoped to avoid what they perceived as the pitfalls of Bleuler's overly synthetic schema. Yet because they relied on an essentially functionalist structure of compensation to explain the origins of abnormal behavior in many cases, that reformulation raised another problem concerning the etiology of schizophrenia. First, by claiming that the dissociation that described schizophrenia was symptomatic of constitutional tendencies, they believed they were refining Bleuler's concept. Borel and Robin summarized:

> The initial trouble is less the daydream than the loss of contact with the environment. It is not because he dreams that the schizoid loses contact. It is because he loses contact with the environment that daydreaming comes to replace an empty reality, frequently in embellished form. As for the rest, it is necessary to recognize that in the present state of our knowledge, this maladaptation to the real is an objective fact [as opposed to an attitude, as Bleuler had conceived it] that most often appears to us as constitutional, inherent in the individual.[22]

But they do not account for these constitutional tendencies or their specificity.

Because compensation was conceived not as a form of repression but rather as an evasion of reality, it could explain schizophrenic

---

[20] M. Montassut, "Les Compensations imaginatives," *EP* no. 4 (1934), 21, 25.

[21] Maurice Mignard and M. Montassut, "Un Délire de compensation," *Encéphale* 19 (1924), 632.

[22] Adrien Borel and Gilbert Robin, "Les Rêveurs," *EP* no. 1 (1925), 164; see also their *Rêveurs éveillés*, p. 99.

behavior only as rational or irrational choices while begging the question of what provoked the choices in the first place. It was therefore not clear how different forms of compensation functioned *unconsciously* (and thus how or why the schizophrenic lost contact with the environment). Thus, Marie B. wanted to be the queen of Spain, but Borel and Robin could not explain what lack or deprivation her desire was compensating for.[23] In other words, they could not explain by which mechanism the memories of infancy were transposed into morbid symptoms. Borel, Claude, and Robin were thus led to a theoretical impasse in which the origins of schizophrenia could be explained only by reference to its symptoms. This tautological account of schizophrenic behavior was linked to the absence of a concept of repression which could explain why that behavior took the form that it did or which could account more clearly for the relationship between dissociation and the subject's personality. In response to this inadequacy, French psychoanalysts formulated a new concept of psychic development, what they viewed as an original explanation of psychosis and an important innovation of Freud's concept of repression.

Scotomization

Edouard Pichon and René Laforgue synthesized the various discussions about schizophrenia under the rubric of psychoanalysis by redefining it as "schizonoia," as a psychogenic process that described a primarily unconscious conflict. Pichon used the concept of "scotomization"—a term he borrowed from ophthalmology—to explain the psychic mechanism that produced schizonoia, a refusal, essentially, to be weaned, to accept moral responsibility.[24]

---

[23] Borel had interpreted a dream of Marie's, in which flowers she wanted to pick withered the moment she extended her hand to pick them, as symbolizing her unfulfilled existence. Her lack drove her further and further into herself and yet at the same time helped her realize her "secret desires"; "It seems that there must exist . . . a will to be ill . . . the psychosis having been a compensation of an existence judged incomplete and having realized in an oblique manner the secret desires of the patient." Henri Claude, Adrien Borel, and Gilbert Robin, "A propos d'une bouffée délirante à contenu symbolique: Essai d'explication biologique et psycholgique d'un désir," *AMP* 81 (1923), 227.

[24] Edouard Pichon, René Allendy, René Laforgue, Raymond de Sanssure, *Le Rêve et la psychanalyse* (Paris: Maloine), p. 207.

The term *scotomization* was originally derived from the Greek word for darkness or obscurity. After 1885 *scotoma* came to refer to a lacuna in the field of vision due to insensitivity at certain points on the retina.

Scotomization was one of the most original contributions of French psychoanalysis to official psychoanalytic theory before the Second World War. It was important because it was opposed to the Freudian notion of repression. Its proponents argued that through scotomization a desire to prolong infantile fusion with the mother was transposed into compensatory fantasies that masked and sustained that fusion into adulthood. The term received some notoriety when it became the object of a lengthy correspondence between Freud and René Laforgue, and Freud himself mentioned the concept in his work on anxiety and inhibitions.[25] Laforgue, an Alsatian fluent in German, published two articles on the subject in the *Internationale Zeitschrift für ärtzliche Psychoanalyse* in 1926, and through the efforts of René Allendy and Laforgue, scotomization was mentioned in *L'Esprit Nouveau*, an avant-garde journal sympathetic to psychoanalysis. As late as 1951 the analyst Michel Cénac referred uncritically to scotomization in a lecture he gave on psychoanalysis and legal issues.[26]

The links between French psychiatric and psychoanalytic concepts of schizophrenia were complex and varied. Here I want to focus on how the theoretical development of scotomization was structured by the psychiatric discussion of schizophrenia in one important respect: Scotomization was in part an elaboration in psychoanalytic terms of the structure of compensation which Montassut had formulated as an alternative to Freud's view.[27] This

[25] Sigmund Freud and René Laforgue, "Correspondance, 1923–1937," *Nouvelle Revue Française de Psychanalyse* 15 (Spring 1977), 235–314.

[26] René Laforgue, "Über Skotomisation in der Schizophrenie" and "Verdrängung und Skotomisation," *Internationale Zeitschrift für ärtzliche Psychoanalyse* 12 (1926), 451–56, 54–65; René Allendy and René Laforgue, "Le Conscient et l'inconscient," *L'Esprit Nouveau* no. 21 (1925), 8; Michel Cénac, "Le Témoinage et sa valeur au point de vue judiciare," *Congrès des Médecins Aliénistes et Neurologistes de France et des Pays de Langue Française* (Paris, July 16–23, 1951), 33. A similar version of Laforgue's first article was published as "Scotomization in Schizophrenia," *International Journal of Psycho-analysis* 8 (1927).

[27] Of course, this entire current of psychoanalytic thought elaborated a complex reading of Freud through French filters which culminated in Lacan's work. It is not my purpose to give a full account of all these developments. See Bercherie, pp. 54–56.

structure was incorporated into the new term. Since in France the concept signified not the return of the repressed but a refusal to repress, the Freudian notion of repression did not entrench itself in France, where it could be assimilated only with difficulty into the intellectual patrimony. Consequently, scotomization seemed a perfectly reasonable and even necessary innovation within French psychoanalytic circles, where it redefined in "psychoanalytic" terms the orthodox understanding of repression as Freud had conceived it. Freud himself, however, greeted the notion with incomprehension, and Elisabeth Roudinesco has even termed the correspondence about scotomization between Freud and Laforgue a "dialogue of the deaf."[28]

Because French psychiatrists had provided no solid explanatory structure by which to judge exactly how and why mental illness "compensated" for a reality manqué and because psychoanalysts rejected the concept of repression as Freud had defined it (which provided such a structure), they were not able to explain schizophrenia in orthodox Freudian terms or to outline precisely how scotomization described an *unconscious* process. Instead, they conceived scotomization—and thus psychosis in general—as a subversion of moral responsibility conditioned by the absence of a proper moral development, the notion, we recall, against which Lacan first argued in 1938.

In an article that appeared in *L'Evolution Psychiatrique* in 1925, Henri Codet and Laforgue incorporated diverse forms of schizophrenic behavior within schizonoia by assigning them a single, though complex causality. Chaslin's discordance, Bleuler's schizophrenia, and Claude's schizomania were all forms of discrepancy between what an individual consciously wanted and what he or she really, unconsciously, desired. Common to all forms of schizonoia was the tendency to create a refuge from reality, described by Bleuler as a desire to be ill, by Montassut as compensation, and by Claude, Borel, and Robin as morbid daydreams. Laforgue and Codet argued that schizonoiac symptoms all represented the same effort to recreate the womb, to substitute some form of autism for the absent mother.[29] The drive to seek this refuge was the consequence

---

[28] Roudinesco, *La Bataille* 1:316.
[29] Henri Codet and René Laforgue, "Les Arriérations affectives: La Schizonoïa," *EP* no. 1 (1925), 102.

of an inadequately developed *oblativité,* the capacity to sacrifice one's needs and desires to social necessities, analogous to Freud's reality principle. Those patients who were incapable of making such a sacrifice scotomized social demands. Laforgue differentiated scotomization from Freud's concept of repression. "Contrary to what happens in normal repression," he wrote, "the mind in spite of outward appearances is really simply trying to evade a situation in which it has to endure frustration and which it apprehends as a castration." In other words, when an individual scotomizes a desire he or she only apparently represses it.[30]

This rather paradoxical concept, in which a desire is only apparently repressed, described a process in which every obstacle to recreating fusion with the mother was removed from the subject's field of vision. The inner retreat of a dreamer represented not so much indifference to the world as an unconscious refusal to make the sacrifices demanded by adult social life.

Laforgue, Pichon, and other analysts wrote about several clinical cases exemplifying scotomization. One essay, which appeared in a collection titled *Le Rêve et la psychanalyse* in 1926, concerned Madame X, a woman paralyzed by the fear of hurting other people. A modern day Penelope, she obsessively undid any work she had accomplished for fear it had been infused with "bad thoughts," and she feared speaking lest she utter something contradictory, less than complimentary, or false. Pichon and Laforgue suggested that Madame X actually wanted to owe nothing to others, and while this desire was consciously impeded, it was unconsciously realized. Thus, she jealously guarded her independence, especially in regard to her husband, whom she treated "like a piece of furniture." In fact, she refused all authority, and "in the end she believed she was above everything and perfect. . . . She cannot admit that anything escapes her; she has to know everything, she has to control everything; she scotomizes her husband, her teachers, and even God the Father."[31]

Apparently, as a child Madame X had terribly resented the birth of her younger brother and her parents indulged rather than disciplined her resentment. His birth coincided with her increasing

---

[30] Quoted in Macey, p. 35. See also René Laforgue, "Schizophrénie et schizonoïa," *RFP* 1 (1927), 13.
[31] Pichon et al., *Le Rêve et la psychanalyse,* p. 184.

sexual desire for her father, even though she was still completely dependent on her mother; consequently, her brother became a rival for her mother's love when the infant should have been rivaling her mother for the love of her father. In order to satisfy her desires, Madame X developed a "masculine" personality, viewing her father with increasing hostility, unable to submit to him and what he represented by way of wisdom and authority. This rejection or refusal to submit became more untenable as she entered adulthood, married, and was expected to assume the obligations of her social role. As Laforgue and Pichon saw it, the camouflage of obsessive altruism functioned as a compensation, or *habillage*, that masked her real desires; it functioned as a distortion that, paradoxically, permitted her true desires to be realized.

Madame X manifested the main characteristic of scotomization as identified by French psychoanalysts. She remained "fixed," as it were, at an anal-sadistic stage of development, replacing her mother with a compensatory narcissism that symbolized the inversion of her desires from the exterior, the social world represented by the father, to the interior, the mother's womb. Her fixation on her mother, coupled with her resentment of her father, was common, they argued, to all schizophrenics, who scotomized authority embodied in language, education, and stages of psychological development entailing a break with the mother and an entry into the "maturity" symbolized by paternal authority.[32]

In another case cited in the same collection, a man resists any form of cultural appropriation, particularly language: "His language is also evidence of his psychic state. It tries to produce in a minimum of time a maximum number of words: he also often swallows half his phrases. They become unintelligible, and the result of this economy is that he is obliged to repeat what he already said."[33] This compensatory mechanism, this linguistic economizing that necessarily wastes words, veils a real refusal to accord others the kind of recognition implicit in speech. In this way scotomization functions as a mechanism to realize a desire that is apparently repressed, instead of as a form of repression. Freudian repression requires an original sighting, as it were, of the thing repressed to set the repressive mechanism in motion (what

[32] Ibid., pp. 201–2.
[33] Ibid., p. 188.

Freud called primal repression), but scotomization represents an original blindness, so that what is being scotomized is not something once seen but something always already masked. "This compensation," wrote Allendy and Laforgue, "differs from sublimation in the sense that . . . it confines itself to masking the primitive tendency without transforming it."[34] Since scotomization masks but does not transform—displace, project, and so forth—unconscious desire, that desire is literally satisfied because it is apparently repressed (Madame X's altruism allowed her to indulge herself), so that the very condition for its satisfaction is its apparent repression.

When the subject scotomizes, he or she only mimics repression; the subject's apparent submission to the law of the father is thus always only the appearance of submission, and desire seems to subvert the normalizing effects of culture. But because unconscious desire and cultural norms cannot be differentiated (Madame X's desire to subvert the law is expressed as lawfulness), unconscious desire has no reference, no origin, except the cultural norms with which it has become continuous. The unconscious is thus at once continuous with and "beyond" culture because it cannot be conceived except in terms of what it is not: because its drives are always already expressed as cultural norms and, in this case, primarily patriarchal ones. The unconscious, then, is not something that can be discovered under layers of repression; it is, quite literally, a blind spot.

Lacan: Psychosis

Scotomization thus shifted the traditional psychoanalytic attempt to understand the content of the unconscious (i.e., to work out the complex links between the primary process and the etiology of sexuality) in a new direction. If scotomization, in Freud's view, led psychoanalysts to an epistemological dead end, it furnished Lacan, in the context of a return to Freud, with a new way of understanding psychosis.

Lacan, as we have seen, criticized the inadequacies of Pichon's use of morality as a criterion to distinguish between normal and

[34] Allendy and Laforgue, "Le Conscient et l'inconscient," p. 3.

pathological development in his 1938 article on the family. There, however, he did not address scotomization directly, though it was the conceptual mechanism Pichon had employed. Despite his criticisms, Lacan did continue to borrow several of Pichon's conceptual innovations, particularly his distinction between the *moi* and the *je*, or between an imaginary self and a "subject of the unconscious," absent in Freud and an impossible distinction to make in German.[35] When Lacan reformulated Freud's own concept of psychosis much later, he turned once again to Pichon.

Pichon, a linguist, began a long effort to find linguistic equivalents for psychoanalytic concepts as early as 1925, when he published an article in *L'Evolution Psychiatrique* titled "Grammaire en tant que mode de l'exploration de l'inconscient." By 1928 he had published a multivolume French grammar with his uncle Jacques Damourette, as well as a few other articles about psychoanalysis and language. Pichon's inspiration was chauvinistic; he believed in the correlation between linguistic and racial (and, as we have already seen, male) superiority and was, as noted earlier, an Action Française supporter. Yet his fascist tendencies did not mitigate the originality of his venture. In the 1928 grammar he linked scotomization with "foreclosure," a grammatical concept of negation: "Language, for those who know how to decode it, is a marvelous mirror of the depths of the unconscious. To regret is to desire that something in the past . . . had never existed. The French language uses the foreclusive to express this wish to scotomize, and in so doing, translates a normal phenomenon" found in an exaggerated form in "mental pathology."[36]

As Pichon defined it, foreclosure designated the second part of negation in French; in that language negation is represented by two words, neither of which can negate by itself. The first is *ne*; the second is one of many possible negative forms such as *rien* (nothing), *aucun* (none), *jamais* (never), and so on. If the *ne* represented

[35] See Roudinesco, *Lacan and Co.*, p. 301. She notes that Lacan "had recourse to the resources of the French language, which allows one to cleave the Freudian *Ich* into an ego (*moi*) and an I (*je*), a move that would be impossible as such in German. The split had already been effected before Lacan by Edouard Pichon." David Macey has also traced Lacan's indebtedness to Lacan (pp. 34–41).

[36] Edouard Pichon and Jacques Damourette, *Des mots à la pensée: Essai de grammaire de la langue française* (Paris: D'Artrey, 1911–50), 2;140. See also Roudinesco, *La Bataille* 1:315.

what Pichon called the *discordentiel*, the second word represented the exclusion of certain things from the speaker's reality. It is this second term he named the foreclusive, and it was the negation implicit in the foreclusive that translated the "blindness" or refusal characterized by scotomization into language.

Pichon died in 1940, some fifteen years before Lacan's seminars on psychosis at the Ecole Normale Supérieure in 1955–1956.[37] By then the xenophobia and anti-Semitism that had tarnished the reception of psychoanalysis in France had been discredited, and Freud's ideas had gained a new prestige. Internal rifts within the Société Psychanalytique de Paris had led to the defection of Lacan and Daniel Lagache and the formation of a new Société Française de Psychanalyse, which sought affiliation with the International Psychoanalytic Association.[38] Lacan did not break away from the SFP until 1964, when he founded the Ecole Française de Psychanalyse, later to become the Ecole Freudienne de Paris.

Lacan had gained notoriety as a theoretician of the first order. By 1953, when he gave the Rome Discourse that was to give birth to a distinctly Lacanian analysis, he had succeeded in linking the different concepts with which he had worked in his revision of the Oedipus complex, the culmination of his work on the mirror stage and family complexes. In the 1953 conference in Rome he officially introduced Saussurian linguistics into the study of the unconscious, and the categories of the imaginary, the symbolic, and the real (among others) into psychoanalytic terminology. When he turned to an analysis of psychosis in 1955 he employed these concepts, referring to Pichon only obliquely, in an admiring and yet critical reference to *Des mots à la pensée*.[39]

In 1954, Lacan had already claimed that foreclosure represented what Freud termed *Verwerfung* (rejection or, more literally, "casting out"). In the Wolf Man case, Freud had made a distinction between *Verneinung* and *Verwerfung* which marked the difference between neurosis and psychosis. Neurosis represented the recovery of something already inserted within the symbolic realm, whereas psychosis described the absence of primary repression. By *Verwer-*

---

[37] Jacques Lacan, *Le Séminaire III: Les Psychoses* (Paris: Seuil, 1981).

[38] For a full discussion of this period in the movement's history, see Roudinesco, *Jacques Lacan*, pp. 151–369.

[39] Lacan, *Le Séminaire III*, p. 253.

fung, Lacan argued, Freud had meant a "symbolic abolition."[40] This symbolic abolition abolished the *nom du père* (name of the father), the architect of the entire symbolic order. What could not be symbolized returned in what he labeled the Real (not to be confused with reality), a prefigurative plentitude that can be conceived only through the mediation of symbolization. Hence he later referred to the real as the realm of the impossible.[41] Lacan worked out his own conception of *Verwerfung*, reconceived as foreclosure, in his reading of the Wolf Man case and the paranoid Daniel Paul Schreber's memoirs, both about which Freud had originally written.

Lacan argued that the Wolf Man lived his fear of castration as "real" (not as symbolized) because he had never adequately situated castration in the symbolic network in which identity was constituted. We recall that for both Freud and Lacan, it is the fear of castration (i.e., the castration complex), symbolic of the father's prohibition of the mother, that causes the boy to renounce his mother and identify with his father. In so doing, it facilitates the normal resolution to the oedipal complex through which the boy's sexual identity is defined. Yet the Wolf Man never passed through this essential stage of development. As a child, he had witnessed a primal scene but had "foreclosed" its meaning, thereby rejecting castration as a signifier for the mother's absent phallus. Since castration had not been "fixed," or attached to a single meaning, it could take on a variety of signified forms. The boy thus never passed through the developmental stage necessary to sexual maturity; because he had not symbolized castration, he did not identify with his father but remained problematically attached to his mother. Furthermore, since castration was never symbolized, this rejection (of castration as signifier) was "lived" through psychotic hallucinations; at age five, the Wolf man believed he had cut off his finger, only to realize, after the initial sighting, that his finger was indeed intact, the hallucination being an oblique "return" of the rejected sighting of castration.

By introducing the concept of foreclosure, Lacan explained in

[40]Lacan, *Ecrits*, p. 388. Parts of the seminars were reprinted in *Ecrits*.

[41]Lacan, *The Four Fundamental Concepts of Psychoanalysis*, trans. Alan Sheridan (London: Penguin, 1979), p. 167. See his discussion in *Le Séminaire II: Le Moi dans la théorie de Freud et dans la technique de la psychanalyse* (Paris: Seuil, 1978), p. 342.

linguistic terms the mechanism by which the psychotic was led to the imaginary recasting of signifiers represented by hallucinations. In so doing, he moved from Pichon's grammar to a theory of the signifier, and from the blind spot that defends against anxiety to a more elaborate casting out of the mother's "castration" from the symbolic order. Lacan suggested that the hallucination was not just a projection but also symbolized a disruption of the whole process of signification. In this case, meaning "slipped" between the (mother's absent) phallus and castration, whose relationship was not fixed but was nevertheless anchored by reference to an event experienced but foreclosed. Lacan conceived psychotic hallucination as an impossible symbolism, as a set of signifiers with no stable referents. The hallucination represented the perpetual discord between meanings and the concepts attached to them. It was full of germs of meaning that had not yet been organized, arranged, and interpreted, and so it expressed the psychotic's suspended relationship with language and culture—with the symbolic order.

Lacan used the paranoid Schreber's howl to describe the psychotic's suspended relationship to the symbolic. Schreber's need to howl came upon him suddenly, and he had to exercise a great deal of control to avoid howling in public. Lacan interpreted the howl as, on one level, a "call for help" (which Schreber addressed to God), but he saw it more profoundly as an image of transparency between words and meaning, as an "asignification" that contained all possible signifiers, so that we can interpret it as a voice that tells without telling, a way of remembering that must always forget because its memories have never been symbolized.[42] It is in this sense that the psychotic is what Lacan termed a *trou symbolique*, a symbolic hole, that is at the same time full of signification.

Because it is at once full of signification and yet nonsymbolic or presymbolic, Lacan continued, psychosis paradoxically offers an "open testimony" of the unconscious. In other words, psychosis represents the unconscious made transparent, whereas neurosis manifests a series of symbolic codes that have to be deciphered. Whereas the neurotic "occupies language," the psychotic "is occupied, possessed" by it. Because foreclosure is a symbolic abolition, it reveals the unconscious as it is lived, like psychosomatic

[42]Lacan, *Le Séminaire III*, pp. 158–59.

symptoms, through the body. Insofar as the psychotic is what Lacan calls a "martyr" of the unconscious, however, insofar as he or she sacrifices psychic stability to the proliferation of meanings, psychosis is unreadable. The lack of symbolic anchorage for the hallucination renders it incomprehensible at the same time that it allows it to be manifested, to be known.[43]

It is with this paradox in mind that Lacan remarked that "the psychotic phenomenon represents the real emergence of a signification that seems unimportant and cannot be anchored, since it has never entered the symbolic system; but it can, in certain conditions, threaten the entire edifice of symbolization."[44] If the psychotic threatens that edifice, it is because she or he bears witness to the symbolic character of what we take to be reality. The psychotic "knows" something we cannot. When Schreber foreclosed castration, he rejected, like the Wolf Man, the father's prohibition of the mother, or what Lacan called the *nom du père*, the law that constitutes knowledge. Psychosis is "the foreclosure of the Name of the Father in the place of the Other . . . the failure of the paternal metaphor, that . . . designate[s] the defect that gives psychosis its essential condition, and the structure that separates it from neurosis."[45]

"Schreber lacks," said Lacan, "according to all appearances, this fundamental signifier, namely, to be a father. This is why it was necessary that he commit an error . . . that he go so far as to think he comported himself as a woman."[46] In Schreber's case, "to be a father" was a suspended signifier. This is why his psychotic crises concerned questions of sexual identity. It is precisely the absence of this signifier that places Schreber outside social (and sexual) order. Hence his confusion about whether or not fathers can procreate (his confusion about the so-called natural components of sexual identity) points to the way in which the introjection of the *nom du père* "creates" reality: "All symbolization is there to affirm that a creature does not engender another creature. . . . In the symbolic, nothing explains creation."[47] Psychosis asks the unaskable—

43 Ibid., pp. 149, 284.
44 Ibid., p. 99.
45 Lacan, *Ecrits: A Selection*, p. 215.
46 Lacan, *Le Séminaire III*, p. 330.
47 Ibid., p. 202.

where do symbols come from? what does it mean to be a father?—
implying that the father is an idea invested with cultural and linguistic meaning rather than a reality that just "means."

Since psychosis is defined by the absence of this original signifier, the psychotic becomes a rift in the symbolic order, a rift that
designates the symbol as symbol, not as truth. Because psychosis
represents a nonsymbolic state, it implies that identity is never
original but the product of a symbolic order into which the psychotic has not been initiated. At the same time, because the psychotic's "knowledge" is nonsymbolic, it cannot be known.

The psychotic is thus a metaphor for what is impossible, un-
knowable, and yet most true about the self: what Lacan calls the
other par excellence—the real. As Shoshana Felman has argued,
the Lacanian unconscious cannot be "discovered" under layers of
repression. "Reading" the unconscious is a "practical procedure,
partially blind to what it does but which proves to be efficient. The
theoretical construction of the unconscious is what, after the fact,
is constructed to account for the efficiency of the practice. But the
practice, the partially unconscious analytic reading practice, pre-
cedes the theory."[48] In other words, for Lacan, the unconscious is
constructed through the very process of trying to understand what
it is and how it works, through the process of accounting for why
"readings" make sense. It is always already normalized or symbolized. At the same time, it is also the blind spot of reading, the
force that directs the reading and yet is itself impossible to read
except in the terms we have constructed to read it. Therefore, the
transferential relationship with the Lacanian analyst does not lead
to a "cure," which would suggest the possibility of eliminating
blind spots. It leads instead to a recognition of the unacknowledged
desire in the analysand's demands, to the recognition, that is, of
the analysand's own blind spot.

But if the unconscious is accessible only when repressed, if
the recognition of the blind spot must itself always be partially
blind, how would the analyst know if he or she got it right? How
would the analyst know that the recognition was not a misrecognition? Wouldn't the blind spot be at the heart, as it were, of the
symbolic itself, wouldn't it render any normative concept of

[48] Felman, *Lacan and the Adventure of Insight*, p. 24.

health impossible, including that guaranteed by the linguistic introjection of the paternal prohibition? Borch-Jacobsen has aptly
summed up the problem: "In fact, if the absolutely last revelation
of being, of desire, and of the subject takes place in erroneous
speech, *what distinguishes it from that other 'error': the alienated
and 'miscognizing' speech of the imaginary ego?* In other words,
what distinguishes *repression,* as the revealing-absenting of desire
in speech, from *resistance,* as the presenting-avoiding of desire
in that same speech?" How, he goes on, "to separate . . . two
types of speech—one of which, now baptized 'symbolic,' is supposed to be more true than the other, which is reputedly 'imaginary.' "[49]

I want to argue that what Lacan called the real or the impossible
represents the conflation of the unconscious and cultural (now
linguistic) norms, a conflation already implicit in the concept of
scotomization. Lacan followed other French analysts in conceiving
the unconscious as always already continuous with and beyond the
symbolic and hence always, in some respect, foreclosed (the real
can never, ever, be "seen," even as it is apprehended).[50] By transforming scotomization into foreclosure, Lacan conceived the blind
spot that disrupts the symbolic as continuous with the symbolic
itself.[51] He thus used the logic of scotomization transformed into
foreclosure to prove the unconscious was structured like a language whose "real" or "true" meaning is always other—located
beyond any place we can "see."

The deviant—whether the psychotic, the criminal, the "liberated" woman—thus symbolizes what cannot be known, structures
a lack into the heart of knowledge. But no deviant can escape the
law of language, which is the law of the father, even as (as is
implicit in Lacan's work) she or he resists it, resists symbolization.

[49] Borch-Jacobsen, p. 116.

[50] For a discussion of the relationship of psychosis to Lacan's concept of the real,
see Roustang, *Lacan,* pp. 66–77. Roustang also notes that the two different meanings of the "real" in Lacan—it both mimics the symbolic and represents what
cannot be known—are reconcilable. This is what I have suggested is already implicit in the concept of scotomization: a mimicry in which the unconscious is at
once present and absent (p. 86).

[51] Martin Jay discusses this conflation between scotomization and foreclosure as
it pertains to Lacan's late critique of ocularcentrism in an unpublished manuscript,
pp. 36–37.

But for Lacan, deviants do point to a place beyond language, beyond culture, which mocks our pretensions to knowledge and mocks in particular those individuals who stake most on its claims—fathers, scientists, professors. In so doing, they give the lie to science. "Psychoanalysis," said Lacan, "is not a science. It doesn't have the status of a science; it can only wait for it, hope for it. It is a delirium. . . . It is a scientific delirium, but that doesn't mean that psychoanalysis will ever be a science."[52] For Lacan, then, knowledge is doomed to be ever incomplete, the desire for it driven by an eternal quest for an ever irretrievable other: "To this mythical representation of the mystery of love, analytic experience substitutes the search by the subject, not of the sexual complement, but of the part of himself, *lost forever*, that is constituted by the fact that he is only a sexed lived being, and that he is no longer immortal."[53]

To go back to the question posed at the end of Chapter 1 and implicitly through this part of the book: If the unconscious—the deviant within—perpetually mocks or undermines those illustrious representations of the law, of "culture," what is the status of expertise, of authority? Or if deviants cannot escape the law of the father, what can possibly be the subversive effect of mockery? First of all, I must concur with feminist critics who stress the extent to which Lacan reinforces the law even though he can hear all the mockery. They argue in different ways that criminals, women, and psychotics can only be emblems of subversion—of truth telling—in a culture in which they already represent otherness. As Alice Jardine notes, Lacan "never moved beyond the male self as absolute metaphor."[54] The "truth" of the self as it is conceived by Lacan thus already represents a cultural construction and appropriation of the other which reinforces the norms he aimed to subvert. The archaic adage he claimed to have pinned to his office wall— "Ne devient pas fou qui veut" (Not everyone has the luck to go mad)[55]—gives us a sense of the side from which he believed we necessarily speak. After all, to want to go mad like the psychotic, to want to be cut off from the symbolic, is to be already securely anchored on the other side of madness, in the culture Lacan equated with fathers. But it is not sufficient to argue that Lacan's work

52 Lacan, quoted in Roustang, *Lacan*, p. 105.
53 Lacan, *Four Fundamental Concepts*, p. 205, my italics.
54 Jardine, p. 161.
55 Lacan, *Le Séminaire III*, p. 24.

replicates normative definitions of the self, not enough to point out what Lacan himself seemed to believe was inevitable. In other words, if Lacan ultimately reinforced the primacy of authorities and of fathers even while subverting and resisting it, if the (male) self was made no less powerful but simply more discreet, how do we *account* for the construction of that primacy as well as its cultural specificity? How do we go beyond the insistence that "regulatory fictions" govern Lacan's revision of Freud to demonstrate how and why those fictions are maintained and take the forms they do?

In the past three chapters, I have described the process by which the self was constructed out of otherness, the process, in other words, by which otherness came to define the meaning of the self, in order to focus on *this* last question. I have traced how Aimée's crime became a metaphor for and shaped the ego; how the "equal but different" (and hence always potentially feminine man) symbolized and shaped the superego; how Madame X's and the psychotic's schizophrenia symbolized and may have structured the real, the id, the impossible. In order to account for the specificity of Lacan's revision of Freud, I have argued that the very rearticulation of the self implicit in these new terms—autopunition, equal but different, and scotomization—was shaped by and itself shaped a new kind of expertise that was reinforced, paradoxically, only through the implicit erosion of its foundations. Whereas psychiatrists and psychoanalysts sought in these new terms to clarify a distinction between self and other, Lacan used them to construct a self that ceased to be referential: one that can be known only once its pleasure has been repressed or symbolized. Thus, while Lacan shared psychiatrists' and psychoanalysts' belief in the otherness of criminals, women, and psychotics, he transformed deviance from a metaphor for what was other into an otherness that was always already symbolized and hence anchored and regulated. That is, the "true" self is at once made into metaphor and deferred, so that its truth is always inaccessible, always bound to be, on some level, a lie.

The "regulatory fictions" that governed Lacan's revision of Freud were thus the product of a historically and culturally specific response to a particular set of questions about the legitimacy of the subject. But Lacan's was not the only model of the nonreferential self to emerge during the interwar and immediate postwar years in

France. To what extent did the processes by which those other selves were defined overlap with the ones I have described? How do we account for the process by which *their* regulatory fictions were constructed *as* fictions? And what more can they tell us about why France has been the home of a certain model of self-dissolution?

PART TWO

SADE'S SELFLESSNESS

Sade was the last of the gallant marquis and the first of the
neurasthenics.
—R. de Bury, *Mercure de France*, 1905

If we go straight to the heart of things, we see that the marquis
de Sade seems more like a victim than an executioner.
—Mark Amiaux, *La Vie effrénée du marquis de Sade*, 1936

For example, if a professor were to force students to read some
of the work of the Marquis de Sade as part of a course on
French society, "it would be actionable," she said.
—"[Catharine] MacKinnon Leaves Yale
  Grads With Tough Talk on Sex Abuse,"
  National Law Journal, 1989

The marquis de Sade (1740–1814) was not known for his
discretion or his philanthopy, and it may seem odd that in a section
devoted to selflessness he should be the central focus. But in the
interwar years Sade's sadistic and not so sadistic crimes, like the
crimes of the "deviants" I have thus far discussed, also became a
metaphor of the self and, more specifically, facilitated the transformation of the self into an other, into a self that is discreetly powerful, apparently selfless.

But even before the Great War, Sade played an essential role in

French medical and literary culture as a metaphor for human evil and for perversion, though his work circulated only covertly until the 1930s. Sade was a prolific writer, but he was perhaps best known as the author of *Justine; ou, Les Malheurs de la vertu* (1791) and *Juliette; ou, Les Prospérités du vice* (1797), two very long and very obscene novels about two sisters who suffer different fates: Justine clings to her virtue in spite of the repeated sexual assaults to which she is subjected, and Juliette grows up to be an immensely wealthy libertine whose erotic imagination knows no bounds. All of Sade's obscene work is peopled by characters for whom human suffering (including, in a limited fashion, their own) is an indispensable sexual stimulant: The giant Minski's castle is furnished with women's bodies contorted into chairs and tables on which sumptuous feasts are served; Juliette sets fire to a full hotel and enjoys the spectacle with her maid from a nearby window; the libertine Clairwil, one of Juliette's closest friends, incessantly demands young men and women to mutilate and murder as her fantasies dictate, and she belongs, as do most of Sade's libertines, to a club that supplies its members with the necessary bodies. In Sade's work other people are merely theatrical props that are discarded and exchanged for others as new erotic fantasies require new decors. His characters are rich and powerful political insiders such as the pope, judges, government ministers—men whose social positions permit them to execute their fantasies with impunity.

The meaning and significance of Sade's works was (and still is) always interpreted in relation to his imprisonment by successive governments, including the ancien régime (under which, although normally immune as a noble, he was charged with poisoning others and with sodomy and condemned to death), the Revolution (whose leaders first released him and later condemned him for moderation), and the Empire. Altogether Sade spent twenty-seven years of his life in prison, both for his crimes and for—as his works were then conceived—writing about them. As Maxime du Camp declared in 1873, "Any man with the courage to leaf through the works of this man . . . would concur that, as arbitrary as it was . . . his imprisonment was justified."[1]

What concerns us in this part is the expression, if not the tri-

---

[1] Maxime du Camp, *Paris: Ses organes, ses fonctions, et sa vie dans la seconde moitié du XIXe siècle*, vol. 4 (Paris: Hachette, 1873), p. 418.

umph, of a markedly less severe attitude toward Sade's deviance in medical and literary circles which emerged during the interwar years. Simply put, doctors and writers began to view Sade as a victim of narrow-mindedness and ignorance.[2] The chapters that follow demonstrate how they transformed Sade from a moral monster into a victim and how that transformation symbolized and shaped a new concept of the self as an irretrievable other. Like the changes documented in Part One, this transformation was framed by a culturally specific dialectic. While the reconstruction of Sade mirrored anxieties about the dissolution of boundaries between the normal and the pathological, it also represented an effort to reinforce those boundaries in new terms.

Chapter 4 describes how that dissolution was cast in terms of an equation of the self with sexual (sadomasochistic) pleasure. It looks at the medical, biographical, and literary reconstruction of Sade as the victim of a moral and legal system that denied nonprocreative sexual pleasure. Chapter 5 analyzes how that denial became, for the writers Pierre Klossowski, Jean Paulhan, Georges Bataille, and in a different way, for Jacques Lacan, itself the source of Sade's own (primarily masochistic) "pleasure." Sade was first conceived as a victim and then reconceived as wanting to be one. This part addresses the nature of that transition from martyrdom to masochism and ventures to give it a historical meaning.

We can link the increasing recognition of sexual diversity in France—the blurry boundary between the normal and the perverted—to psychiatric ideologies and psychoanalysis, but only as they were conceived and defined in relation to *Sade's works*. Thus,

---

[2] This argument was used in 1956 in the obscenity trial of Jean Paulhan and Jean-Jacques Pauvert, who were accused, respectively, of distributing and publishing Sade's works. The defense lawyer in the case, Maurice Garçon, summed it up in his closing remarks. He did not directly refute Sade's deviance but declared that his reputation had been "so immeasurably deformed and vulgarized that today still, if we had not discovered the original dossier [documenting Sade's crimes] in the National Archives, we would remain petrified with horror." He pleaded with the judges to recognize to what extent ignorant, superstitious, and philosophically narrow moral leaders of the past had interpreted Sade's "hardly serious" crimes as the acts of a madman. Since, he argued, moral conventions change over time, the greatness of Sade's works could be recognized today by truly modern individuals unencumbered by the weight of religious conviction or archaic moral judgments. Not only was Sade "hardly dangerous," he was a great writer whose works had been unjustly accorded the status of pornography by a more restrictive era. Jean Paulhan, *L'Affaire Sade* (Paris: Pauvert, 1963), pp. 98–100.

whereas elsewhere the "scientific" discourses about sexuality rescued the self from both too much pleasure and too much repression, in France, where Sade became the emblem of liberated pleasure, they led to the self's dissolution. I want to define the dual
ideological and cultural process by which Sade's crimes came to be
equated with the self's pleasure, by which Sade's self was defined
and redefined as other through the construction of nonprocreative
sexuality as a morally acceptable, even necessary, pleasure.

Chapter Four

The Virtue of Crime

In 1886 Richard von Krafft-Ebing, the father of sexology, explained perversion as a congenital defect. His views were echoed by most fin-de-siècle medical works about Sade, even by those—and they constituted the bulk of those published—concerned to liberate Sade from the metaphorical prisons of the moralizers, written by men who overcame the prejudices of their epoch to recognize in Sade a phenomenon worthy of scientific and literary attention.

In 1885 an anonymous piece about Sade was published in *La Revue Indépendante.* Two years later a lengthier version was published as "La Vérité sur le marquis de Sade." Its author was Charles Henry, the director of a physiology laboratory at the Sorbonne, who was not identified until the critic Lucien Descaves revealed his name in an article in *Le Journal* in 1930.[1] Henry's article signaled the first attempt to rehabilitate Sade as an important thinker in spite of or even because of his perversion, but his text was not isolated. In 1899 Claude Tournier, writing under the pseudonym Dr. Marciat, published an important article. It was followed in 1901 by two pseudonymous books, one by Iwan Bloch, writing as Eugen Duehren, and the other by a certain Jacobus X.[2]

---

[1] Maurice Heine, *Le Marquis de Sade* (Paris: Gallimard, 1950), p. 105. Descaves's essay is reprinted in this collection.

[2] Claude Tournier [Dr. Marciat, pseud.], "Le Marquis de Sade et le sadisme," in Dr. Alexandre Lacassagne, ed., *Vacher, l'eventreur, et les crimes sadiques* (Lyon: A. Storck, 1899), pp. 185–243; Iwan Bloch [Eugen Duehren, pseud.], *Le Marquis de Sade et son temps* (Paris: A. Michalon, 1901), first published as *Der Marquis de Sade und seine Zeit* (Berlin: H. Barsdorf, 1900); Jacobus X, *Le Marquis de Sade*

Dr. Marciat and Jacobus X explained the marquis's sadism as the result of an overwrought imagination stimulated by years of prolonged imprisonment and hence prolonged chastity, insisting that these misfortunes produced a kind of "genital perversion," to use Marciat's term, which explained Sade's obsession with eroticized violence. Marciat denied that Sade was a madman "in the exact sense of the term" and claimed that he was afflicted by "moral insanity" (folie morale).[3] Jacobus X, for his part, divided Sade's literary works into readable and unreadable texts, maintained that he was a precursor of French naturalism, and argued that "he is a very particular writer, but a writer all the same." He considered the characters in Sade's novels no more immoral than those in Zola's but still found Sade to be an "inverted degenerate" and thought his works (presumably his "unreadable" ones) should be subject to censorship lest they fall into the hands of a "born sadist."[4]

Another expert on perversion, Dr. Emile Laurent, titled a chapter in his book about sadism and masochism "Sadism and Literature" and claimed that even though Sade's sadism was provoked by hatred of women, heredity was "the real origin of this sexual monstrosity."[5] Other doctors made similar assertions.[6] While most of them were

---

devant la science médicale et la littérature moderne (Paris: Charles Carrington, 1901).

[3] Tournier [Marciat], pp. 185, 216.

[4] Jacobus X, pp. xiii, xii, 225.

[5] Laurent, p. 30.

[6] While sharing Jacobus X's verdict, Iwan Bloch, the first transcriber of Sade's Les Cent-vingt Journées de Sodome, found scientific merit in Sade's work as a catalog of perversions even though he considered it primarily a mirror of the depraved morals common to late eighteenth-century France. Jacobus X took offense at this assertion, as did French patriots during the Great War, who criticized it strongly. See Paul Voivenel, "Les Allemands et le marquis de Sade," excerpt from Progrès Médical, January 16 and February 17, 1917, pp. 12–13, in Bibliothèque Nationale (Voivenel cites Octave Uzanne, "Le Divin Marquis et le sadisme germain," La Dépêche [June 1916] but does not gives pages), and the pamphlet Comment le docteur Boche [Boche was a derogatory word for a German], pour justifier à l'avance les infamies allemandes, accusait de sadisme sanglant les Français en général et les Parisiens en particulier," published in 1918, copy in Bibliothèque Nationale. The pamphlet was a direct attack on Duehren. In one of Louis Morin's illustrations Duehren is portrayed on his knees worshiping a commemorative monument to the marquis de Sade: the monument represents a man stabbing a young woman whose hands and feet are bound. All these articles claim that it is not the French but the Germans whose "race" is most imprinted with sadism, and Voivenel goes so far as to list examples of the faithful couples Duehren overlooked in his analysis of the "debauched" lives of eighteenth-century French aristocrats.

concerned to establish that Sade was not "mad" in any technical sense and so to establish the interest and, in some cases, the legitimacy of Sade's writings, they never questioned the assumption that Sade was pathological. Instead, they tried to understand that pathology in nuanced, if not new, terms capable of illuminating the relationship between Sade's pathology and his writing.

But scientific opinion about deviance had evolved considerably since the Congrès International de Médecine de Paris had hosted Krafft-Ebing and some of his disciples in 1900. The Sade scholar Maurice Heine referred to that conference, as well as to the works of Marciat, Duehren, and Jacobus X, as the intermediate period in the understanding of Sade and sexuality in general.[7] Heine looked to such pioneers as Havelock Ellis and especially to the German Magnus Hirschfeld for inspiration. Both had insisted that sexuality be approached as objectively as any other topic in science and that "inversion" (homosexuality) was an innate, congenital disposition. Ellis implied that it was cruel and even socially unhealthy to repress "perverts"; instead, they needed to be approached with compassion and to be "helped" only if they so desired.[8]

In Germany, Hirschfeld formed the Medical Society of Sexual Sciences with the collaboration of Iwan Bloch, among others. In 1921 he convoked the first International Congress for Sexual Reform, one of whose objectives was the removal of legal proscriptions on homosexuality. This conference inspired Edouard Toulouse to inaugurate the Association for Sexological Studies in France in 1931—late, to be sure, compared to other European countries.[9] That same year, in his preface to the French reissue of Krafft-Ebing's *Psychopathia sexualis*, Pierre Janet criticized Krafft-Ebing's assumption that all sexual activity not destined for procreative ends was necessarily pathological and noted accordingly that "sexual life should not always be judged from such a severe point of view."[10] It was also at this time that Hirschfeld moved his

[7] Maurice Heine, *Recueil de confessions et observations psychosexuelles* (Paris: Editions Jean Crès, 1936), p. v.

[8] See Paul Robinson, *The Modernization of Sex* (New York: Harper and Row, 1976), pp. 1–42.

[9] See Toulouse's preface to Angelo Hesnard, *Traité de sexologie normale et pathologique* (Paris: Payot, 1933), p. 10.

[10] Pierre Janet, Preface to Richard von Krafft-Ebing, *Psychopathia sexualis* (Paris: E. Laurent and Sigismund Csapo, 1931), p. 7.

Sexual Sciences Institute from Berlin to Paris and began soliciting supporters in France.[11]

Most of the doctors who wrote about sadism during the interwar years sought to provide a philosophical interpretation of what Magnus Hirschfeld had called the "meaning and essence" of sexuality.[12] They also tried to be less judgmental than their predecessors in their analysis of the sadistic instinct. They repudiated any morally inspired rejection of perversion as evidence of a depraved self and even questioned to what extent sadism was pathological. The young Dr. Salvador Sarfati, who wrote a medical thesis on Sade in 1930, declared that however dubious its other merits, Iwan Bloch's book *Le Marquis de Sade et son temps*, written under the pseudonym Eugen Duehren, had the distinction of being the first to note that sadism did not necessarily require a *passage à l'acte:* that it was first and foremost a thing of the mind and not the organism or the instinct. Sarfati outlined a hierarchy in which unconscious sadism would be considered normal, conscious sadism a psychological problem, and active sadism (*sadisme du fait*) cause for medico-legal concern.[13] Another writer, summing up the medical literature on Sade, agreed that "sadism has its degrees. It can be imaginative, and it is as such that it predominates in at least half the human race; as the psychoanalysts say, if to imagine a thing is to live it, then the majority of individuals can think of the marquis de Sade as a sort of unhypocritical fall guy."[14]

[11] See letter from Hirschfeld to Heine on August 5, 1933, in which Hirschfeld responds to Heine's earlier request for one of his "questionnaires psychobiologiques," which Heine finished translating into French by December of that year. Heine's papers also contain the announcement of the opening of the Institut des Sciences Sexologiques on April 7, 1934, at 24 Avenue Floquet, 75007, Paris. In the announcement the institute declares itself to be a "center of scientific investigation and instruction complete with archives and a specialized library, whose core collection will be formed from the remains of the library closed down in Berlin." (The Nazis burned Hirschfeld's library and closed down the Berlin institute in 1933.) In addition, Hirschfeld wrote that the central bureau of the International League for Sexual Reform, founded in 1928 by Havelock Ellis, Auguste Forel, and Hirschfeld himself, was also being transferred from Berlin to Paris. Bibliothèque Nationale, MS 24397.

[12] Magnus Hirschfeld, *Perversions sexuelles* (Paris: Editions Internationales, 1931), p. 35.

[13] Dr. Salvador Sarfati, *Essai médico-psychologique sur le marquis de Sade* (Lyon: BOSC Frères, 1930), pp. 8–9, 12.

[14] Jean Desbordes, *Le Vrai Visage du marquis de Sade* (Paris: Editions de la Nouvelle Revue Critique, 1939), p. 81.

One of the commonest arguments made during the interwar years was that sadism was a normal part of the sexual act insofar as the "act of possession is an often bloody act of violence," as L. Pierre Quint would have it; that, in the words of Gilbert Lély, "during sex the comportments of the man and of the woman are, respectively, those of sadism and masochism."[15] Sadists, said others, often became surgeons, nurses, butchers, or hunters, and masochists sometimes became prostitutes.[16] One doctor reiterated Havelock Ellis's argument that sadism was nature's way of stimulating sexual activity when a man lacked the necessary sexual "energy."[17] In such arguments the pervert was reconceived as a victim and reintegrated into humanity through a critique of the society whose rules he or she transgressed. "Only recently," mused one psychiatrist, "in treating all vice as perversion, we held its victim responsible without trying to cure him. We condemned whoever departed from an ordinary way of life and thought no more of it."[18] The anarchist Ernest Armand, following medical opinion, clamored for a "revision of sexual morality" in one of his many political pamphlets, claiming that "the observations of impartial experts have demonstrated that perverts and inverts are no different, physiologically or psychologically, from normal people."[19] In fact, the increasing volume of "lay" medical literature about liberalizing sexuality prompted one psychiatrist, who mourned the loss of religious discipline, to accuse his colleagues of encouraging a kind of spiritual laziness and of promoting an "excessive cult of the erotic."[20] He had in mind popular works like La Psychologie du vice, in which its author, Dr. Pierre Vachet, admitted, "Speaking honestly, it is not easy to determine where vice begins or ends,

---

[15] L. Pierre Quint, Le Comte de Lautréamont et Dieu (Marseilles: Les Cahiers du Sud, 1929), P. 75; Gilbert Lély, Prologue to D. A. F. Sade, Morceaux choisis (Paris: Seghers, 1948), p. xxi.

[16] Dr. Octave Béliard, Le Marquis de Sade (Paris: Laurier, 1928), p. 283; Dr. René Allendy, "Les Conceptions modernes de la sexualité," Crapouillot (September 1937), 38. See also Louis Perceau [Louis Helpey, pseud.], Le Marquis de Sade et le sadisme (Sadopolis: Imprimé spécialement pour l'auteur et quelques amis, n.d.), pp. 36–37.

[17] Dr. J. R. Bourdon, Perversions sexuelles (Paris: Editions Internationales, 1931), p. 10. On Ellis, see Robinson, p. 24.

[18] Bourdon, p. 7.

[19] Ernest Armand, La Revision de la morale sexuelle (Paris: L'En Dehors, 1930), pp. 15–16.

[20] Wilhelm Foerster, Morale sexuelle (Paris: Librairie Blond and Gay, 1930), p. 163.

because the distinction between the normal and the abnormal" is so difficult to determine.[21] (For a contemporary example of this kind of thinking, see Figure 1.)

Perversion was thus not always conceived as the product of an individual's moral weakness; often it was seen as arising from a culture's religious and moral hypocrisy, from an unnatural repression of a "natural and universal instinct," wrote Jean Galtier-Boissière, "a principle of life."[22] Hirschfeld referred most explicitly to the problem of condemning perversion out of hand in *Le Tour du monde d'un sexologue,* a "sexual ethnology" in which he claimed that the diversity of sexual morality and the institutions established to regulate it in different cultures provided substantial proof that what was considered perverse varied from culture to culture. Studies of sexuality should therefore be based not on assumptions about sexual instinct but on an analysis of how cultural institutions shape instinct, on "a scientific and objective knowledge of man and his sexuality" which would be capable of laying the basis for "rational sexual reform."[23]

To "help" the pervert, French doctors believed they had to cut through the archaic religious notions of original sin and moral weakness in order to address the individual through an appeal to reason rather than fear. They had to insist upon the naturalness of sexual behavior in order to prevent, as Vachet put it, "any precocious deviations of the sexual instinct." Vachet also suggested that boys should be disuaded from going to brothels not by instilling in them the fear of God but by making them aware of all the risks of venereal disease.[24] The sexologist's role was above all to encourage "normal sexual evolution" through an objective analysis free of the religious and moral censure that had heretofore made it impossible for men and women to accept and understand what was most fundamental about themselves. "If we replace the mystery of sex with the truth of sex," argued the psychiatrist-cum-psychoanalyst Angelo Hesnard, "the dangerous chastity of ignorance,

[21]Dr. Pierre Vachet, *La Psychologie du vice* (Paris: Librairie Blond et Gay, 1934), p. iv.
[22]Jean Galtier-Boissière, "Contre le mensonge et contre l'hypocrisie," *Crapouillot* (September 1937), 2.
[23]Magnus Hirschfeld, *Le Tour du monde d'un sexologue* (Paris: Gallimard, 1938), p. xiv.
[24]Pierre Vachet, *L'Inquiétude sexuelle* (Paris: Grasset, 1927), p. 202.

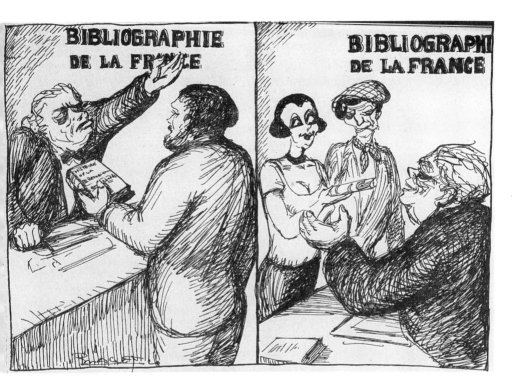

Figure 1. Moral dissolution after the Great War. From *Le Grand Guignol*, no. 33 (December 1926). Courtesy Bibliothèque Nationale.

—You say that the President of the Republic has sent his compliments to the author of *The History of the Third Republic*? I refuse to publicize such tendentious books! This book just won the International Grand Prize for Literature at Geneva? So what of it! All the important daily newspapers publicize it? I say to hell with them!

—Monsieur the Director, we bring you the plates for the publicity of our book *Carnal Paradise; or, The 128 Positions of Coitus*, modern follow-up to the *Kama-Sutra*, written by a masseuse-procuress during her stay at St. Lazare.
—Oh! Very well, my friends! I don't know how to thank you enough in the name of all my colleagues in the Cercle de la Librairie. Only have the kindness to put aside a few copies for us!

which, knowing nothing, invents everything, will make way for the serene chastity of science."[25] The revelation of that truth would in turn make possible, said Galtier-Boissière, a "radical transformation of social justice."[26] Perhaps the most blatant appeal for the rational control of sexuality came from none other than Edouard Toulouse: "Only the certain knowledge of these [sexual] facts can aid us in understanding that the sexual act should not be of an exclusively private order, that it must submit to collective surveillance and control."[27]

The humanization of the pervert thus did not simply expand the boundaries of what was considered normal. Instead, many doctors no longer believed that perversion should be brutally repressed because they insisted that repression *caused* perversion. They shifted the burden of controlling perversion away from the state (the courts, the prisons) to medical men, and repudiated the nineteenth-century belief in a depraved and hence necessarily recidivist pervert in favor of a new emphasis on rehabilitation, on a gentler and more rational medical regulation of sexual instinct. It is no coincidence that doctors in the postwar period were obsessed with the determination of sex. This obsession was a response to the blurring of sexual boundaries—of masculinity and femininity and of normality and pathology—effected at the end of the nineteenth century and exacerbated by the war. Doctors' efforts to wrench sexuality in an "appropriate" direction to ensure that it remained "healthy,"[28] their stepped-up attempt to regulate sexuality in medical (rather than moral) terms, reflected (as in the parallel medical discourse we have thus far explored) their efforts to redefine and control the pervert's "dissolving" character. The new discourse on Sade, like the discourse on criminals, women, and psychotics, thus mirrored and generated shifts in the deployment of medical power and hence in the construction of sexuality itself.

[25] Hesnard, *Traité*, p. 697. It should perhaps be noted that the respected psychiatrist René Binot referred to Hesnard's book in 1948 as the "classic work in the French language" on perversion. See his preface to *Médecine et sexualité* (Paris: Convergences, 1948), p. 16.

[26] Galtier-Boissière, "Contre le mensonge," p. 2.

[27] Toulouse, Preface to Hesnard, *Traité*, p. 10.

[28] See, for example, W. Boven, *Adam et Eve; ou, La Question des sexes* (Paris: Delachaux et Niestlé, 1933); Edouard Pichon, *Evolution divergente de la génitalité et la sexualité dans la civilisation occidentale* (Paris: Editions Denoël, 1939), pp. 5–6. I cite the pamphlet (copy in the Bibliothèque Nationale); the article originally

The Biographical Portrait: Recovering the Self

These new assumptions about the regulation of the sexual instinct structured the interwar reinterpretation of Sade's life and works, which was largely the product of doctors (especially psychiatrists) turned biographers. The quest of biographers, essayists, and novelists for the "real" Sade methodologically replicated the scientific quest for the meaning and essence of sexuality, of whose complexity Sade's desire, in its obsessiveness, its variety, and its cruelty, was highly symbolic. But whereas some medical men asserted that sexual expression was healthy but that some expressions were less healthy than others, Sade's biographers, as well as other medical men and writers, reinterpreted Sade's sadism itself as a healthy form of sexual expression.

This transformation of all sexual expression, including Sade's, into something healthy was thus consistent with the idea that sexual, even perverse instinct informs the most normal kinds of behavior. At the same time, it repudiated conventional medical efforts to establish a hierarchy of instincts and sexual practices on a continuum from healthy (i.e., monogamous marriage) to unhealthy (e.g., deviations such as homosexuality) and, in so doing, represented another stage in the "liberation" of sexuality which still informs normative assumptions about sexual expression.

Even in the context of a so-called liberation of desire, Sade's truth became inseparable from new normative assumptions about the truth of sex. But how did sadism become part of what was considered healthy sexuality and what were the ideological bases of that development? How did Sade, this chronicler of what most writers before the twentieth century deemed the most unspeakable human evil, become a metaphor for a normal, healthy, even sublime desire? How did the man whose contemporaries described him as dangerous, and not without reason, come to symbolize what was most fundamental (sometimes unpleasant but most often exhilarating) about human nature? How did Sade's liberation, in other words, become a metaphor for the recovery of the self? Here the fact that Sade was a writer becomes crucial. That is, Sade was not

---

appeared in *RFP* 10 (1939), 461–70. Both these authors argue that sexuality was no longer so much the mirror of instinct as the product of a correspondence between sex (instinct) and gender. This correspondence they wanted regulated appropriately.

only a sadist but a man who wrote about sadism. Writers in the nineteenth century did not pay much attention to the distinction between Sade's life and his fiction, but by the interwar years, that distinction constituted the basis for a reinterpretation of Sade's desire.

Most of the evidence doctors and writers used against Sade during the nineteenth century, as his defenders were quick to point out, was not gathered through an objective appraisal of each incident or a careful reading of documents (which were then for the most part unavailable) but was sought instead in his scandalous novels, considered ample testimony to his guilt. The "objective" and "scientific" observers of the early twentieth century, by contrast, chose to evaluate the nature of Sade's sadism through an investigation of the relationship between his life and his writing, between Sade's real crimes and the sexual rituals described in his novels. They vowed not to be influenced by rumor or by preconceived notions about what was or was not normal, but to suspend judgment (thus following doctors' advice as to the most constructive means of investigating and treating perversion) in order better to get at the truth.

Their efforts were aided by the documents and texts Maurice Heine's labors had made available during the interwar years. Heine, who undertook the publication, distribution, and analysis of Sade's oeuvre, devoted nearly his entire life to recovering the truth about Sade by combing archives all over France, nearly ruining himself financially through the purchase of the marquis's manuscripts. He committed himself to offering an "authentic" version of Sade for public consumption, undertaking the wearisome task of transcribing Sade's minuscule handwriting and thus preparing his unpublished manuscripts for publication.

Heine was born in 1884 in Paris and trained to be a doctor. He renounced his profession after six years of residency, when his parents, who had opposed his original desire for a literary vocation, died. He then moved to Algeria and became a writer for various anticolonial journals, eventually becoming the editor of *La France Islamique*, in which he defended the rights of Algerians to claim French citizenship. Heine joined the Socialist party in 1919, went over to the Communists after the schism at Tours in 1923, but was eventually excluded from the party for his opposition to the antidemocratic policies of the Third International, which had established Soviet domination over the European parties. Heine spent the rest of his life as a free-lance writer, turning out articles for journals such as the *Nouvelle Revue Française, Hippocrate,* and *Minotaure,* among others, articles generally concerning his hero, the marquis de Sade.[29]

Along with some of Sade's other admirers, Heine created the Société du Roman Philosophique in 1923, which had as its principle aim, said Gilbert Lély, to "create a link between researchers and bibliophiles interested in Sade."[30] Their main objective was to "publish and edit [but not to sell] Sade's manuscripts, to encourage and publish works about Sade, and to publish a periodical bulletin in order to keep the literary public informed."[31] They also celebrated the anniversaries of Sade's birth and death regularly from at least 1927 to 1933. Although financial problems prevented the society from living up to all its promises, it was able to finance the editing and publication of Sade's *Historiettes, Contes, et Fabliaux* in 1926 and *Les Cent-vingt Journées de Sodome,* which appeared in three volumes from 1931 to 1935.[32]

This widespread dissemination of his work sparked numerous biographies and other commentaries that sought to tell the truth about Sade. Their authors chiseled away at the archaic fears and superstitions that had congealed, as contemporaries saw it, into the legend of the divine marquis. The publication of Sade's letters in 1929 greatly aided researchers, as did many of the manuscripts and trial proceedings Heine had transcribed during the 1920s and 1930s. Modern scientific research on perversion was employed to shed a more sophisticated light on the documents at hand.[33]

[29] A short autobiography can be found in Heine's papers and was published in an edited version by Gilbert Lély in his tribute to Heine. See Lély's appendix to D. A. F. Sade, *Oeuvres complètes* (Paris: Tête de Feuilles, 1973), 2:668–69.

[30] Ibid., p. 667.

[31] Bibliothèque Nationale, ms. 24397.

[32] Lély, appendix, p. 667. On Sade's birthday, members of the society would dine at the Cochon au Lait, a restaurant near the Théâtre de l'Odéon situated on the site where the Hôtel de Condé, Sade's birthplace, had once stood.

[33] D. A. F. Sade, *Correspondance inédite,* ed. Paul Bourdin (Paris: Librairie de France, 1929). This effort, it should be noted, was not limited to Sade. The infamous sadist Gilles de Rais, condemned in the fifteenth century for the murder of some eight hundred children, was the subject of several studies that sought either to rehabilitate him by seeing him as a victim of church politics or to decry the legend that had transformed him into a romantic hero because of his nobility and his close relationship to Joan of Arc. See Fernand Fleuret, *De Gilles de Rais à Apollinaire*

Dr. Octave Béliard's 1928 biography of Sade was typical. He insisted that Sade was really no different from many men of the present epoch, that a veil of bourgeois hypocrisy concealed our own complicity with Sade's desires.[34] Most of Sade's "biographers" echoed this opinion, as did those authors who used him as a mouthpiece for various points of view. Sade was most often conceived as a victim of bourgeois hypocrisy, as a martyr who had the courage to express with conviction all the force of his imagination, who had, like all prophets, been misunderstood. This opinion was substantiated by "scientific" proof derived from graphological and literary analyses, but writers' most common reference, as I have said, was to the apparent discrepancy between Sade's life and the tales he told in his works, a discrepancy that was interpreted as concrete proof that the true Sade was not a monster but indeed a paragon of virtue. This discrepancy became the foundation for a transmutation of Sade into the noble victim of his own prophetic vision, a sort of latter-day Cassandra. The quest for the real Sade, as Jean Desbordes put it, was inspired by a desire to "unmask the face . . . [of the man] who was both a victim and a visionary."[35] The writers who participated in this unmasking thus already had a pretty good idea of who they would discover under the mask.

Louis Perceau's little pamphlet *Du marquis de Sade et le sadisme* exemplifies this kind of literature. Although Perceau was a writer interested in erotic literature, rather than a scientist or a biographer, he structured his essay according to a "scientific format," dividing it into three parts. He began with the legend about Sade, challenged the legend with the "reality," and finished with a summary of modern opinion on sadism, which expressed the general view that sadism was a matter, as he put it, of "degrees" and pathological "only when manifested by a woman."[36]

Perceau attacked the moralist Jules Janin's famous condemna-

(Paris: Mercure de France, 1933). The first essay on Gilles de Rais is, with slight revisions, a reprint of his "Essai de réhabilitation," published in *Le Procès inquisitorial de Gilles de Rais.* Fleuret claims Gilles was entirely innocent. See also Emile Gabory, "La Psychologie de Gilles de Rais," *Revue du Bas Poitou* 3 (1925), 16. Sade, however, was the center of this kind of discourse, and his significance derives from the fact that he was a writer.

[34] Béliard, p. 110.

[35] Desbordes, p. 7.

[36] Perceau, p. 37. Perceau was one of the editors, along with Guillaume Apollinaire and Fernand Fleuret, of the catalog of the *enfer* of the Bibliothèque Nationale, the section containing licentious books.

tion of Sade, which had appeared in the *Revue de Paris* in 1834. He accused him of "romantic exaggeration linked to a narrow mind and reactionary stupidity" and denounced Janin's opinion as the relic of a superstitious age, declaring, "Jules Janin speaks of Sade as a Breton peasant woman speaks of the devil." After a long discourse on sexual freedom, Perceau summarized: "The marquis de Sade was a man like any other, with virtues and vices. If it is difficult to congratulate the author of *Justine*, it is not necessary to make him out to be a monster or a madman."[37]

The conception of Sade as Everyman was reiterated in countless medical accounts, which also emphasized the gap between the legend about Sade and the "reality" of his desire. Dr. Sarfati claimed that although Sade may have seemed in his novels to be a "master of voluptuousness," a man who "knew how to extend the accepted circle of sexual variations," in reality his "desires required nothing beyond that which a woman normally offers to a man."[38] Indeed, Sarfati went on to argue that the only "authentic" representation of Sade was to be found in the writer Jean-Jacques Brousson's characterization of him as a mute and powerless martyr. In *Les Nuits sans culottes*, Brousson makes Sade the victim of his own disciples during the Terror in 1793. He is incapable of participating in an orgy they assume he will orchestrate and is consequently subjected to an endless array of insults, accused of being "but a lover of the pen," a "satyr of writing but not of desire," and a "hypocrite." His most ardent disciple, exasperated, has the last damning word: "You heat the oven but never dare to put yourself in it!"[39] This image of Sade as incapable of desire or even of speech (he remains mute throughout the incident), his passivity in the hands of his female pupils (Sade is, in addition, dressed as a woman in order to conceal his identity from the revolutionaries hunting him), resembles the majority of portraits of Sade during the interwar years, conveying the image of a noble and tragic victim of injustice. Dr. Augustin Cabanès claimed that the "bloody eroticism of the divine marquis was more virtual than real" and that he expressed himself "through his writings rather than his acts."[40]

[37] Ibid., pp. 6, 9, 24.

[38] Sarfati, p. 123.

[39] Jean-Jacques Brousson, *Les Nuits sans culottes* (Paris: Flammarion, 1930), p. 185.

[40] Dr. Augustin Cabanès, *Le Cabinet secret de l'histoire* (Paris: Albin Michel, 1925), 3:418. This was a revised edition of a book originally published in 1900.

Paul Bourdin argued that Sade was "cruel only when caught up in the paroxysms of an unregulated and unwholesome imagination, while in real life he was just an insidious hypocrite."[41] And finally, though he by no means exhausts the list, Dr. Otto Flake declared with emotion that "the monster he seems to be in his books hardly corresponds to the man he was in reality. In Sade the intellectual element predominated, and his great spiritual energy corresponded to his violent sexual temperament."[42]

In order to validate this perception of Sade as an innocent, as Everyman, writers in particular turned to the documents pertaining to Sade's trials. Heine made the transcripts of both legal proceedings against Sade available in 1933.[43] The first concerned his abuse of Rose Keller, the widow of a pastry maker, on Easter day in 1768. She accused Sade of offering her a job as a domestic to lure her to his home. When they arrived, Sade bound, raped, and beat her and, according to the testimony, made incisions in her thighs, back, and buttocks, into which he poured melted wax. She managed to free herself and fled through an open window. Keller accepted a monetary settlement made out of court and dropped the charges. Much was made of this incident, which was circulated in many different versions.

In the second case, in which Sade was condemned to death in absentia and hanged in effigy at Aix-en-Provence in 1772, he had orchestrated an orgy at a brothel in Marseilles at which he distributed Spanish fly, an aphrodisiac (which was known popularly as *pastilles de Richelieu*). After trying to sodomize the prostitutes, who refused to comply, Sade sodomized and was sodomized by his valet. Eventually some of the women began to vomit and believed they had been poisoned. They later brought charges against Sade, and he and his valet were sentenced to death for sodomy and attempted murder through poisoning. Sade managed, with the help of his powerful family, to flee to Italy, and his sentence was eventually commuted.

[41] Bourdin, Introduction to Sade, *Correspondance inédite*, p. xlii.

[42] Dr. Otto Flake, *Le Marquis de Sade*, trans. Pierre Klossowski (Paris: Grasset, 1933), p. 31.

[43] Maurice Heine, "Le Marquis de Sade et Rose Keller; ou, L'Affaire d'Arcueil devant le Parlement de Paris," *AML* (June 1933), 309–437; Heine, "L'Affaire des bonbons cantharides du marquis de Sade," *Hippocrate* no. 1 (March, 1933). Both are reprinted in Heine, *Le Marquis de Sade*, pp. 155–210, 120–54.

Most of the stories about Sade revolved around these two episodes, though Sade was involved in others that lent themselves less easily to the stuff of legend.[44] The countless versions of each story obscured his actual behavior. Some chroniclers claimed the women in Marseilles had been poisoned and died; some said they jumped out the window, preferring certain death to the "appalling" scene (i.e., anal intercourse between the marquis and his valet) unfolding before them. Some said Keller had managed to escape through an open window; others insisted that she was discovered by a crowd who heard her cries as they passed the house in which she was held captive.[45]

No one during the interwar years denied that Sade had actually raped, beaten, and sodomized women and men; what they questioned were the precise nature of the events, the gravity of the

[44] He was imprisoned for two months for the abuse of Jeanne Testard and was accused of abusing at least five young women from Lyon and Marseilles (in December 1774–75), whom he had hired to work as domestics at his castle, La Coste. The father of one of the young women is supposed to have shot Sade, nearly killing him. These incidents were never brought to trial, however. See the hagiographic biography by Gilbert Lély, *The Marquis de Sade* (New York: Grove Press, 1970), pp. 169–89.

[45] The death of two of the prostitutes was reported in Bachaumont's *Mémoires secrets* in 1772. See *Anecdotes piquantes de Bachaumont, Mairobert etc. pour servir à l'histoire de la société française, à la fin du règne de Louis XV (1762–1774)* (Brussels: Gay et Doucé, 1881), pp. 162–163. The least sensational eighteenth-century account of the incident was reported in a letter in *Correspondance de Madame Gourdan* (Brussels: Henry Kirtenmaecher, 1866), pp. 255–66. Brière de Boismont recounted that Keller was saved by a crowd that heard her moans. His 1841 account is reproduced in Dr. Paul Moreau de Tours, *Des aberrations du sens génésique* (Paris: Asselin, 1880), pp. 59–60. Paul Lacroix declared that Keller had saved herself by escaping through a window (the origin of the story was a letter from Mme du Deffand to Horace Walpole printed in 1812 in Mme du Deffand, *Lettres à Horace Walpole écrites dans les années 1766 à 1780* [Paris: Treuttel et Wuetz, 1812], 1:227), and he repeated Bachaumont's version of the Marseilles affair, claiming one woman jumped to her death. See Paul Lacroix [P. L. Jacob, pseud.], *Curiosités de l'histoire de France* (Paris: Adolphe Delahays, 1858), pp. 236–37 and, on the Marseilles affair, p. 240. Lacroix's book reprints an article titled "La Vérité sur les deux procès du marquis de Sade," which appeared in the *Revue de Paris* 37 (February 1837), 135–44. Janin's version of what happened between Sade and Rose Keller is reported in Janin, *Les Catacombes* (Paris: Werdet, 1839), pp. 177–78. Janin also claims she escaped. See also Alcide Bonneau, *La Curiosité littéraire et bibliographique* (Paris: Liseux, 1882), pp. 131–76. For an extensive review of (and excerpts from) the many different versions of these stories and others, see Françoise Laugaa-Traut, *Lectures de Sade* (Paris: Armand Colin, 1973), pp. 6–27. Laugaa-Traut views these articles as part of a fantasy about sadism couched in moral terms.

charges, and whether they merited the punishment Sade had received. The inquiry reflected the profound transformation of moral values to which Pierre Janet had alluded in his preface to *Psychopathia sexualis*.[46]

By comparing Sade's documented behavior with his works, writers reached different conclusions about Sade's guilt from those espoused in the nineteenth century. With some exceptions, Sade's crimes had been interpreted in those years as a mirror of the moral decay prevalent in the late eighteenth century—part of the attempt to use a medical model of degeneracy to analyze the social body— or as evidence of his own physical or psychic deterioration.[47] Most summaries of Sade's life referred to his crimes severely as "disorders." The critic Jules Janin's 1834 piece in the *Revue de Paris* attacking Sade as a *honte sociale*, as a satyr who maimed and tortured innocent women, was among the most frequently cited. Janin emphasized the danger posed by the increasing availability of Sade's works and reiterated an eighteenth-century view of Sade as a moral monster.[48] The *Grande Encyclopédie* in 1895 described Rose Keller as "an unfortunate woman" who escaped in the morning, dramatically drenched in her own blood, and in Restif de la Bretonne's famous, though much earlier account she was portrayed as the helpless victim of a monster who sought to use her body for

[46] Janet, Preface, pp. 6–7.

[47] Duehren's work on Sade is the classic example. Other works reflecting this general analysis include Henri d'Almeras, *Le Marquis de Sade: L'Homme et l'écrivain* (Paris: Albin Michel, 1906); Paul Englisch, *L'Histoire de l'érotisme en Europe* (Paris: Editions Internationales, 1903). Sade's behavior is generally conceived as an example of eighteenth-century libertinism, itself conceived as evidence of spiritual and moral deterioration. This kind of argument tends to be more characteristic of German turn-of-the century texts than French ones, though French commentators often reiterated some of these themes. It is significant that Otto Flake, a German, begins his study of Sade in 1930 by refuting the thesis that the eighteenth century represented decadence and dissolution. He argued instead that it represented the birth of a new world, an "explosion of elementary forces," which Sade's behavior reflected. Flake, pp. 16–17.

[48] Janin, *Les Catacombes*, pp. 136, 160–71. Janin claimed his own interest in the marquis was inspired by the torment Sade's works produced in a boyhood friend of his who had accidentally opened a volume found in his uncle's library. The boy's character, Janin reports, was transformed overnight. A gentle, unassuming, and likable individual, after reading Sade he became bizarre, lifeless, and was unable to communicate. He was diagnosed as an epileptic until the maid found a copy of one of Sade's works hidden in his bed and the community was informed of the real origin of the boy's illness.

an anatomy lesson. Henri d'Alméras referred to her as a poor woman driven by misery to prostitution.[49] In 1912 Remy de Gourmont recounted an anecdote he must have borrowed from Alcide Bonneau's 1882 account of the Keller incident, in which Sade is caught by the police in the process of roasting a prostitute alive. Gourmont's story is ironic (he reminds us that Sade did not drive the brochette through his victim but merely attached her to the roasting equipment), but his image of Sade accords with most nineteenth-century accounts.[50] To be sure, writers' attitudes shifted depending on whether they wrote at the beginning or the end of the century or according to their own moral beliefs, but none contested the marquis's fundamental *evil*. Whether they were horrified or pretended to be horrified by it (Bonneau, Janin) or, like Gourmont and Flaubert, were fascinated, was a matter of temperament.

In contrast, writers during the interwar years used the same narrative strategies over and over to render Sade's crimes the consequence of a natural desire, an example of natural behavior—in short, to integrate them into a comprehensible context of human motivation. Thus while most writers claimed that it was their intention not to rehabilitate but to understand Sade, the methods they employed transformed him into a victim by demonizing the women he victimized and the religious and moral values that "protected" them. Moreover (and I will clarify the significance of this portrayal further on), these writers also described the revolutionaries to whom Sade had at one time lent his support as pathological specimens.

Writers tended to point to the dubious reputation of the women Sade had abused as a way of excusing him. Whereas in most nineteenth-century texts, as we have seen, Rose Keller was depicted as a poor, bereft, if "fallen," woman, by the twenties and thirties she had metamorphosed into a self-serving slut. Writers downplayed

[49] *La Grande Encyclopédie* (Paris: Société Anonyme, 1895), 29:46–47; Restif de la Bretonne, *Nuits de Paris* (London, 1778), 6:2566–70; Alméras, *Marquis de Sade,* pp. 58–59.

[50] Remy de Gourmont, *Mercure de France,* February 1, 1912, cited in Cabanès, p. 419. Another typical nineteenth-century opinion of Sade is expressed by Fernand Drujon: "In this infamous work [*Justine*] Sade has pushed atrocity to its limit." *Catalogue des ouvrages, écrits, et dessins de toute nature poursuivis, supprimés, ou condamnés depuis le 21 octobre 1814 jusqu'au 31 juillet 1877* (Paris: Edouard Rouveyre, 1877), p. 215. According to Drujon, *Justine* was destroyed by royal order on May 19, 1815.

her rape and mutilation and emphasized Sade's literary greatness, as if one kind of suffering (the pain of being misunderstood) were comparable to or outweighed the other. In fact, Sade's "pain" obliterated (whatever we can imagine to be) the pain of his victim. But how did their different torments become comparable and by what criteria? How can literary greatness excuse sadistic behavior? And how, we might justifiably ask, can we be made to feel sorry for, even to admire, a man whose sadism is, so to speak, on the record?

First, how exactly did commentators during the interwar years transform Rose Keller into a self-serving slut? To begin with, Dr. André Javelier did not pardon the marquis entirely but insisted that "the victim was not very interesting, if indeed there was a victim." He went on to claim with confidence that she was "hardly more than a vamp" and to declare that her testimony was only "a work of the imagination, an erroneous interpretation of the facts owing to the obvious strength of her tactile over her visual perception."[51] Dr. Béliard and the writer Emile Henriot claimed that Rose Keller was of doubtful morality and believed, along with several other writers, that Keller's use of the compensation Sade paid as a dowry for her subsequent marriage confirmed their judgment.[52] Jean Desbordes claimed that Keller would not have found Sade's demands unusual and could not possibly have regretted her experience since it provided her with the means to marry.[53]

The writer Louis Perceau, to whom I have already alluded, tried to reconstruct the "facts" in order to present a more comprehensible version of the Keller affair. Perceau's version deserves to be cited in full:

The story can be quite easily reconstituted. The prostitute [fille de joie] Rose Keller was brought home by Sade to participate in an orgy. She was beaten [and here Perceau adds a footnote assuring the reader that "beating was common at the time in order to supplement erotic scenarios"]. Then, as she was a bit simpleminded, he could not resist

---

[51] Dr. André Javelier, Thèse pour le doctorat en médecine: Le Marquis de Sade et les "Cent-vingt Journées de Sodome" devant la psychiatrie et la médecine légale (Paris: Librairie le François, 1937), p. 20.

[52] Béliard, p. 107; Emile Henriot, "La Vraie Figure du marquis de Sade," in Courrier littéraire, XVIIIème siècle (Paris: Marcel Daubin, 1945), 1:187. This article was originally published in Le Temps in February 1930.

[53] Desbordes, p. 83.

the desire to play with her credulity and . . . told her she was going to be dissected.

This story, which the girl told to the police, circulated rapidly, and that is why the marquise du Deffand was able to report it with such precision. But in fact the marquise's letter only reiterated Keller's version, the version of the girl who had been fooled, a version itself deformed and vulgarized by public rumors.

Today this kind of testimony would no longer be accepted except for the records.[54]

Perceau's account uses many different and by now familiar rhetorical strategies to diminish Sade's criminal responsibility. Perceau portrays Keller as fundamentally complicitous and, in so doing, manages to accuse *her*, implicitly, of bad faith. He represents Sade's behavior as so innocent and acceptable that it is not at all clear what Keller had to complain about.[55] Finally, he dismisses Keller's testimony on legal grounds, blaming not just Keller's simplemindedness but the archaic legal system that supported and accepted her testimony.

Jean-Jacques Brousson's novel, to which I have also alluded, effects perhaps the most remarkable transformation of the Keller story. In his account, Keller has completely ceased being a victim; indeed, she has actually become the perpetrator of the crime. Although Brousson does not mention her by name, it is clear that he is referring to Keller when he speaks of Sade's most enthusiastic "disciple." After being beaten by the marquis in circumstances resembling Keller's, this woman discovers what pleasure really is and subsequently opens a *couvent sadique* both as a tribute to her master—calling it a convent of course indicates that it is a place of worship—and in order to have a secluded meeting place where the disciples of the sadistic "order" can indulge their most extraordinary fantasies (though it is never clear whether Keller's inspirational first encounter with Sade is real or her own fantasy).[56] The Keller figure later saves Sade from the guillotine and brings him back with her to the convent, expecting him to be delighted by her efforts, but remember that in this account it is Sade who is the

[54] Perceau, pp. 18–19.

[55] Some accounts of the Keller incident claim other individuals participated: other prostitutes, Sade's valet. Nevertheless, Keller accused Sade of abusing her.

[56] Brousson, *Les Nuits*, p. 179.

unwilling participant, berated by Keller's all-female entourage. Brousson's book in this way absolves Sade of any crime (and emphasizes instead his sensitivity to the evil lurking in others) by portraying Sade as Keller's victim.

This attitude toward Keller and toward Sade himself was perhaps most succinctly expressed by Maurice Heine. "Why all the fuss over a spanking?" he asked, not concealing some exasperation. In his typically cautious effort to be fair to everyone involved, Heine suggested that no one was to blame and pointed his finger instead at an archaic and repressive moral code; Sade, he argued, could not admit to the courts he went as far as he did, and Rose Keller could not admit her desire to go all the way with him. Sade could own up to his desires within certain limits, but if Keller had confessed her penchant for libertinism, she would surely have been put in a hospital.[57] Heine was clearly not fond of double standards, and his skewed thinking about Keller is all the more troubling because it makes explicit that she simply did not count in his (and others') reevaluation of Sade.[58]

[57] Heine *Le Marquis de Sade*, pp. 203, 207. Jean Paulhan used similar words, remarking, "It seems established that Sade gave a spanking to a whore in Paris: does that fit with a year in jail?" Paulhan, "The Marquis de Sade and His Accomplice," in D. A. F. Sade, *Three Complete Novels: Justine, Philosophy in the Bedroom, Eugénie de Franval, and Other Writings* (New York: Grove Press, 1965), p. 7.
Andrea Dworkin has already noted the extent to which the reality of Sade's crimes has been denied. She links this denial to the structure of patriarchal domination, however, without analyzing it as part of a historical moment in the restructuring of patriarchy. Dworkin explains that denial ahistorically by reference to an intrinsically violent male sexuality. In her work on pornography, Dworkin in fact affirms from a feminist perspective what writers in the twenties affirmed from a quite different point of view: that Sade is Everyman. Sade's importance, she declares, "is not as dissident or deviant: it is as Everyman, a designation the power-crazed aristocrat would have found repugnant, but one that women, on examination, will find true. In Sade, the authentic equation is revealed: the power of the pornographer is the power of the rapist/batterer is the power of man." Dworkin thus uses the same essentialist framework as those writers she criticizes. Only, she judges Sade's "essential" nature to be evil instead of innocuous or an emblem of human freedom. Dworkin's analysis recalls nineteenth-century feminist tracts that presume an intrinsically aggressive male nature. Andrea Dworkin, *Pornography: Men Possessing Women* (New York: Putnam, 1981), pp. 70–100. For a nonfeminist but equally critical (and more compelling) analysis titled "The Vogue of the Marquis de Sade," see Edmund Wilson, *The Bit between My Teeth* (New York: Farrar, Straus, and Giroux, 1965), pp. 158–227.
[58] Rose Keller tended to be the focus of this kind of discussion, but the prostitutes in Marseilles do not fare much better. Dr. Sarfati complained that abusing pros-

The cruelty of arranged marriages was used by Sade's apologists to explain and to justify his hatred of women (and hence his crimes against them). Sade had been forced to marry a woman whom he did not love, and it tormented him all his life. Dr. Marciat (Claude Tournier) had already made this argument in 1899, and in the 1920s it became the center of an overall analysis of Sade's misogyny. After he had completed seven years of military service in 1766, Sade's father forced him to marry Renée de Montreuil, a woman from a very rich and a very respectable family. Although Sade at first objected, he was threatened with disinheritance and finally acceded to his father's wishes. His wife, who remained devoted to him in spite of his moral transgressions, was not, however, portrayed as a "saint of conjugal love," as Paul Ginisty had called her at the end of the nineteenth century.[59] Instead, she was seen as a masochist who longed to be abused.

Louis Perceau mocked Janin's image of Renée de Montreuil as "a poor, gentle, pretty, virtuous, timid girl" and argued that Sade's unhappy marriage justified his hatred of his wife: "The Marquis de Sade had to obey [his parents] but he bore a hatred for his wife from which he was never able to free himself. He may have been unjust, but he had his reasons, especially given the hateful act of his parents, who negotiated his marriage like a business affair, with no regard for the opinions of those involved."[60] And Dr. Ivan-Claude Larouche applied a term coined by Dr. Edmond Locard to describe Renée de Montreuil: No longer perceived as virtuously persevering, she was transformed into an "enclitophile," someone who was obsessively attracted to criminals because of an essential masochism.[61]

Others refrained from explicitly accusing her of masochism but

---

titutes should hardly be considered a serious offense, and Jean Desbordes argued that only the prostitutes of Marseilles, more prudish than most, would have been shocked by Sade's provocative suggestions. Sarfati, pp. 39–40; Desbordes, p. 111.

[59] Paul Ginisty, *La Marquise de Sade* (Paris: E. Fasquelle, 1901), p. 27.

[60] Perceau, p. 22. Balkis too claimed that Sade's unhappy marriage explained his general hostility to "wives." Balkis, *Pages curieuses du marquis de Sade* (Paris: Les Bibliophiles Libertins, 1928), p. 11.

[61] Ivan-Claude Larouche, *Prestige du crime* (Paris: Société Parisienne d'Edition, 1946), p. 102. He claimed that "never, in spite of his crimes, did this infernal man, whose very name scorched the delicacy of some, inspire the least repulsion in his wife. The marquise never ceased to love her corrupt husband, and her devotion in fact constitutes an example of enclitophilia."

nevertheless enlisted the reader's sympathy on Sade's side against
the oppressive countenance of his wife. Dr. Octave Béliard attributed Sade's hatred of women and his sadism in general to his
marriage, and in his biography of the marquis included a fictional
reconstruction of Sade's first encounter with his wife's younger
sister, with whom he fell in love. In his account, Sade, who mis-
takes Louise de Montreuil for her older sister, his wife-to-be, is
enchanted by her beauty and her youth. Sade returns home love
struck and announces his happiness to his father. The father is
puzzled by his son's reaction, and the contrast between his father's
befuddlement and Sade's enthusiasm is the mystery on which the
"biography" centers its dramatic tension. When the reader finally
learns with Sade that the woman with whom he has fallen in love
is not in fact his future wife, when Béliard describes his fiancée
Renée as older and unattractive, she feels Sade's tragic misfortune
as her own and is subtly entreated to endorse Sade's stealing away
with Louise in a later part of the book, which is in fact its most
touching, romantic, scene. Sade emerges as the romantic hero, and
Renée de Montreuil as an unsympathetic obstacle to his happiness.[62]

Not bothering with this kind of lengthy biographical explanation, Otto Flake declared simply that "Sade's misogyny" was natural: "He hated in Renée and in women in general a being subject to
the whims of sentiment, to whom truth is not accessible."[63]

As Sade's sexual crimes were purged of their criminality, the
rewriting of his relationship to the French Revolution transformed
his fantasies about crime into the refusal of crime. Writers, as they
had always done, linked Sade's work to the bloody excesses of the
French Revolution, but what captured their imagination during
the interwar years was not the proximity of Sade's fantasies to

[62] In fact, in most biographical reconstructions of Sade's life, Sade is the gallant
marquis unfairly treated by vengeful women (thus paralleling the treatment of
Keller by Brousson). In a novel by Sylvain Bonmariage, Sade is a man no woman can
resist. He gallantly affects indifference to all the women in the village where he is
staying in order not to offend any of them. When a certain Madame d'Oigny tries to
entice him into her bed in order to make all the other women jealous, Sade "told her
that he hated to have his hand forced even if the card in question was the Queen of
Hearts . . . and he excused himself for having to take leave of her." Sylvain Bonmariage, *La Seconde Vie du marquis de Sade* (Lille: Mercure de Flandre, 1927),
pp. 158–59.
[63] Flake, p. 82.

the Terror but instead the fact that Sade had condemned political violence.

In the century preceding the Great War, Sade was often discussed in conjunction with the French Revolution in order to condemn the monstrosity of both the writer and the revolutionaries through the comparison. One of the most colorful anecdotes in this vein was circulated by Charles de Villiers in 1797 and found exponents throughout the nineteenth century. In a famous letter published about *Justine* in *Le Spectateur du Nord*, Villiers linked Sade with Robespierre:

> It is said that when this Robespierre, and when Couthon, St. Just, and Collot, his ministers, were tired of murders and convictions, when some small remorse penetrated those hearts of steel and, at the sight of the numerous judgments they had to sign, the pen fell from their fingers, they went and read a few pages of *Justine* and came back to sign. I cannot guarantee the authenticity of the anecdote, but it is told far and wide and it is believed in France.[64]

In the course of the nineteenth century, this linkage between Sade and the Revolution was reiterated in different, more sophisticated terms, which recognized the satirical quality of Sade's work and rooted his subversiveness in a kind of iconoclasm characteristic of the dandy. Sade was an iconoclast who nevertheless respected the rules, a noble committed to exposing the hypocrisy of the very society he gathers around him, a true believer difficult to distinguish from a cynic and necessarily hypersensitive, elegant, and effeminate. Sade's ideas were consequently less in advance of his time (as his interwar enthusiasts were to assert) than an ironic (and hence critical) mirror of it. In a much cited passage from their 1862 work *La Femme au XVIIIe siècle*, the Goncourt brothers suggested that the maimed and mutilated bodies in Sade's novels expressed the weariness of a century that, tired of torturing souls, had turned to the novel pleasure of torturing bodies.[65]

[64] Quoted in Perceau, p. 15. Also quoted in a much longer excerpt in Laugaa-Traut, p. 75. I have used the English translation in Maurice Blanchot, "The Main Impropriety," in *Literature and Revolution* (Boston: Beacon Press, 1970), p. 59.

[65] Edmond and Jules de Goncourt, *La Femme au XVIIIe siècle* (Paris: Flammarion, 1982), p. 176. In *La Maison Philibert* (1904), Jean Lorrain draws an analogy between the legal immunity of aristocrats in Sade's works and the corruption of Third Re-

By the interwar years Sade had become not an iconoclast but a humanitarian, whose compassion was underscored by the fact that the Revolution had finally condemned him for moderation. Even Sade's political satire *Philosophy in the Bedroom*, whose epigraph parodied a passage from a pornographic pamphlet directed against Marie Antoinette in 1791, was interpreted not as a prescription for but as a mighty tirade against the Revolution and the Terror in particular. Hence writers during the 1920s and 1930s made much of Sade's remark in the section of the *Philosophy* headed "Yet Another Effort, Frenchmen, If You Would Become Republicans": "An already old and decayed nation which courageously casts off the yoke of its monarchical government in order to adopt a republican one, will only be maintained by many crimes; for it is criminal already, and if it were to pass from crime to virtue, that is to say, from a violent to a pacific, benign condition, it should fall into an inertia whose result would soon be its certain ruin."[66] They claimed that Sade had been a revolutionary, one of the rare aristocrats who prophesied the fall of the monarchy and understood the merits of democratic government; he had not condoned any sort of tyranny, whether in the name of monarchy or democracy.

In the new accounts Sade was made out to be reflective and human, while the revolutionary leaders who directed the guillotine's systematic and senseless labors were demonized, portrayed as a blood-hungry mob driven by a fanatical desire for truth. In *Les Princesses de Cythère*, Pascal Fely described Sade as "a lamb compared to the other enthusiasts of the guillotine; they were fanatics, he was only a dilettante, a poor devil of an intellectual to whom has been attributed, after his books, more ingenious crimes than this grand seigneur, rotten with literature, would have had the audacity to commit. Sade would have at the most been an Adolphe de Cantacuzène or a Robert de Montesquiou, precious poets."[67]

---

public liberalism, in which a high position similarly guaranteed immunity from the law. Lorrain's work both imitates Sade's satire and implicates Sade himself in the very corruption he parodies. Through the voices of the prostitutes in the novel, Lorrain equates Sade's talent for both writing and evasion with those of contemporary politicians. Jean Lorrain, *La Maison Philibert* (Paris: Librairie Universelle, 1904), pp. 277–79.

[66] D. A. F. Sade, *Philosophy in the Bedroom*, p. 333.

[67] Pascal Fely, *Les Princesses de Cythère* (Paris: Jean Fort, 1920), pp. 166–67 (originally published in 1913). Adolphe de Cantacuzène was the author of, among others, *Sourires glacés* (1896); Robert de Montesquiou, author of *Hortensias bleus* (1896), was the model for Proust's Charlus.

This book, which presents itself as a chronicle of French sentimental life (hence the reference to Cythère, the mythical island of love celebrated in Watteau's famous painting) views the revolutionary period as a tragic turn toward "ferocity" and endlessly cites anecdotes of atrocities committed by fanatical revolutionaries whose crimes were "more horrible than anything the mind of that lubricious poet could ever have conceived." Indeed Fely's work is an open apology for Sade, who, he declared, should be "acquitted" of his infamous reputation because of the "attenuating circumstances" constituted by the malicious whisperings of "mediocrities who could not have appreciated his tremendous intellectual force." "This blood lover was, after all, a great artist, and his atrocious dreams were sublime; the torturers of Nantes were only vulgar rascals."[68]

Sade's compassion was further verified by one of the letters published in Bourdin's edition, in which the marquis denounced the spectacle of the guillotine. Sade himself had been put on a list of "moderates" to be executed and was unfortunate enough to be locked in a prison cell with a direct view of the guillotine where other moderates perished. He was saved when Robespierre fell from power.

Sade's opposition to capital punishment was thus implicit in his work and personal testimony, and sympathizers played on the irony of this attitude in a man who unwittingly gave his name to sadism. They used this romantic contrast as the basis for a fantasy about Sade's humanitarianism and his prophetic powers. Brousson's Sade deplores the indiscriminate use of the guillotine and declares, "You are all sadists without knowing it."[69] In fact, in most interwar writing, it is Sade who "knows" and who is persecuted for knowing. Maurice Heine reproached Dr. Sarfati and other Sade critics for accusing him of pettiness and avarice when in fact he had even saved his enemies (in particular his mother-in-law) from the guillotine. Sade, Heine went on, was altruistic, a true humanitarian.[70] Jean Desbordes pointed out that Sade could easily have asked to become a commissar of the people during the Revolution in order to live out his fantasies under the sanction of the law, but chose not to.[71]

[68] Fely, pp. 175, 167, 76.
[69] Brousson, Les Nuits, p. 154.
[70] Heine, Le Marquis de Sade, p. 109.
[71] Desbordes, p. 31.

If some disputed his humanitarianism, it was generally agreed that Sade was a prophet. This interpretation of Sade was indebted to the horrors of the Great War and especially, in the early thirties, of Hitler's rise to power. Sade became more than a pornographer or a dandy; he was a visionary whose works had prophesied the Apocalypse. In the Great War, "his conclusions [about human nature] were finally verified," wrote Heine. They might, if readers had listened more carefully, even have prevented the tragedy brought about by Hitler, said Gilbert Lély. The critic René de Planhol called Sade a clairvoyant and, citing the famous remark from *La Philosophie dans le boudoir* I quoted earlier, claimed that he had "diagnosed the exact law of all revolutions."[72]

Thus, through the distinction between Sade's life and works, he was transformed into a noble, virtuous, and innocent victim who had the courage to speak of the monster in all of us without himself committing any crime. In the first reading, Sade's sexual violations of women were conflated so completely with consensual sex that Sade, *in spite of* the evidence, was judged to have done nothing out of the ordinary, nothing that other aristocrats had not done more discreetly, nothing that men and women permitted to act according to their natural impulses would balk at doing, nothing that was not just sex. In the second reading, Sade was acquitted not in spite of but because of the textual evidence. Here Sade's sadism was conflated so completely with his prophetic virtues that his work not only was not criminal but refused criminality. So Sade was normalized and mythologized.

This paradox whereby Sade's crimes were seen as unreal (normal) even as they described what was most fundamentally real about human nature (its pathology) thus oddly transformed his criminality into a virtue, into the most profound kind of humanitarianism. This transformation was made possible, however, precisely because these writers severed the link between his life and his work, between (in any case highly contested) interpretations of his life and fiction. The first step was to exonerate him of whatever crimes he had really committed. Then his work could speak to us about crime without being criminal; Sade's crime was defined no

[72]Maurice Heine, Preface to D. A. F. Sade, *Historiettes, Contes, et Fabliaux* (Paris: Simon Kra, 1927), p. vii; Lély, Prologue to Sade, *Morceaux choisis*, pp. xxxiv–xxxv; René de Planhol, *Les Utopistes de l'amour* (Paris: Garnier Frères, 1921), pp. 196–97.

longer by what he did to others but by the fact that he tells us something we don't want or can't bear to hear. Hence he is a prophet, sublime. Most curiously, his very proclamation of crime guarantees him to be no criminal. In a contradictory move, Sade was purged of his sadism and yet given status as a writer because he was a sadist. Writers and critics played out this contradiction to revamp Sade's image during the interwar years, exonerating him of crime through a reconstruction of the "facts," revising his status as a writer and thinker, examining how his work was connected to and yet something more than his desire. They moved away from primarily pseudoscientific evaluations of Sade (medical, biographical, historical) to literature. How does literature replicate this purging of Sade's sadism?

The Literary Portrait

Mario Praz's 1933 classic, *The Romantic Agony*, was the most extensive discussion of Sade's influence on nineteenth-century writers that had then been undertaken. Praz, an Italian, devoted an entire chapter of his work to the literary influence of Sade on some of France's greatest writers. He quoted a famous remark made by the critic Charles Sainte-Beuve in 1843: "I will dare to affirm that Byron and Sade . . . have perhaps been the two greatest inspirations of our modern writers; the first, accessible and visible, the second clandestine, but not too clandestine. In reading some of our more fashionable novelists, if you want the . . . secret stairway to the alcove, never lose this last key."[73] But, as Heine pointed out in his review of the book, Praz declared that Sade "did not even possess the most elementary qualities of a writer," that he was a "pornographer," even as he argued that the marquis exercised a tremendous influence on writers from Stendhal through Flaubert and the Goncourt brothers. Praz was thus primarily interested in the "spirit" of the Sade revival reflected in these works. Heine's own criticism of Praz's work lacked rigor and yet better expressed the changing assessment of Sade's literary status in the 1920s and 1930s: "How can M. Praz reconcile the negative character of this

[73] Mario Praz, *The Romantic Agony* (Oxford: Oxford University Press, 1970), pp. 82–83.

author with the positive influence he recognizes he had over an entire century?"[74]

Sade was most often conceived as a sadist, not always as first and foremost a writer. In the nineteenth century the interest in Sade coincided with a revival of interest in the Christian tradition, said Praz, "with the ensuing stress on martyrdom and the lives of the saints into which sado-masochism strikes its deepest roots."[75] Most of the various literary interpretations of Sade's work focused on sadism, and in popular perception Sade was still deemed a madman of sorts. For example, in 1895 the *Grande Encyclopédie* declared that "his works are unreadable," his writing "extravagant," and his imagination "delirious."[76] But Huysmans, Flaubert, Stendhal, Barbey d'Aurevilly, and other writers linked his sadism in a more sophisticated way to a kind of Catholicism *à rebours*, identified it as a sacrilege inspired not by a refusal of God but by the weight of God's presence, not by a lack of spiritual commitment but by a drive to lose one's self in what Praz called a "joy tempered by fear," and hence in a most spiritual, Catholic debauchery.[77] For romantic writers in particular, Sade became a fascinating and unspeakable character, hero and victim of a Luciferian revolt, the prototype of the *maudit* (damned) figure. Sade's sadomasochism represented the ecstatic self-dissolution characteristic of martyrdom, especially as conceived in a century that envisioned itself as undergoing painful moral deterioration, a century that had transferred its allegiance from God to Satan but was no less Catholic for all that. Sade was perceived as a mirror of the fin de siècle's own latent Catholicism, its own malaise; as Gustave Flaubert remarked at a dinner he attended at the Goncourts', Sade had uttered "the last word of Catholicism."[78]

[74] Heine, *Le Marquis de Sade*, pp. 272, xxi.

[75] Praz, p. xxi n.

[76] *La Grande Encyclopédie* 29:14. See also the "Avis des éditeurs" in the 1881 edition of Sade, *Les Crimes de l'amour*: "The style of his work is detestable; if the author was mad, he was no writer." (Brussels: Gay et Doucé, 1881).

[77] See the discussion of Huysmans in Praz, pp. 320–21.

[78] Flaubert, quoted by Edmond and Jules de Goncourt, *Journal, 1858–1860* (Monaco: Fasquelle et Flammarion, 1956), 3:213. The image of Sade as a martyr is common to many nineteenth-century texts, especially Petrus Borel's *Madame Putiphar*. The linkage between sadism and Catholicism is a Decadent theme, elaborated most extensively by Huysmans in *Là-Bas* and given perhaps its most literal rendition in the Decadent classic, Joseph Péladan, *La Vertu suprême*, vols. 14–15 of *La Dé-*

Several imaginary portraits and lithographs—since we have no life portrait of Sade—attest to this vision. In a well-known 1829 lithograph reproduced in Guillaume Apollinaire's work on Sade (1909), as well as in Paul Ginisty's 1901 work on the marquise, Sade cuts a young and elegant figure: the portrait is framed by a *bonnet de folie* on the top and a satyr on each side (see Figure 2). Underneath is another, vaguer sketch of a man in a prison cell at a writing desk. Sade's mouth is twisted, his eyes look off into the distance, his head is held high. In spite of Sade's refinement the portrait is somewhat sinister: Sade's face actually mirrors the face of the satyr to the right, and the satyr to the left corresponds to the softer, blurrier image of the writer below. The image is hence ambiguous but sinister in its very ambiguity, in its refusal to tell the viewer which man is the real Sade, in subtly insisting that the tenderness of the man writing and the madness of the man gazing are inseparable.

In later portraits, Sade incarnates the so-called dissipated soul of the fin de siècle—refined and elegant but impotent, weary, and prey to his own weakness (Figure 3). Paul Lacroix described Sade (after Sade's self-description in a letter) as "plumpish, with blue eyes and blond, curly hair. . . . His least movement betrayed a perfect grace and his harmonious voice penetrated women's hearts." The *Grande Encyclopédie* depicts him as having beautiful white hair and a very soft voice, as being of an exquisite *politesse* that concealed the "disorder of the brain," as a "robust man without infirmities." The writer Alphonse Gallais notes that "what is most striking about the marquis de Sade is the way he joins a most pleasing exterior to all his vices."[79]

In *Les Confidences d'une aïeule,* Abel Hermant described Sade (who appears as a character in the novel) in similar terms:

> He was large and slim, and seemed young even though his hair was all white, a white that made him look even younger and appeared to be pure *coquetterie*. I suspected for a moment that he was powdered. That made me notice the elegance of his costume. . . . He was dressed

---

cadence latine (Geneva: Editions Slatkine, 1979), pp. 298–331. Sade was an important influence on all nineteenth-century French (and many English) writers. For further reference, the reader should look to Praz, as the subject is inexhaustible.

[79] Lacroix, quoted by Marciat, p. 187; *La Grande Encyclopédie* 29:15; Alphonse Gallais, *Les Enfers lubriques* (Paris: J. Fort, 1909), p. 237.

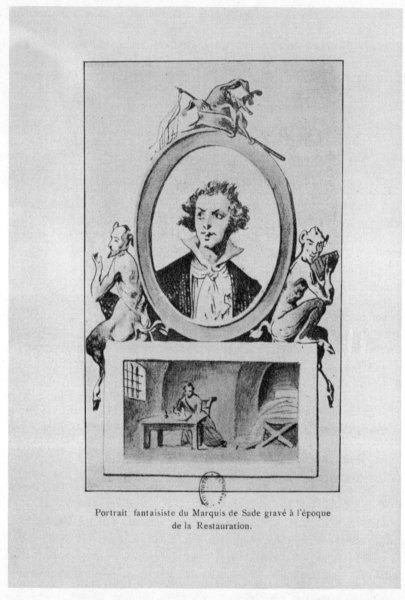

Portrait fantaisiste du Marquis de Sade gravé à l'époque
de la Restauration.

Figure 2. Whimsical Portrait of the Marquis de Sade. From Guillaume Apollinaire,
L'Oeuvre du marquis de Sade. Paris: Bibliothèque des Curieux, 1909. Courtesy
Bibliothèque Nationale.

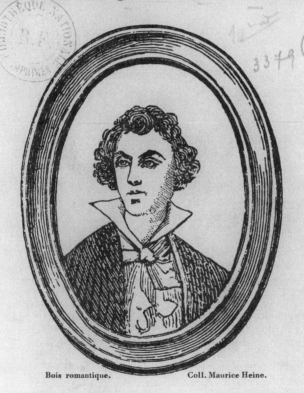

MARK AMIAUX

LA VIE EFFRÉNÉE
DU MARQUIS DE SADE

Bois romantique.   Coll. Maurice Heine.

LES ÉDITIONS DE FRANCE

Figure 3. The Unbridled Life of the Marquis de Sade. From Mark Amiaux, *La Vie effrénée du marquis de Sade.* Paris: Editions de France, 1936. Courtesy Bibliothèque Nationale.

not in blue [the Republican color] like Robespierre but in black; and
this color gave him a sinister look without taking away from the
gentleness of his features. He had the most beautiful eyes in the world
and a look that caressed you.[80]

Sade's clothing, as in other novels, provides a sinister hint, especially in contrast to his innocuous appearance.[81] In Hermant's
work Sade is a sort of amateur psychologist who deplores the mechanical vulgarity of the guillotine (even though the occasion for
his discourse is an execution at the Place de la Révolution). Hermant uses the image to convey Sade's refinement as an illustration
of an aesthetics of vice, but also to condemn the savage, primitive
blood that presumably flowed in Jacobin veins.

Hermant's portrait was reproduced in descriptions of Sade left by

[80] Abel Hermant, *Les Confidences d'une aïeule* (Paris: Editions de France, 1933),
pp. 49–50. The novel was originally published in 1909. Heine later accused Hermant of plagiarizing Sade in another novel. Maurice Heine, "Actualité de Sade," *Le
Surréalisme au service de la Révolution* 2 (1930), 4–5.

[81] For example, Fernand Fleuret, *Histoire de la bienheureuse Raton, fille de joie*
(Paris: Gallimard, 1926), describes Sade as "dressed in black plush." Fleuret's book
was written in the twenties but paints a very belatedly dandyish portrait of Sade. In
texts throughout the interwar years Sade retains this dandyism. In Sylvain Bonmariage's portrait, Sade is so self-assured that "nothing bothered him"; even when
interrupted in the course of an encounter with the gardener's daughter, he knows
how to handle the situation gracefully. In regard to women, Sade knows the power of
his charms but refuses to abuse them, preferring to "affirm his independence above
everyone." He offers the narrator of the story this piece of wisdom: "I deduced that
Sade was not as crazy as all that the day he told me that one can make women suffer
without beating them." Bonmariage, pp. 162, 259.
   Charles Méré's play *Le Marquis de Sade*, which had a run at the Grand Guignol in
1921, also portrayed the marquis in nineteenth-century terms as a noble and tragic
character whose authority is explained by his gentleness: "How to explain the
power I have over them, my empire?" the marquis declares to one of the asylum
keepers. "Gentleness! I obtain more from them through gentleness than others
do . . . with a straitjacket!" Sade incarnates authority exercised with grace, manifests an aristocratic paternalism toward the madmen at Charenton, who are mere
projections of Sade's own literary "kingdom": an amoral Jacobin, a hysteric named
Justine, a shrew named La Dubois. In a still from the play, Sade is portrayed amid
the madmen, protecting another madwoman from their rage. He is almost larger
than life, his arms are extended on each side to hold back his subjects in a seemingly
effortless and almost elegant concentration of force. His gesture is repeated again as
he tries gallantly to save one woman from the assaults of another, until he abandons
himself almost reluctantly, guiltily, to the pleasure he derives from watching them.
Charles Méré, *Le Marquis de Sade*, reprinted in *Le Théâtre* (Paris: Christian Bour-
gois, 1969), pp. 142–44. To these texts one could also add Georges Maurevert, *La
Plus Belle Fille du monde* (Paris: Flammarion, 1922), p. 233.

men who had encountered (or claimed to have encountered) the marquis in prison. Charles Nodier described Sade at the end of his life as obese, with "weary eyes that still kept, somehow, something refined and brilliant which would come to life from time to time like the dying spark of an extinguished coal." Ange Pitou said he "trembled at the idea of death" and was horrified at the sight of his white hair; "sometimes he would shed tears . . . [crying] why am I so horrible and why is crime so charming?"[82]

Apollinaire effected the transition from this nineteenth-century literary mythology of Sade to another sort of mythmaking which culminated in the surrealist work of the 1920s. He published *L'Oeuvre du marquis de Sade,* a selection of Sade's works he had discovered in the section of the Bibliothèque Nationale reserved for licentious books, the *enfer.*[83] In this book Apollinaire set Sade up as the emblem of the century to come: "This man, who seems to have counted for nothing during the whole nineteenth century, might become the dominant figure of the twentieth."[84] He refuted the nineteenth-century view of Sade as a martyr representing the essential depravity of human nature as well as what that conception owed to psychiatric notions of perversion as a symptom of bad blood. Sade was no incarnation of original sin, said Apollinaire; he was a "modern spirit" who represented the variety, complexity, and liberty inherent in human nature, a writer whose works anticipated Freud and Krafft-Ebing "by at least a hundred years," an advocate of women's liberation and of radical political ideas.[85]

The link Apollinaire forged between Sade's sadism and human liberty in fact became the interpretative norm for the generation of avant-garde thinkers to come. Much has already been written about the surrealists' rehabilitation of Sade and a host of other

[82] Guillaume Apollinaire, *L'Oeuvre du marquis de Sade* (Paris: Bibliothèque des Curieux, 1909), pp. 12–13, 13–16. Apollinaire added a brief biography that includes these portraits.

[83] See Pascal Pia's catalog *Les Livres de l'enfer, du XVIe siècle à nos jours* (Paris: C. Coulet and A. Favre, 1978).

[84] Apollinaire, p. 22.

[85] Ibid., pp. 21–22. Apollinaire identified Justine as an example of traditional womanhood, "miserable, submissive, and less than human," and Juliette as the "new woman" who will remake the universe. Sade chose women as his heroines, in Apollinaire's view, because he wanted to demonstrate that women should be as free as men. Apollinaire's uncharacteristic naïveté in this regard is quite remarkable, for Juliette, even if a caricature, is a relentless murderer. The point is that Apollinaire seems to take her "freedom" quite literally.

marginal literary figures. Here I am interested primarily in how their reconstruction of Sade participated in a more general literary transformation of Sade's sadism into a new vision of the self. The interwar literary portraits, most of them surrealist inspired, were indebted to the fin de siècle, but they transmuted the nineteenth-century image of a dandy to another vision. In fin-de-siècle portraits Sade's aristocratic manners and his cruelty were contrasted to and yet linked with his impotence and obsequiousness; in the interwar years his gentleness was instead contrasted to and linked with his irony, his playfulness, to convey an image of beauty and power, of a cynical and hence compromised but forceful purity. The new portrait thus invested Sade with an extreme gentleness, with a boundless love and an extreme nobility that contrast with his otherwise "feminine" features. This portrait humanizes Sade not by making him gentle instead of sinister but by synthesizing the two qualities. Writers attributed to Sade a noble masculinity that integrates but supersedes his feminine characteristics and in fact gives those traits their allure; his sadism is recast as a depth of character, usually conveyed by Sade's eyes, whose lucidity and wisdom give the softness of the portrait an intellectual dimension that underscores its power and constitutes its truth. But Sade's gaze is no longer the opaque and weary gaze of the dandy; it is the forceful stare of the man who bears his knowledge heavily and proclaims it out loud (see Figure 4).

This new portrait of Sade retains some features of dandyism, in particular its insistent masculinity. The dandy was necessarily male because it repudiated all that was natural, symbolized by the feminine. His masculinity was linked to an image of deterioration, of weariness, because the dandy's maleness represented the self cultivated *as* image, perpetually and exhaustingly taking up new poses that emptied identity by doubling and multiplying it. Barbey d'Aurevilly called them "double and multiple natures, of an undecidable intellectual sex, in whom grace is still more graceful as strength and strength appears again as grace; Androgynes of History, no more of the Fable, of whom Alcibiade was the most beautiful in the most beautiful of nations."[86] The new image of Sade's mas-

---

[86] Barbey d'Aurevilly, "Du dandysme et de George Brummell," in *Oeuvres romanesques complètes*, vol. 2 (Paris: Bibliothèque de la Pléiade, 1966), p. 718. This essay was first published in 1845.

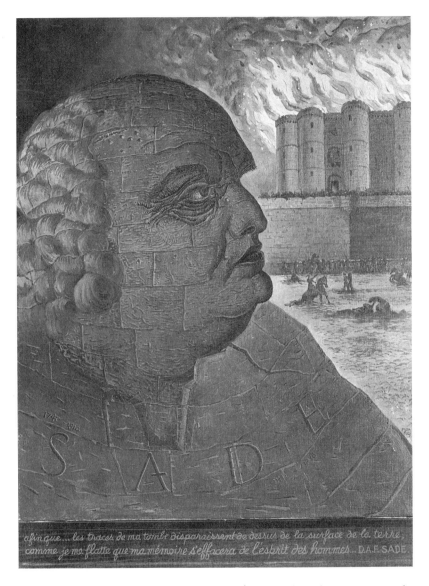

Figure 4. Man Ray, *Imaginary Portrait of the Marquis de Sade*, 1938. Copyright 1991 ARS, N.Y./ADAGP. Courtesy of Lauros-Giraudon. ". . . so that . . . the traces of my tomb disappear from the face of the earth, as I flatter myself that my memory will vanish from the minds of men."

culinity in fact reversed and transformed this celebration of artifice and androgyny (that horror of all that is deemed natural). It is an image of grace mingled with force, but less that of a gallant iconoclast than that of a sweet prophet committed to changing the world; it is the celebration of sadism as a natural rather than a perverted desire. Sadism (and instinct itself) was reinterpreted as a kind of male spirituality that bursts forth as a healthy, powerful, even revolutionary force.

The rapid diffusion of Apollinaire's enthusiasm by surrealist publications, as well as (if more discretely) by popular medical books, provoked Paul Bourdin's angry claim that "all the new canons of psychiatry and sexual psychopathology invite amateurs to excuse [Sade] by virtue of his very defects."[87] His comments were aimed at the likes of André Breton, who had declared: "Sade's oeuvre can pass for the most authentic precursor to Freud and all of modern psychopathology."[88]

Through the 1920s, the surrealists, like Sade's biographers, developed an image of Sade as both victim and visionary and made his name synonymous with a persecuted truth. They used him as an emblem of the affirmative force of the libido and as a tragic symbol of the power of censors and of bourgeois defenders of the state and the family in particular. The surrealists sought to liberate what they believed to be the potential and truth of human nature from its moral and rationalist (and, after their affiliation with the Communist party in 1930, social and political) confines; the movement thus both poeticized and politicized Sade. He emerged as one of the major figures in the surrealist pantheon, at once a prophet, a pioneer, and a martyr to modernity.

Essential to this rehabilitation was the claim that there was nothing realistic about Sade's novels. André Breton maintained in the *Manifeste du surréalisme* that "Sade is surrealist in sadism," stressing precisely that Sade's excesses are primarily imaginary, unreal or "surreal." Paul Eluard, celebrating Saint Justine's Day in the journal *La Révolution Surréaliste*, summarized this view: "All the figures the imagination creates must become absolute mistresses of the realities of love." He added that Sade "wanted to

[87] Bourdin, Introduction to Sade, *Correspondance inédite*, p. x.
[88] André Breton, *Anthologie de l'humour noir* (Paris: Pauvert, 1972), p. 39.

celebrate the amatory imagination."[89] In the surrealist golden age of sexuality, there is room for sadism, for a mix of *amour fou* and *humour noir*, mad love and black humor, sex and freedom, blessed with the infinite possibilities opened up by the imagination.[90]

In André Breton's eyes, therefore, Sade was no longer the "last of the Catholics" but the first in a long line of revolutionaries including Arthur Rimbaud, Raymond Roussel, and the comte de Lautréamont (Isidore Ducasse) who, like Sade, were all misunderstood visionaries; Sade's crimes were the expression of love and liberty, "perhaps the most crazy, the most indescribable means of loving." Gilbert Lély, Sade's most important biographer and a surrealist fellow traveler, declared that Sade's voice represented the "perpetual movement of liberty," and he coined a phrase, shocking in its naïveté, which still adorns paperback editions of Sade's work today: "Tout ce que signe Sade est amour," which could be loosely translated as, "Sade means love."[91]

Most surrealists and those inspired by them linked Sade's sadism to crime reconceived as a glorious and subversive truth. In a famous talk he gave at the Surrealist Exposition in 1936, Paul Eluard

[89] André Breton, *Manifestoes of Surrealism*, trans. Richard Seaver and Helen R. Lane (Ann Arbor: University of Michigan Press, 1972), p. 26; Paul Eluard, "D. A. F. Sade, écrivain fantastique et révolutionnaire," *La Révolution Surréaliste*, December 1, 1926, p. 9.

[90] The surrealists often repeated an apocryphal anecdote first reported by Victor Sardou in the *Chronique Médicale* in 1902, a story that became emblematic of ironic social protest and was reproduced in many surrealist and nonsurrealist texts during the interwar years. The image of Sade it conveyed was sardonic, playful, innocuous, and scandalous all at once. Sade, the story went, would dip roses in the sewage streams of the Charenton asylum, a smile always on his lips. Breton referred to the story in the *Second Manifesto of Surrealism* in 1930, painting a picture of a noble man full of scorn for the cultural symbol of sweetness. "Even," Breton declared, "if [the story] is not completely apocryphal, [it] would in no way harm the impeccable integrity of Sade's life and thought, and the heroic need that was his to create an order of things which was not dependent upon everything that had come before him." Breton, *Manifestoes*, p. 186.

[91] André Breton, *L'Amour fou* (Paris: Gallimard, 1976), p. 138; Lély, Prologue to Sade, *Morceaux choisis*, first page. This is a late example, but is testimony to the remarkable staying power of this vision of Sade, which has survived until the present in Annie Le Brun's and Jean-Jacques Pauvert's work. Two more recent examples, though more tempered in their enthusiasm, are Raymond Jean's *Portrait de Sade* (Paris: Actes Sud, 1989); and a film, Henri Xhonneux's 1989 production *Marquis*. The film is parodical and the biography is not hagiographic, but both emphasize Sade's visionary heroism.

described the sadism of Sade and Lautréamont as the murderous instinct of victims responding to a a silence born of neglect or refusal, a "calm that will cover them with ashes," the proper sentiment of martyrs to truth. Eluard's image of the birth of the modern world out of Sade's ashes transformed the marquis into the glorious embodiment of freedom stifled by moral hypocrisy, a vision reiterated in Eluard's polemic against two very disparaging articles about Sade published in the *Figaro* in 1926.[92]

In these articles the critic Maurice Talmeyr had insisted on Mme Sade's love for her ungrateful husband. Eluard defended Sade's "greatness" against Talmeyr's "hypocrisy." Then, in another article in the same vein, published in 1927, he maintained that there had never been enough evidence to convict Sade for the crimes for which he had been imprisoned, that Sade had been the victim of "false accusations" that made it difficult to decipher the truth about his life.[93]

Maurice Heine, for his part, applauded the liberation of Sade as the liberation of a truth that had heretofore "perished in the prison of moral conformism."[94] In his preface to the 1930 edition of Sade's *Infortunes de la vertu*, dedicated to his surrealist friends, Heine argued that Sade's sadistic fantasies were not the cause but the result of his imprisonment. They denied his isolation and thus represented the triumph of desire over objective reality. Though he is "physically a prisoner, a small amount of ink and paper will suffice to free his mind." No sooner did Sade start writing than the Bastille turned into the "tower of Liberty."[95] Sadism, here, has nothing to do with real pain inflicted on real bodies; it has been reduced to another innocuous surrealist game, conflated with imagination and the pleasure principle.

In a poem published in 1934 in the surrealist review *Documents* (not to be confused with Georges Bataille's by-then defunct review of the same name), Maurice Heine constructed an image of a Sade who feminizes himself and, in so doing, becomes all the more

[92] Paul Eluard, *L'Evidence poétique* (Paris: Chez GLM, 1937), publication of conference in London on June 24, 1936.
[93] Eluard, "D. A. F. Sade, écrivain fantastique et révolutionnaire," pp. 8–9; Eluard, "L'Intelligence révolutionnaire: Le Marquis de Sade, 1740–1814," *Clarté* no. 6 (February 1927), 180.
[94] Heine, *Confessions*, p. xxiii.
[95] Heine, *Le Marquis de Sade*, p. 64.

manly. "The Sade we admire," "Sade whom we love," and "Sade whom we exalt"—so begin the three verses, in a rising crescendo that sweeps us from noble to ever nobler sentiment—is the man who renounces his noble birth with pride, the man who calls his valet M. le marquis and asks to be called Lafleur (the flower), who is delighted to be burned in effigy and by virtue of all his qualities becomes "the conqueror of nature," the "liberator of sex," a "rebel," and finally, Sade, reduced to himself by preeminence as liberator, conqueror, and revolutionary. Sade is also portrayed as "delicate" and without "arrogance" and is said to amuse himself "playing games" with the "whores of Marseilles." He is a military man who nevertheless knows that the arrogance of the military is more dangerous than the pride of thieves who kill in order to steal. Heine's poem not only renders Sade's sadism innocuous, it makes it the very condition of his glory, of his humanity.[96]

These various portraits of Sade as hero, martyr, and victim, this surrealist translation of the marquis into a pure image of heroism made more heroic by his oppression, was part of the general re-creation of Sade as a Gioconda-like figure with a tranquil smile on his lips and a gaze that conveyed purity and lucidity. Gilbert Lély retained of Sade only "the rays of an invisible smile" rising over the ruins of La Coste (Sade's castle), evoking the timelessness (if not the subtlety) of the Gioconda's smile as well as its inaccessible wisdom. His portrait also alluded to Sade's wisdom in a more literal fashion: "Your real splendor is born from the song of your desires and the movement of your thought."[97] Heine's "Hommage" considered Sade's persecution a consequence not of his sadism but of his "cold reason." Sylvain Bonmariage claimed that Sade's greatest virtue was knowing how to "elevate the most primitive sensations to the heights of an idea." Thus it is not surprising that in a review of *Les Infortunes de la vertu* in 1930, Jean Paulhan noted that it

[96] Maurice Heine, "Hommage," *Documents* no. 1 (June 1934), 26–27.

[97] Lély, Prologue to Sade, *Morceaux choisis*, first page. Walter Pater's description of the Gioconda as a sadistic figure is strikingly similar to this equation of her smile with Sade's. "Hers is the head upon which all 'the ends of the world are come,' and the eyelids are a little weary. It is a beauty wrought out from within upon the flesh, the deposit, little cell by cell, of strange thoughts and fantastic reveries and exquisite passions. . . . She is older than the rocks among which she sits; like the vampire, she has been dead many times, and learned the secrets of the grave." Pater, *Leonardo da Vinci* (London: Phaidon Press, 1971), pp. 11–12. Martin Jay called this passage to my attention.

was as a writer that Sade wanted to be and should be remembered. Sade was important, said Paulhan, not for the "novelty" he represented—that people take pleasure in the suffering of others—but for "the rigorous and absolute spirit that shapes and composes that sentiment and knows how to impose on us its novelty."[98]

Writers in the 1930s thus considered Sade significant less for his sadism than for having written about it. His apologists discerned in his work evidence that the beauty of great literature could derive as much from the most gruesome descriptions of pain and suffering as from the aesthetics of a romantic agony. Sade's work was not pornography but the expression of a theme great writers from Shakespeare (e.g., *Othello*) to Zola (e.g., *La Bête humaine*) had explored in countless ways: passion turned from love to violence, the violent man's humanity. As Paulhan put it some years later, "For literature halts, and so almost does language, before an event (which is sometimes called animal, or bestial) wherewith the mind seems to have nothing to do," but not Sade's writing. Or as he said even later, at his own obscenity trial in 1956, Sade's writing "is an example that cannot be followed."[99]

Paulhan was not alone in praising Sade's style. The recognition accorded his genius was widespread and focused on what René Planhol called his "imperturbable logic."[100] Psychiatrists, however, were less inclined to take Sade for a great writer. They had long since accepted his sanity: Sarfati, for example, claimed Sade had "never suffered from any kind of delirium," and Voivenel asserted that Sade's imprisonment could not have been occasioned by any "alteration" of his faculties.[101] His literary merit, however, was in dispute. Whereas Dr. Otto Flake, keeping in mind the objections of his colleagues, insisted that "whether we like it or not, Sade belongs to literature," and Dr. André Javelier declared that next to Sade "Balzac seemed like a pathetic plagiarist," most psychiatrists diagnosed Sade as sane but boring and repetitive.[102]

[98] Heine, "Hommage," p. 27; Bonmariage, p. 8; Jean Paulhan, review of *Les Infortunes de la vertu*, in *Nouvelle Revue Francaise* (September 1930), 417.

[99] Paulhan, "The Marquis and His Accomplice," p. 18; Paulhan, *L'Affaire Sade*, p. 52.

[100] Planhol, p. 187.

[101] Sarfati, p. 173; Dr. Paul Voivenel, *Le Génie littéraire* (Paris: Felix Alcan, 1912), p. 200.

[102] Flake, p. 85; Javelier, p. 42. Among those who disparaged Sade's literary merit, see Béliard, p. 288.

Writers tended to be more generous in their assessments. Jean Desbordes called Sade a "writer of genius." The critic Georges Lafourcade analyzed Sade's literary influence on the English writer Swinburne, Heine considered his works a precursor of the *roman noir*, as gothic novels were called in France. Paulhan compared him to Stendhal and Restif de la Bretonne. Lély, with typical hyperbole, claimed that only Shakespeare's poetic genius compared with Sade's.[103]

This transposition of desire into reason—into an "icy eroticism," as one writer put it[104]—this acceptance of his work in the canon of great literature, normalized Sade because it disassociated his sadism from madness or perversion and made it the very force of his reason. As in the biographical portrait, Sade's works were no longer defined as the outpourings of a madman or the embodiment of human evil but as the literary vengeance of a man whose life had been brutally stolen from him, as the perfectly rational reaction of a man powerless before the successive regimes that saw fit to censor his desire. Transforming his sadism into the rationale of great literature made Sade above all a writer by turning him into the most lucid thinker of all time, into a genius whose literary works gave evidence of a man who by virtue of his suffering saw farther and deeper than ordinary men and whose tragedy was not what he saw but that what he saw was censored. Sade was thus remade in the image of a surrealist hero: a sensitive, mystical, almost childlike man whose reason transgressed the acceptable boundaries of rationality, pushed beyond them to another, "truer" or more authentic world.

Through his suffering Sade became both compassionate and reflective. He was a man able to remain above or distant from other men because he was so profoundly and so compassionately Everyman. Writers during the interwar years in this way restored to Sade the manliness that Dr. Flake claimed was his most distinctive char-

---

[103] Desbordes, p. 241; Georges Lafourcade, *La Jeunesse de Swinburne* (Strasbourg: Publications de la Faculté des Lettres, 1928), pp. 264–65; Heine, *Le Marquis de Sade*, p. 231. (This piece originally appeared in the *Nouvelle Revue Française* [August 1933], 190–206, as "Le Marquis de Sade et le roman noir," and was also published in a medical journal, *Le Courrier d'Epidaure*, in 1938); Lély, Prologue to Sade, *Morceaux choisis*, p. xxxvi. See also René-Louis Doyon, *Du marquis de Sade à Barbey d'Aurevilly* (Paris: La Connaissance, 1921), pp. 96–98; and Fély, p. 176.

[104] Jean-Jacques Brousson, "Le Dossier Sade," *Les Nouvelles Littéraires*, March 1, 1930, p. 3.

acteristic: "What is so interesting about Sade is the . . . acuity with which he knows how to free himself from the sentimental constraints that mask the profundity of things. He distances himself from them impatiently, as from the useless duties befitting the masses and women. He seems so radically male that he can find no other relationship to God or to women, to morality or to the world, than a cynical one."[105] Unlike the "hysterical exaggerations" of Rose Keller, which resulted from stupidity or malice, Sade's "obvious overstatement[s]," Breton wrote, "allow the reader to relax and to think that the author is no dupe."[106]

It was Sade's "reason" and his courage to articulate it that earned him the status of a wise and noble victim common to both the biographical and literary transmutations of his image. In both these discourses Sade's nobility was thus linked not to his crime but to his refusal of and warning against crime. Writers in this way purged Sade of all guilt because they saw his sadistic fantasies as the consequence of a glorious self-sacrifice, of his insistence on speaking to a world that refused to listen. Because Sade's work originated in pressure from outside which grew so unbearable that the "real" Sade exploded onto pages and pages of manuscript, because Sade's desire was forced out of him under pressure, it became sadistic after the fact. It was thus not Sade's desire (which was normal) that caused his fantasies but his being punished for it. Sade's punishment, as it were, drove his writing, lent it its force, freed his mind, conflating his punishment and his sadism so completely that his sadism could be accounted for only as the desire to be punished, that is, as the desire to be free.

This mythologizing of Sade by the surrealists and many others thus came close to the nineteenth-century myth of true love and self-sacrifice, the idea that love was inevitably bound up with self-annihilation. In this romantic imagery, Sade's "love" for humanity led to self-annihilation, but it also, of course, as with all martyrs, led to immortality. Sade's writing was the product of a selflessness, of a self-sacrifice, that revealed humanity to itself; Sade, in other words, died for our sins.

But however much it may seem to resemble the nineteenth-century idea of his martyrdom, this romantic reading doesn't quite

---

105 Flake, pp. 32–33.
106 Breton, *L'Anthologie de l'humour noir*, p. 39.

qualify Sade for saintliness. We might say it is because the evidence required for canonization disappears. As I have argued, this reading of Sade as a martyr was rooted in the surrealist contention that texts were not necessarily mirrors of reality, that Sade's crimes were the stuff of fiction. In the threefold process by which writers transformed his sexual crimes into consensual sex, transformed his literary "crimes" into the refusal of crime, and reinterpreted his desire as reason, Sade's crimes were not just made into metaphor but entirely suppressed or, in Lacanian parlance that is quite apt, "foreclosed." Accordingly, much like the doctors and psychiatrists whose pronouncements they despised, the surrealists suppressed an important question about the meaning and essence of sexuality or, in this case, of Sade's sexuality: What was Sade's desire, or better, where was it? If he was not a criminal but wrote about crime, if he was not a pervert but wrote about perversion, and finally, if he was selfless but his writing was the ultimate expression of the modern self, from whence originated his words? This is the question writers after the surrealists put to Sade, and both the question and its answer were already implicit in the dual transformation of Sade's sexual self into his truth and Sade's truth into his martyrdom. Although doctors and writers in the interwar years were the first to argue that Sade's words could not incriminate him, they also argued that he had to be incriminated in order to produce words.

Chapter Five

The Pleasure of Pain

$\mathbf{W}$here did Sade's words come from? The surrealists had given an ambiguous answer: Sade's words were the expression of his free, radical spirit, *and* they were the result of his punishment. Of course, it is possible to have it both ways. The marginal man simply becomes increasingly indignant, increasingly lucid, increasingly committed to his criminality once he is punished for it. But this answer still suggests that the state's refusal to let Sade speak is the source of his words. It doesn't explain why he proclaimed his criminality so loudly in the first place, in spite of all the odds.

The surrealists, along with the writers who concern us in this chapter—Georges Bataille, Pierre Klossowski, Jean Paulhan, and Jacques Lacan—agreed that Sade was compelled to write. But in contrast to the surrealists, these writers sought to account for and explain that compulsion. How did they explain it and why did they explain it the way they did? How did they account for what most of them referred to as Sade's "secret"?

The Tragic Man

Georges Bataille was raised in Reims. He entered the prestigious Ecole de Chartes in 1918, where he studied medieval history and literature and subsequently qualified as a librarian. In 1924 avant-garde writer and surrealist fellow traveler Michel Leiris introduced him to the painter André Masson and the surrealist circle. Later

Bataille claimed not to have been impressed by the surrealists, though he was indebted to them. During the interwar years, he worked at the Bibliothèque Nationale and was the center of a group of disaffected writers, including Raymond Queneau, Leiris, and Pierre Klossowski.[1] In 1929 Bataille founded the short-lived anti-surrealist review *Documents*. The following year he was "ex-communicated" from the surrealist movement, and in the *Second Manifesto* Breton singled him out for a particularly virulent attack, evidence of their intense personal as well as ideological rivalry.[2]

In an implicit repudiation of the surrealists' adherence to the Soviet-directed Communist party, Bataille joined Boris Souvaraine's Trotskyist Cercle Communiste Démocratique (whose members included Simone Weil and Colette Peignot). He remained a member from 1931 to 1934 and published several articles in the group's periodical *La Critique Sociale*. By 1936, alienated from surrealism, disillusioned by the triumph of fascism and the failure of (Soviet) Marxism, Bataille, along with Pierre Klossowski and Georges Ambrosino, formed an alternative secret society he dubbed Acéphale (headless), and the society began printing a periodical by the same name. Obeying a logic at once Sadeian and Nietzschean, the society (in which Lacan too was said to have participated)[3] rejected the established church in favor of a *contre-église*, a church, as it were, without God and hence "headless." Theirs was a politics conceived in religious terms. "If there existed a virulent religious organization, new and uncouth from head to toe, one sustained by a spirit incapable of a servile structure," wrote Bataille, "a man might learn . . . that there is something else to love other than this barely concealed image of financial necessity that one's country is when up in arms."[4] Thus, the first issue of *Acéphale* quoted Kierkegaard: "What looks like politics and imagines itself to be politics, one day will show itself to be a religious movement."[5]

[1] Pierre Klossowski, "Le Corps du néant," in *Sade mon prochain* (Paris: Seuil, 1947), pp. 169–70.

[2] Surya, p. 26. See also Georges Bataille, "Notice autobiographique," *Oeuvres complètes*, vol. 7 (Paris: Gallimard, 1976), p. 460.

[3] Surya, pp. 256–57.

[4] Bataille, Introduction to Roger Caillois, "Brotherhoods," in Denis Hollier, ed., *The College of Sociology*, trans. Betsy Wing (Minneapolis: University of Minnesota Press, 1989), p. 149.

[5] Quoted in Hollier, *College of Sociology*, p. xxv.

With Acéphale and with the founding of the Collège de Sociologie in 1937 (about which I have more to say in a later chapter), Bataille thus intended to map a new path to spiritual renewal by repudiating the utilitarian structure of either capitalist or communist societies in favor of human existence. At that time Bataille thus fashioned himself upon what he dubbed the "tragic man," the spirit that refuses to be reduced "to the condition of a slavish instrument" and is "unable to stop itself from the movement of self-destruction that is its peculiar nature."[6]

Pierre Klossowski, at that time a Catholic, shared Bataille's (originally Marxist) critique of capitalist reification. He had read widely (as had Bataille) in existentialist philosophy, including Kierkegaard and Schelling, and had translated a host of German works. He was involved with the left-wing Catholic review *Esprit*, the first issue of which was published in 1932. *Esprit*'s adherents sought a "third way" between capitalism and communism in what its leader, Emmanuel Mounier, termed "personalism." They rejected above all the submission of the human spirit to the utility and materialism represented, as they saw it, by Marxism, capitalism, and fascism.[7]

In Bataille's and Klossowski's work during the 1930s, Sade emblematized the tragic man with whom they identified. Above all, he symbolized our culture's inability to hear what a marginal man said. In their conception, the defenders of bourgeois morality believed Sade's works were dangerous because they *meant* exactly what they said; the surrealists believed his works were innocuous, even liberating, because they *could not mean* what they said.

Though the surrealists' position represented an apparent improvement over the censorious mind of the bourgeois legislator, their praise of Sade in fact had an equally deleterious effect. The surrealist leader André Breton, Bataille charged, in celebrating Sade, made it impossible for us to hear him. In a posthumously published polemic against Breton, written in 1929 or 1930, he argued that the surrealists "place[d] these writings [Sade's] (and with them the figure of their author) above everything (or almost everything) that can be opposed to them, but it is out of the question to

[6] Georges Bataille, "The Sorcerer's Apprentice," in Hollier, *College of Sociology*, p. 13; 148.
[7] Emmanuel Mounier, *Manifeste au service du personnalisme* (Paris: Editions Montaigne, 1936), p. 151; See also Paulette Mounier-Leclercq, ed., *Mounier et sa génération* (Paris: Seuil, 1956), which contains Mounier's letters; and Jean-Loubet del Bayle, *Les Non-conformistes des années trentes* (Paris: Seuil, 1969), pp. 121–52.

allow them the least place in private or public life, in theory or in practice. The behavior of Sade's admirers resembles that of primitive subjects in relation to their king, whom they adore and loathe, and whom they cover with honors and narrowly confine."[8] In rehabilitating Sade, the surrealists had placed him distinctly above ordinary men and women, elevated him to a heavenly realm. Thus they had effaced his desire, made it unreal or, more appropriately, sur-real. Bataille put it even more succinctly in his 1935 novel *Le Bleu du ciel*. The narrator, referring to the surrealists, says to his lover: "Listen to me Xénie. You've been involved in literary goings-on. You must have read De Sade. You must have found De Sade fantastic. Just like the others. People who admire Sade are con artists, do you hear? con artists!" And he asks her, in an implicit criticism of the surrealists' celebration of sadism, "So have you eaten shit, yes or no?"[9]

The surrealists' celebration of Sade's words thus begged the question of why Sade felt compelled to speak and hence of the meaning of his words. Klossowski sought to explore that question in terms of what he later called Sade's "limit-position," his paradoxical inability to be heard even as he spoke.[10] Klossowski argued that Sade's insistence on speaking against all odds was inseparable from the triumph of the tragic man over the world of "economic and military necessity" and "fascist domination." According to Klossowski,

> The more successful an individual, the more he concentrates the diffuse energies of his epoch, and the more dangerous he is for that epoch; but the more he concentrates within himself these diffuse energies in order to bring them heavily to bear on his own destiny, the more he liberates his epoch. Sade took the virtual criminality of his contemporaries for his personal destiny. He wanted to pay all alone, in proportion to the collective guilt his conscience had invested.[11]

[8] Georges Bataille, "The Use Value of D. A. F. de Sade (an Open Letter to My Current Comrades)," in *Visions of Excess*, trans. and ed. Allan Stoekl (Minneapolis: University of Minnesota Press, 1985), p. 92.

[9] Georges Bataille, *Blue of Noon*, trans. Henry Matthews (New York: Urizen Books, 1978), p. 68.

[10] Klossowski, *Sade, mon prochain* (1947), p. 169.

[11] Pierre Klossowski, "The Marquis de Sade and the Revolution," in Hollier, *College of Sociology*, p. 221. See also Bataille, Introduction to Caillois, "Brotherhoods," p. 148–49.

This willingness to "pay all alone," to act as the repository of human guilt, was the only viable means of asserting the claims of human existence in a world that turned human beings into things.

Klossowski explored this admittedly rather Christian desire to suffer alone for the sins of humanity more specifically in a series of articles in the early thirties. In a 1935 article he repudiated the notion that Sade's texts were simply the metaphorical expression of his rage, a righteous and beautiful testament to Sade's lucidity: "If the trial [of charges brought against Sade by his wife's family] must necessarily turn him against human justice, must we believe that this trial is only the projection of his inner trial, the trial that his conscience inflicts upon him? Maybe the punishment procured for him by his unconscious will, this iniquitous punishment, was necessary precisely in order to win his inner trial?"[12] Klossowski, as we will see, interpreted Sade's works as the tragic tale of a desire to challenge God, a crime that inevitably fails, indeed, that results in nothing but a profound longing for his authority. In his work Sade longs, impossibly, for a virtuous world in which God is manifest.

In Sade, he argued, the Enlightenment's substitution of nature for God, the assertions of La Mettrie, d'Holbach, and Helvétius that nature is in a state "of perpetual movement," led not to happiness but to tragedy, to "the conscious and willing acceptance of tragedy."[13] For to admit that the world is in a state of perpetual movement, Klossowski argued, is to admit that the natural state of the universe is always in the process of dissolution as well as creation and that all creation is hence ephemeral. Similarly, while the romantics harbored a nostalgia for the maternal breast which they transposed into visions of a golden age, in Sade nature is cruel and indifferent, in a state of "perpetual movement" that abandons man to the law of the jungle, where the guilty sacrifice the innocent, where the strong dominate and tyrannize the weak. In fact, Klossowski wrote in a 1933 article about Sade's mother hatred, Sade reconstructed nature in the image of a father rather than a

[12] Pierre Klossowski, "Le Mal et la négation d'autrui dans la philosophie de D. A. F. Sade," *Recherches Philosophiques* 4 (1934–35), 268. It is perhaps worth noting that Lacan was affiliated with this publication in 1935–36. It was a periodical of the phenomenological movement, edited by Alexandre Koyré, among others. Lacan wrote a review of Eugène Minkowski, *Le Temps vécu*, in 5 (1935–36), 424–31.

[13] Klossowski, "Le Mal et la négation d'autrui," p. 278.

mother. The mother represents all the foolish romantic illusions about the plentitude of nature; she embodies the hypocritical veil cast over the truth that nature is indifferent to, even promotes, human suffering. "In Sade's eyes," he claimed, "the image of the father symbolizes the realization of all the passions with which nature has invested man, an image to which Sade desperately aspired."[14]

But Sade could never live up to this image—the one in which the surrealists had molded him. Instead, Klossowski transforms Sade from a symbol of wisdom, force, and reason into the image of a man plagued by a rift deep in his interior, who nobly, because tragically, bore the burden of knowing who he could never be. Sade's works were not a fantasy about who he could be if he were liberated; rather, they depicted the man he could never be, his impossible and hence "desperate" aspirations. This inner rift was rooted in the libertine's fruitless quest for God's love. Sade's "religion of evil," Klossowski claimed, "exalts the necessity of God's injustice. . . . Could not all the evils with which God overwhelms humanity be the ransom in exchange for which God would accord to man the right to cause suffering and to be infinitely vicious? Such that one could see in God the original guilty one, the one who would have attacked man before man attacked him."[15]

Klossowski argued that Sade retained moral categories even while rigorously professing his atheism. Evil is justified not because there is no God but as a means of avenging man against an evil God. It is consequently the cruelty of God that justifies, even necessitates, the cruelty of man, abandoned by a father who ravages, abuses, and condemns his children to destroy their own creatures or be destroyed in turn. Sade did not invert the world by making Satan triumph; he subverted the Manichean notion of good and evil by replacing it with a paradoxical one: an evil God or, as Klossowski put it, an "absent God." The structure is assimilated into the "enlightened" or naturalist conscience: "The atheistic spirit who hurls the anathema against nature thus wanted to render absurd this reproach that he cannot repress and which escapes

[14]Pierre Klossowski, "Eléments d'une étude psychanalytique sur le marquis de Sade," *RFP* 6 (1933), 465, 458. For an image of nature as a phallic mother in Sade, see Jane Gallop, *Thinking through the Body* (New York: Columbia University Press, 1988), pp. 61–66.
[15]Klossowski, "Le Mal et la négation d'autrui," p. 274.

him in spite of himself. Conscience, while accepting Nature's supremacy, has not yet renounced the mechanism of moral categories which, in its struggle with God, it had deemed necessary and useful to maintain: it could wreak vengeance upon God."[16] The libertine's atheism is not a denial of God but an angry attempt to force God to manifest himself. His (for in Sade the libertine is either literally or symbolically male) revolt takes the form not of absolute renunciation of God but of sacrilege, profanation unbefitting the real atheist, for whom all forms of sacrilege are meaningless since he does not invest the sacred with any value. It is thus precisely because the libertine values God that he revolts.

Because it is his love of God that motivates the libertine's hatred, his revolt is in fact a quest for divine love which is a reaffirmation of God's power. In a vicious circle the libertine aims to provoke God by denying him, to make God manifest himself by repudiating his presence. The libertine thus addresses a perpetual reproach to God destined to remain without a response. The paradoxical structure of God's present-absence reproduces itself in the present-absence of the libertine's revolt, "which revolts without any other hope than to remain a revolt" and therefore manifests itself as a transgression against God which will always be bound to his laws.[17]

Nor has the libertine been able to renounce the moral categories, the moral conscience, that binds him to other human beings in spite of himself. Because the libertine, in Sade most often acting as a sadist, requires evidence of others' misery in order to feel pleasure in his own fortune, he is dependent on others for his status as master. Through this need to define his own mastery in terms of others' suffering, "the libertine's debauched conscience remains complicitous, even while inverting these moral categories that the atheistic conscience will denounce as forged by the weak."[18] If the libertine renounces a Christian denunciation of the jungle, he nevertheless remains imprisoned in the Christian categories of

---

[16] Ibid., p. 280.

[17] Ibid. Klossowski expressed another version of this Kojèvian/Nietzschean formulation in a lecture he gave at the Collège de Sociologie in 1939. He argued that revolutions do not offer the promise of liberation but trace a vicious circle in which the liberator inevitably becomes a tyrant in turn. "The Marquis de Sade and the Revolution," pp. 221–25.

[18] Klossowski, "Le Mal et la négation d'autrui," p. 276.

good and evil because he inverts rather than transgresses them. Because he remains within a dialectical struggle of mutual recognition, the *prochain*'s (fellow man's) suffering is necessary to his experience of mastery. Since the *prochain* is a mirror without which he cannot experience, identify, or "see" himself, the sadist cannot destroy her without risk to his very mastery, without ensuring his own self-annihilation. In this way the libertine only reproduces in his own evil the state of dissolution proper to the "perpetual movement" of nature.[19]

Man's attempt to subvert God in the end always confirms divine laws. No matter what the crime, no matter what its gravity, it will never measure up to God's (or nature's) supreme indifference. Because the libertine's revolt against God only manifests his desire for God's recognition, his crimes can be only simulacra of God's original crime against man, repeated without end: "divine aggression," wrote Klossowski, "would be so incommensurate that it would legitimate forever the impunity of the guilty and the sacrifice of the innocent."[20] The libertine's revolt is thus really only a masochistic reenactment of God's original indifference toward man. Like the child who is being beaten, the libertine desires a beating that will be interpreted as proof of God's love: "What was originally a motive for suffering [God's indifference] becomes, on a metaphysical level, the very compensation for this suffering. The experience of deception is lived a second time as a universal law: Nature does not love her creatures."[21]

In his fantasies the sadist insists on God's absence; he tries, through his impersonal and perpetual exchange of dead bodies for living ones to be indifferent to suffering and, like God, to possess no moral conscience. Yet insofar as the sadist depends upon others for his sense of "mastery" (Hegel's word, to which Klossowski alludes), he cannot eliminate his moral conscience without eliminating a consciousness of his own mastery. Klossowski, borrowing Sade's own term, called this elimination of conscience "apathy"; the sadist's desire to be master is inseparable from a desire for self-

---

[19] Klossowski reproduces a Kojèvian interpretation of Hegel in this argument. I am less interested, however, in linking it to Kojève (already done by more than one scholar—for example, Hirsch, pp. 17–21) than in demonstrating how it participates in a broader transformation in the reading of Sade.

[20] Klossowski, "Le Mal et la négation d'autrui," p. 274.

[21] Klossowski, "Eléments d'une étude psychanalytique," p. 474.

liquidation, from a desire to be a "pure organ of experience" without consciousness, and hence from a desire for a "pure" emptiness.[22] Or consciousness, becoming conscious of one's mastery, is none other than the apathetic state proper to crimes committed in the most absolute indifference, with a sangfroid that is the summit at once of indifference and *jouissance*.

The libertine's desire to be master can be realized only in Sade's fantasies, in Sade's literary works. Fantasy functions as a kind of closure against the loss of mastery intrinsic to sadistic desire; it provides the illusion of a bridgeable gulf between desire and its object by making that desire (as apathy) livable, communicable, by arresting the sadist's paradoxical movement toward self-annihilation. Sade's fantasy no longer signifies, as it did for the surrealists, a drive to liberation, a sort of will to pleasure, but instead represents a drive to mastery which will always already be a drive to self-liquidation, a desire not to be guilty which painfully evokes the pangs of moral conscience again and again. Sade's revolt against God and against the human justice that conceived itself in his image was therefore destined to cleanse his soul.

Jean Paulhan: Sade's Secret

Jean Paulhan was not, strictly speaking, one of those who articulated Sade's "secret" in terms of a limit-position. Nevertheless, his preface to *Justine* was highly influential, in part because it made explicit many of the themes that concerned writers who read Sade just before and after the Second World War. Paulhan's piece was written shortly after the war, but it in fact straddled the prewar and postwar discourses about Sade. Above all, Paulhan insisted with Klossowski (if from a quite different point of view) that Sade's writing was a metaphor of aspiration to an ideal he could never live up to. And once again, masochism was a metaphor for that failure, that irreparable rift between real and ideal.

Paulhan had been the editor of the *Nouvelle Revue Française* since 1925, a literary adviser to Gallimard, and a prominent critic. In 1941 he published his most influential book, *Les Fleurs de Tar-*

---

[22] Klossowski, "Le Mal et la négation d'autrui," p. 292.

bes, in which he analyzed the status of literature in terms of the tension between the modern desire to shed rhetorical conventions and a classical adherence to them. Paulhan came out on the side of rhetoric against those whom he called "terrorists," including the surrealists, who naïvely thought they could render language "direct and innocent," authentic and uncontaminated.[23] Paulhan did not reaffirm the virtues of classicism, but he rendered all claims to truth problematic, including what he called the "commonplaces" of rhetoric. If we all agreed on the ambiguity of rhetoric, he argued, we would reach a consensus that meanings are always bound to be ambiguous and so would free ourselves from the quest for innocence.[24]

Paulhan's 1946 preface to *Justine* also implicitly repudiated the surrealists' effort to use Sade's work as an emblem of authentic thought unencumbered by the weight of convention, rhetorical or otherwise. Instead, Paulhan emphasized Sade's ambiguity. He suggested that it was easy enough to portray Sade as good instead of evil but that doing so sidestepped what was important, what was most "real" about Sade. As with ordinary criminals, what was most striking about him was not his evil but his apparent normality. Paulhan put it this way:

> Criminals are in general curious people, more curious than law-abiding people. I mean unusual, giving more food for thought. And though it may happen that they utter nothing but banalities, they are more surprising to listen to—owing precisely to this contrast between the dangerous content within and the inoffensive appearance without. Of all this the authors of detective stories are very aware: no sooner do we begin to suspect the honest country lawyer or the worthy pharmacist of having once upon a time poisoned a whole family, than the slightest thing he says warrants our most avid attention, and he needs but predict a change in the weather for us to sense he is meditating some new crime.[25]

[23] Jean Paulhan, *Les Fleurs de Tarbes* (Paris: Gallimard, 1941), pp. 151–52.

[24] As Maurice Blanchot noted in his 1941 review of the book, Paulhan's proposal did not solve the problem of how to determine originality in literature but affirmed the paradox that originality is always already an interpretation. Maurice Blanchot, *Comment la littérature est-elle possible?* (Paris: J. Corti, 1942).

[25] Paulhan, "Sade and His Accomplice," p. 5.

This contrast between the "inoffensive appearance" and what lies deeper within speaks to our most profound conflicts about evil, he says. We admire criminals for their daring, and yet we are frightened by them at the same time. Sade is not a monster (we admire him for refusing the hypocrisy implicit in so many lofty expressions of virtue), and yet he is a monster, a man whose behavior and whose writing we would hardly want to encourage. Sade's writing is difficult to understand because of that dual experience of affinity and alienation, because Sade is not a monster and yet his writing is beyond the comprehension of any "normal" individual.

Paulhan thus insisted that we cannot give Sade our unmitigated approbation. Perhaps Sade was a victim, a martyr, as the surrealists said. But Paulhan asked precisely how Sade's compulsion to write about crime could also be a compulsion to virtue, to self-sacrifice. In other words, Paulhan tried to account for Sade's originality (the unspeakable cruelty in his works) by examining what appears to be a rather commonplace literary quest for virtue.

Paulhan began his study by suggesting that Sade's work, the work that had occupied the minds of the greatest writers for an entire century, had a secret.[26] That secret, it turns out, has to do with the origins of the work's inspiration. Paulhan argued that Sade's martyrdom was less the result of political injustice (though of course he admitted it was that too) than psychological necessity, that the myth of Sade's martyrdom was as much his fantasy as our own. Sade's work, he contended, was motivated by a masochistic desire for self-destruction, so that his reason for writing was not a cry for freedom but a yearning for punishment.

To support his argument, Paulhan claimed Sade used his most virtuous character, Justine, as a mouthpiece. The novel whose title bears her name, published in many different versions during Sade's lifetime, has often been referred to as his most scandalous work and was renounced in self-defense by its author, who claimed not to have written it. The novel recounts the trials and tribulations of a young orphaned and abandoned girl who clings to her virtue in spite of all the evidence that it will do her no good. This evidence is, as it were, inscribed on her body through repeated rapes and beatings and etched into her soul through repeated betrayals by the very individuals whom she believes she can trust: When she saves

[26] Ibid., p. 3.

a man from a gang of criminals, he rapes her and steals the only money she had; when she goes to a monastery seeking solace in religion, the monks imprison her in the convent, which has been transformed into an elaborate series of torture chambers from which none of the women who enter escape alive. Justine—and this is the absurdity of her fate—does escape, only to be raped, beaten, and betrayed again. She never learns.

And neither, according to Paulhan, did Sade. How else to explain the fact that he spent twenty-seven years of his life in prison, that he denounced political regimes at his own peril, provoked the courts time and time again by consistently abusing their moral precepts? Does this obduracy not suggest, Paulhan asked, that Sade himself did not learn, refused to learn, from experience? Does it not imply that Justine is a metaphor for Sade's own experience of persecution, that, as Paulhan put it, "Justine is Sade himself."[27] Sade, in fact, did not see what he saw. He insisted on telling the truth in spite of what he knew to be the consequences; he refused to act according to what he knew about man's fundamental evil. This masochistic insistence on the merits of virtue in a world in which he knew virtue reaped no rewards shaped his personality and his writing and made Sade a moralist, a weaver of fairy tales whose messages owe their power to a profound consciousness of human evil. Sade thus refused the lie that man is good.

If the fairy tale is the fantasy of a guilty conscience, or at least a tale with a moral, Sade's *Justine* represents its highest art. But Justine is a metaphor not simply for Sade's virtue but for the psychological impasse represented by his masochistic desire to be virtuous, for an impossible virtue, for "the sole passion," Paulhan wrote, "that cannot be thwarted without encouraging it, punished without rewarding it. Perfectly incomprehensible: absurd. What remains to be said? Only that the critic can turn this absurdity into a rationale."[28] The only means of satisfying masochistic desire is by denying it satisfaction. That is why Sade refused to see what he saw; that is Sade's rationale.

But by making virtue a metaphor for masochism Paulhan reconstructed a new image of Sade's subversiveness at the expense of Sade's social criticism, his black humor. He discussed what Sade

[27] Ibid., p. 35.
[28] Ibid., p. 36.

saw as the absurdity of the guilty conscience not in social but in psychological terms, not in terms of the hypocrisy in bourgeois virtue but as masochism. In so doing, he made Sade complicitous with the very culture he parodied, and he reinterpreted *Justine* as a morality tale in which her virtue is impossible (because people are evil) but nevertheless remains an ideal. Even though Justine's virtue is absurd or impossible, even though its rationale becomes less and less convincing as each new adventure turns into a deadly struggle from which she escapes in the nick of time, it is inseparable from a social condition that Sade mocks rather than idealizes.

Sade demonstrated to what extent the "naturalness" of (female) masochism is linked to a social condition that makes it seem like a natural and hence ideal or viable choice. As Angela Carter has argued, Justine believes in the naturalness of her virtue, she believes she has made a choice to be virtuous and that her rigorous defense of moral purity has a rationale that transcends her: "Justine's virtue, in action, is the liberal lie in action, a good heart and an inadequate methodology."[29] She also incarnates the myth of femininity which Sade deconstructed: the absurdity of her virtue mirrors the absurdity of the feminine condition, which paradoxically defines self-integrity in terms of self-denial.[30]

Sade's own desire to be virtuous (if that is indeed his desire) is inevitably of another order entirely. Unlike Justine, Sade knows

[29] Angela Carter, *The Sadeian Woman* (New York: Pantheon, 1978), p. 55.

[30] There is a lot of debate among feminists over whether Sade's work is a parody of social norms or a mirror of his life and so a prescription for how men do or should treat women. I have been stressing, instead, the way Sade is represented by various writers. Thus, while there is no "correct" reading of Sade, no Sade to "get right," there are clearly more or less valuable or useful readings of his work. Of course, those readings are less about Sade than about the politics or the fantasies of the people who read him. My own view is that Sade's work is parody, and yet it also reiterates and reinforces normative assumptions about gender roles. Negotiating these terms is the difficult task of anyone asking critical questions of literature and, of course, of anyone analyzing pornography as a cultural product. I cannot possibly address these kinds of questions here. I am reading Sade's work as parody, but I do not want to suggest that he is a feminist or even, as does Angela Carter, a "moral pornographer." On the question of how to think about pornographic works that have been canonized (or, more generally, about the often ambiguous boundaries between art and pornography), see Susanne Kappeler, *The Pornography of Representation* (Minneapolis: University of Minnesota Press, 1986); and Susan Gubar's essay "Representing Pornography: Feminism, Criticism, and Depictions of Female Violation," in Gubar and Joan Hoff, eds., *For Adult Users Only: The Dilemma of Violent Pornography* (Bloomington: Indiana University Press, 1989), pp. 47–67.

that virtue does not coincide with divine purpose but consists in obeying an arbitrary set of rules (he sees). His own desire to be virtuous is a consequence of his unnatural deprivation of freedom, his masochistic desire not to be free, so that Sade (in contrast to Justine) submits to no one's desires but his own, his desire to write. Thus Sade's masochism was not in his blind virtue but in his insistence on living virtuously even though he knew virtue was a sham. Justine's virtue leads to the logical fulfillment of her masochism: She is killed by a lightning bolt. Sade's virtue leads to the psychological impasse Paulhan conceived as masochism: He keeps writing. Sade's parody called the idea of virtue into question by demonstrating to what extent it is part of an insidious and oppressive cultural logic; Paulhan criticized virtue by making it pathological (i.e., masochistic) at the same time as he idealized it as the driving force of great literature, as the impossible truth of who Sade would have wanted to be. He did not transgress the moral categories Sade parodied but reinforced their power by making virtue the metaphor of an impossible ideal, by transposing Sade's black humor into the tragedy of a rationale that will never make any sense. Sade's writing thus possesses a secret that is revealed and yet never, ever, betrayed.

The Postwar Discourse: Klossowski

After the war, the course of Bataille's and Klossowski's reflections shifted from this stress on the psychological, the psychoanalytic, the metaphysical, or even the sociology of limit-positions (what others could not hear Sade say) to another use of Sade which emphasized what he said. Bataille and Klossowski and many other French writers now turned to Sade not because (after Theodor Adorno's question) it was no longer clear what artists could say after Auschwitz but because after the war it became even more imperative to understand better what Sade had said. As Simone de Beauvoir wrote in 1952, "He is trying to communicate an experience whose distinguishing characteristic is . . . its will to remain incommunicable." Or as Raymond Queneau put it in 1945, "That Sade wasn't personally a terrorist . . . that his work has profound human value . . . will not prevent all those who had adhered in some respect to the theses of the marquis from being forced to envision, without hypocrisy, the reality of the concentration camps, with their horrors no longer located in the mind of a man but practiced by thousands of fanatics. Mass graves are the logical conclusion of philosophies, as unpleasant as that may be."[31]

In the 1967 reissue of *Sade, mon prochain*, Klossowski renounced his earlier Catholicism, revised several of the essays, and eliminated two others, including "Le Corps du néant," in part criticism and analysis of the group Acéphale that had formed around Bataille in 1936.[32] Denis Hollier has noted that at this time Klossowski was concerned with the issues Walter Benjamin had first articulated in "The Work of Art in the Age of Mechanical Reproduction," with which Klossowski was familiar. He looked to Sade, Hollier notes, to analyze how "mechanical reproduction was . . . to lead to the standardization of voluptuous emotion through industrial exploitation."[33] Here I want to ask how Sade's guilty conscience—the source, as I have argued, of his "voluptuous emotion"—was, so to speak, standardized or rationalized. Or to put it another way, how was that rationale of which Paulhan spoke, the masochism that could never make sense, now given a meaning (a use value) other than its own senseless revolt against the master or ideal it strives so desperately to be? How, in other words, can Sade's guilt be said to have consequences, to say something whose meaning is not always elusive, not necessarily something that cannot be heard?

In the revised version of *Sade, mon prochain* and more specifically in the new essay "Le Philosophe scélérat," Klossowski argued that Sade's writing and desire were meshed in a paradoxical relationship he called an "ecstasy of thought"—the infinite and monotonous repetition of sexual crimes in a state at once of delirium and sangfroid. This repetition manifests a kind of voluptuousness in sangfroid which expresses the libertine's capacity to delight in murder. It constitutes what Klossowski called Sade's "unreadability," his monotony, a submission of desire to reason. He noted

[31] Simone de Beauvoir, "Must We Burn Sade?" in D. A. F. Sade, *The 120 Days of Sodom and Other Writings*, trans. Austryn Wainhouse and Richard Seaver (New York: Grove Press, 1966) p. 12; Raymond Queneau, *Bâtons, chiffres, et lettres* (Paris: Gallimard, 1965), p. 216.

[32] For an in-depth discussion of differences between the two editions, see Jane Gallop, *Intersections: A Reading of Sade with Bataille, Blanchot, and Klossowski* (Lincoln: University of Nebraska Press, 1981), pp. 67–112.

[33] Hollier, *The College of Sociology*, p. 219.

that in Sade *jouissance* is inseparable from an idée fixe, whereas the true libertine's power is defined precisely by freedom from prescriptive rules. Klossowski located this paradox in the act of writing itself, so that the rules of language structure the very experience of *jouissance*, the very transgression of language.[34]

In *Sade, mon prochain*, Klossowski in fact substituted for the paradox of an "absent God"—that which made the libertine eternally virtuous in his evil, masochistic in his sadism—the notion of what might be called an absent text. Sade's relationship to his writing parallels the libertine's relationship to God; Sade "never transgresses [in this case, the] laws of language except in the gesture whereby he reproduces them *in* their transgression." (In the same way, in Klossowski's earlier version, the libertine reproduced moral categories in his revolt against God). Desire is in the text and yet dissimulated by the very language that represents it. Sade's texts, Klossowski said, "slyly invite the reader to see outside what does not seem to lie in the text—whereas nothing is visible anywhere except in the text."[35]

The texts thus invite the reader outside at the same time as they cordon off the exterior, close all the doors. Since Sade's writing reproduces the laws of language in its very transgression of language, the effect of his work is what Klossowski called a "foreclosure of language by itself." The text's transgressive meaning is thus both present and uncannily absent: "Foreclosure means that something remains outside. That which remains outside is, once again, the act to be done. The less it is perpetrated the more it raps on the door—the door of literary vacuity. The blows struck on the door are Sade's words, which, if they now reverberate within literature, remain nonetheless blows struck from without."[36]

Sade's writing thus pursues a secret always foreclosed. As Klossowski put it in a passage he left unrevised, that pursuit is tantamount to an impossible quest for Justine which parallels the libertine's impossible desire to be God, to be absolute master:

In Sade's eyes Juliette is a Justine whose secret has been torn from her but who has remained in fact ungraspable. One crime, or two, or a

[34] Pierre Klossowski, *Sade, My Neighbor*, trans. Alphonso Lingis (Evanston, Ill.: Northwestern University Press, 1991), pp. 40. French edition: *Sade, mon prochain* (Paris: Seuil, 1967), p. 51.
[35] Klossowski, *My Neighbor*, pp. 40, 41; *Mon prochain*, pp. 53–54.
[36] Klossowski, *My Neighbor*, pp. 41–42; *Mon prochain*, p. 53.

hundred are not enough to reveal this secret; she must be pushed into ever greater crimes, crimes commensurate with the infinite purity of her sister, Justine. In narrating her adventures, which have no reason ever to come to an end, Sade wishes to forget the vexation that the loss of the unpossessable Justine causes him.[37]

Sade thinks he can have Justine, but in thinking so, he affirms she is forever lost. For this attempt to equal her "infinite purity," to attain a consciousness bleached of the memory of crime, and hence to attain a pure or absolute mastery (in which the consciousness of mastery is eliminated), takes the form of committing crime. Justine is foreclosed, forever lost, because the desire to efface crimes is always already the desire to commit it (that is why Juliette's adventures will never end).

Sade's writing is thus driven by a desire to forget that he can never be absolute master, to forget, then, that he can never be an empty and "pure organ of experience without consciousness," because to live absolute mastery requires that one have consciousness, that one be as calculating as Juliette (rather than as unconsciously virtuous and hence as pure and empty as Justine). It requires, in short, that one have language. It is because language must be used to communicate an essentially incommunicable experience that "nothing is visible anywhere except in the text," and all that is outside must necessarily be foreclosed by the language required to bring it to life (language that itself has consequently foreclosed something else—hence the phrase the "foreclosure of language by itself"). Thus, if Sade's crimes are always a drive to absolute mastery which is bound to fail (an effort, finally, to forget or efface crime which cannot help but evoke its memory), then Sade's work is a metaphor for a mastery always really deferred; the work allows him to live his desire for absolute mastery. Sade's works are, to use a Klossowskian term, simulacra of absolute mastery.

The crime is thus still a paradoxical drive to self-annihilation which is inevitably arrested. But now the emphasis is less on the subject's foreclosed and tragic lack than on how that lack is lived, on how the subject *lives* his own drive to suicide without in fact dying. That is, Klossowski has shifted his emphasis from the trag-

[37]Klossowski, *My Neighbor*, pp. 105–6; *Mon prochain*, p. 149.

ic, because senseless, rationale of the libertine's revolt to a contemplation of its lived effects, from the tormented psyche of the marginal man to the politics of mass murder, from the senseless guilt that renders human beings dysfunctional in a functional, utilitarian world to the foreclosed guilt that keeps the world functioning.

The Postwar Discourse: Bataille

Bataille referred to what Klossowski called Sade's "crimes" as the violence he saw at the very foundation of civilization itself, although human beings persist in seeing it as outside of culture. Violence exercised or justified in the name of the state, such as capital punishment or war (forms of legal murder), is simply not perceived as violence; all violence manifested in rational or institutional structures is dissimulated. Violence obviously exists in so-called civilized cultures, but as a secret. Violence, according to Bataille, is essentially a "profound silence . . . which never declares it exists, and never affirms the right to exist, which exists without declaring it exists."[38] Sade's work deconstructs this cultural fantasy that violence is outside or elsewhere because it gives violence a voice. In so doing, Sade's work refuses what Bataille called the "trickery" of the state because it names violence, refuses to pretend that it is somehow outside of the proper limits of what we refer to as civilization, and insists, on the contrary, that violence structures all our political and social institutions. But to the extent that Sade spoke to others, he partook in the very civilization that dissimulates the violence at its foundations. "If Sade's characters had really lived, they would have lived silently," said Bataille. "The violence Sade expressed transformed violence into what it was not, into something to which it was necessarily opposed: into a reflective, rationalized violent will."[39]

Because it names violence, Sade's language is not that of the state, of the executioner, but that of a victim who could not keep silent about the injustice done to him.[40] And unlike the execu-

---

[38] Georges Bataille, *L'Histoire de l'érotisme,* in *Oeuvres complètes* 8:209.
[39] Ibid., pp. 210, 213.
[40] Ibid., p. 211.

tioner, the state that commits murder in the name of justice, Sade doesn't try to fool anyone. By refusing to hold his tongue he betrays the solipsism proper to the libertine and speaks not in the name of justice but in the name of an impossible desire for justice, impossible, Bataille argues, because it is both proclaimed and silenced by language, because Sade names violence but by naming it also transforms it into "what it is not."

Sade certainly did not keep quiet. And yet, as Bataille saw it, Sade's writing was compelled by a death wish, an impossible desire to be "released" through self-destruction: "In an endless and relentless tornado, the objects of desire are invariably propelled towards torture and death. The only conceivable end is possible [sic] desire of the executioner to be the victim of torture himself. In Sade's will . . . this instinct reached its climax by demanding that not even his tomb should survive: it led to the wish that his very name should 'vanish from the memory of men.' "[41] Like Klossowski, Bataille believes that Sade's writing forecloses the drive to self-annihilation which compels it and enables Sade to live what real human beings could live only silently. Because to live as absolute master, one would have to be dead—to be, we recall from Klossowski, a "pure organ of experience without consciousness." Sade's absolute mastery is thus made metaphor, lived, and yet infinitely deferred. The transgressive, self-dissolving potential of violence (if we are to believe Bataille) is never realized, because it is always transposed into a "reflective, rationalized violent will" that depersonalizes human interaction, turns human beings into executioners. Here Bataille, like Klossowski, chose to stress not Sade's tragic lack but how it was lived.[42]

[41] Georges Bataille, *Literature and Evil*, trans. Alastair Hamilton (New York: Urizen Books, 1973), pp. 98–99, 95.

[42] It is interesting to note Gilles Deleuze's strikingly parallel reading: "Pornological literature is aimed above all at confronting language with its own limits, with what is in a sense a 'nonlanguage' (violence that does not speak, eroticism that remains unspoken). However this task can only be accomplished by an internal splitting of language: the imperative and descriptive function must transcend itself toward a higher function, the personal element turning by reflection upon itself into the impersonal." Deleuze, *Masochism: Coldness and Cruelty*, trans. Jean McNeil (New York: Zone Books, 1989), pp. 22–23. This image of depersonalization also resonates well with Borch-Jacobsen's discussion of Lacan's ego-world in terms of a "statue man": "The ego-world is a statue: as hard as stone, as cold as ice, it is standing in front of the ego that is petrified there—that is, in the ego-world it both

Toward Lacan

In Sade, according to Bataille and Klossowski, mastery is the effacement of pleasure, a drive to pleasure which is livable only as reason. In order to experience pleasure the libertine must, paradoxically, turn himself into a machine: That is, he cannot feel. At the same time, both Bataille and Klossowski emphasized a moment always already foreclosed in Sade, a tragic emptiness or lack at his core which Maurice Blanchot rejected and Albert Camus discussed from a very different point of view.

Blanchot argued that Sade's libertines achieve mastery.[43] Insofar as desire was always mediated by (what Sade called) apathy, Blanchot contended, it maintained the libertine above the law; apathy—*insensibilité,* as Blanchot termed it—made possible the perpetual annihilation of others, unmediated by the recognition of God or the *prochain* which the early Klossowski had found implicit in the libertine's atheism. Blanchot's libertines are not bound up in a dialectic of recognition (or a drama of foreclosure) but are instead self-same. Blanchot insisted that if we follow Sade's logic, it leads to the ruin of all moral categories and therefore away from the moral conscience (the recognition of others) to the "unique man," "solitary" and "insouciant": "it seems only fair to leave to [Leopold von] Sacher-Masoch the paternity of masochism, and the paternity of sadism to Sade. The pleasure Sade's heroes find in degradation never lessens their self-possession, and abjection adds to their stature. Shame, remorse, a penchant for punishment, all such feelings are foreign to them."[44]

Camus viewed Sade as an iconoclast whose revolt was inspired

gazes at and petrifies itself." One could easily argue that Sade's self resembles this statue man: an always already foreclosed self that, like Juliette, is perpetually in search of what it has lost but can never attain. Borch-Jacobsen notes, furthermore, that "the eye of paranoid knowledge, in its tireless self-curiosity, rises up against itself in a monstrous, persecutive erection, and it must be castrated with a vengeance." Borch-Jacobsen, p. 60. For a discussion of Bataille on Sade, see Jean-Michel Heimonet "Recoil in Order to Leap Forward: Two Values of Sade in Bataille," *On Bataille: Yale French Studies* 78 (1990), 227–36.

[43]Blanchot's analysis is also close to Michel Foucault's reading of Sade, which sees the lightning that strikes and kills Justine as a metaphor for Juliette's criminality: "The light of an instant which nature draws out of itself to strike Justine is only one and the same thing as the long existence of Juliette, who will herself disappear." *Histoire de la folie à l'âge classique* (Paris: Gallimard, 1972), p. 554.

[44]Maurice Blanchot, "Sade," in *Justine, Philosophy in the Bedroom,* p. 52.

not by moral conviction but by the absence of any moral sentiment whatsoever, whose identity was defined not through inner conviction but in response to an anonymous hostile "outside."[45] Like the dandy's, Sade's revolt was about self-fashioning. His dream of total omnipotence was therefore only an inversion of his inner void, his inner emptiness, the mirror of a place where he alone existed in and for himself. It represented the absolute negation of the world, a metaphysical revolt masquerading as a political one.

If Lacan, too, chose to emphasize Sade's adherence to the law, to a space in which it is "psychically impossible to breathe,"[46] instead of the transgressive (even if failed) moment in Sade's work emphasized in particular by Bataille, he nevertheless did not see Sade as a proto-Fascist, as self-same. Lacan explored Sade's relationship to the law by analyzing another relationship, between Sade and Kant, in "Kant with Sade" (1962). In Kant's case, reason guides and guarantees the exercise of morality (the categorical imperative), and in Sade's, it guarantees and justifies immorality.[47] In Kant, legal-rational structures prove compatible with moral ones, and in Sade they are compatible with immoral ones. Lacan used the declarations of the French revolutionaries to explore the legitimacy of both claims, but in the process took a detour—as he always did—through Freud.

The unrestrained desire supposedly unleashed by the Revolution upset proper lineages—paternities, to be exact—of all sorts. Sade, too, broke all the rules. At the same time, the image of the evil father after which Sade (according, we recall, to Klossowski) fashioned himself is different from the image Lacan painted of him in "Kant with Sade." There he attempted to undermine the lineage drawn by Maurice Heine and the surrealists as well as by that tradition in French psychiatry born, like Kant, of the Enlightenment, which saw Sade as Freud's precursor and, by implication, Lacan's as well. He rejected the idea that Sade's cataloging of perversions in any way preceded Freud's own recognition of the libido, disparaging the notion as that kind of progressive thinking that

---

[45] Albert Camus, The Rebel (New York: Knopf, 1957), pp. 36–54.

[46] Jacques Lacan, L'Ethique de la psychanalyse (Paris: Seuil, 1986), pp. 236–37.

[47] It should be noted that Max Horkheimer and Theodor Adorno also compared Kant with Sade, in The Dialectic of Enlightenment (London: Verso, 1979), pp. 81–119.

would equate the naming of desire with some sort of liberation.[48] It was instead precisely the naming of desire that sanctified the law, and it was through this sanctification, Lacan argued, that Sade could be linked to Kant, that legislator par excellence.

In fact, the only common ground Lacan discovered between Sade and Freud is that each is too distant from his own evil; "Sade is not close enough to his own evil to meet his fellow man there. A trait that he shares with many and notably with Freud."[49] It is this inability to live up to one's own evil, actually, that circumscribes Sade's rebellion, for it is impossible to will evil and be evil, as much as one might try: "A work which wills itself to be bad [méchante] cannot permit itself to be a bad [méchante] work, and it must be said that the *Philosophy* [*in the Bedroom*], by a whole side of good work, lends itself to this witticism." And more: "For Sade we see the test of this . . . in his refusal of the death penalty, which history, if not logic, would suffice to show is one of the corollaries of charity."[50]

Lacan in this way attempted to relocate Sade in his proper "place"—with Kant—in order to explore the conditions of what turns out to be a compulsion to virtue, and thus to distinguish Sade's sadism from the sadism that does not have a place in thinking because it does not obey the law. But Sade—and this, Lacan claimed, was the proof of the pudding—could and did: "A fantasy is indeed quite upsetting since one does not know where to set it, because it is there, wholly in its nature as fantasy which only has reality as discourse and expects nothing from your powers, but demands that you set yourself straight with respect to your desires."[51]

It is fantasy, Lacan suggested, that constitutes the limits of Sade's own sadism; fantasy makes desire possible because it "intervenes to sustain *jouissance* by the very discord to which it suc-

[48] Jacques Lacan, "Kant with Sade," trans. James B. Swenson, Jr., *October* 51 (Winter 1989), 55.
[49] Jacques Lacan, *Ecrits* 2 (Paris: Seuil, 1971), p. 147. Jane Gallop quotes this passage in *The Daughter's Seduction*, pp. 86–87. I have used her translation. I also want to note the peculiarity of Lacan's comment: It is not clear how "evil" Freud was.
[50] Lacan, "Kant with Sade," pp. 72 (translation slightly modified), 74.
[51] Ibid., p. 66.

cumbs."[52] Fantasy stops the inevitable annihilation that results when the right to *jouissance*, as in Sade's work, becomes the law. Sadistic desire constitutes a paradox in which the absolute right to rule annihilates the rules, in which turning the right to pleasure into law essentially means the "freedom" to die of desire.

In this way Sade's texts replicate the revolutionary desire that struggles that "the law be free, so free that it must be a widow, the Widow *par excellence* [the guillotine]."[53] But the law, of course, cannot both be free and be law, cannot, in other words, generate new fathers, which is why such a fight for freedom must be waged by a widow. When men try to live their desire as the law, Lacan argued, they can be only tragic paternities, paternities to which such men as Jesus are compelled, men who really know "how to kill." Lacan quoted Ernest Renan's *Life of Jesus*: "Masterpieces of fine raillery, [Jesus' ironic remarks] are written in lines of fire upon the flesh of the hypocrite and the false devotee. Incomparable traits, worthy of a son of God. A god alone knows how to kill after this fashion."[54]

But Sade, said Lacan, was no Jesus: His flesh was simply too weak. "Sade thus stopped, at the point where desire is knotted together with the law." For if Jesus died in the name of the law, if he laid down his life in order to live his desire as the law, Sade had no such integrity. Sade tried desperately to pretend he was "sinful beyond measure" (and hence, like Jesus, free of conceivable sins, a pure master), when he was only an ordinary sinner who would not venture to "throw the first stone."[55] He was just a braggart:

> Listen to him bragging of his technique, of immediately putting everything which occurs to him into operation, thinking moreover, by replacing repentance with reiteration, to have done with the law within. He finds nothing better to encourage us to follow him than the promise that nature, woman that she is, will magically always yield to us more.
>
> It would be a mistake to trust this typical dream of potency.[56]

[52] Ibid., 62.
[53] Ibid., p. 71.
[54] Ibid., pp. 73–74.
[55] Ibid., p. 74.
[56] Ibid., pp. 74–75.

But for all his bragging, for all his claims about wanting to disappear without a trace, we are left with an enormous quantity of words that can be found in "every respectable library."[57] In fact, even though Sade himself didn't know it, he kept invoking the law not to fulfill his aspirations to absolute mastery—to "be" the law—but to uphold it: "The apology for crime only pushes him to indirect avowal of the law." It is all there, said Lacan: If Sade really saw himself as absolute master, why don't his victims ever consent? No, the victims resist, and resist unto death. And why did Sade take the "educational" function of his work so seriously? Why did he refuse to recognize "the impotence in which the educative intention is commonly deployed" (as any *really* scandalous book would have)?[58] Criminals who make Sade's claims usually do not have such good intentions.

Lacan's answer to this mystery is that Sade upheld the law not because he desired absolute mastery but because he *repressed* that desire, accepted what he lacked.[59] "Of what Sade is lacking," Lacan wrote, "we have forbidden ourselves to say a word. One may sense it in the gradation of the *Philosophy* toward the fact that it is the curved needle, dear to Bunuel's heroes, which is finally called upon to resolve a girl's *penisneid*, and quite a big one." Sade may have tried to pretend he lacked nothing, but his very adherence to the law, in spite of his best intentions, suggests instead that in fact he accepted his lack. That is why, at the end of *Philosophy in the Bedroom*, he "closes the affair with a *Noli tangere matrem*. V...ed and sewn up, the mother remains forbidden. Our verdict upon the submission of Sade to the Law is confirmed." It is why the *Philosophy* is a "good work."[60]

Sade's work thus represents the expression of a lack always deferred, a desire to be the father the man has accepted he can never be. We recall that entry into the symbolic order splits the ego and defuses the aggressive potential in the mirror stage, with its refusal of the alterity of the other. Lacan implied that Sade in fact learned to compensate for the loss of the (m)other through his incessant

[57] Ibid., p. 66. As the translator, James Swenson, notes, this reference is to Jules Janin's slightly hysterical assertion that Sade could be found "everywhere," in "all the libraries."

[58] Ibid., pp. 74, 72–73, 72.

[59] Ibid., p. 68.

[60] Ibid., p. 75.

demands (his capacity to name), which are really only demands for the (forever) lost object of desire called now by other names, other demands. Sade's compulsion to write (his bragging, his reiterations) thus represents a lack expressed as a demand that can never ever get what it wants.

Lacan thus leaves behind what he called "existentialist custom tailoring" and "personalist ready-made" (an indirect attack on Klossowski)[61] to maintain that no desire can be free and be articulated as desire, that all desire owes its articulation to the law, so that Sade, for all his claims to the contrary, must be beholden to it: "If happiness is the uninterrupted agreeableness, for the subject, of his life . . . it is clear that it is refused to whomever does not renounce the path of desire."[62] Desire is thus constituted through the renunciation of desire; to be the father one must renounce being the father. In other words, to fulfill one's desire one must, in effect, repress (or rather, symbolize) it; Sade's dreams of absolute mastery could be fulfilled, paradoxically, only when he submitted to the law. Mastery is thus always only the illusion of mastery, a mastery lived and yet infinitely deferred. Sade can be a master only to the extent he is not one.

Thus, although Lacan sought to distance his Sade from what he conceived as Klossowski's (as well as Bataille's and Paulhan's) saintly or even somewhat psychotic Sade, it is not at all clear how they are different. Of course, Lacan insisted, pace Bataille and Klossowski, that Sade is not always unconsciously begging for punishment but seeks to avoid it by (unconsciously) adhering to oedipal law. But if to adhere to the law means to be fulfilled by remaining unfulfilled, what distinguishes that adherence from the dialectic of self-punishment? Is there really any difference between the foreclosure of absolute mastery and the symbolic deferral of it? Aren't both equally illusions of mastery that arrest the self-annihilation proper to absolute mastery?[63]

What definitely does distinguish Bataille's and Klossowski's

---

[61] Ibid., p. 65. Simone de Beauvoir argued that Sade's "denial of others" was rooted not in metaphysical anxiety, as Klossowski maintained, but in a deeply personal effort to clear his conscience (his consciousness of his sexual otherness) by turning that denial into an ethic. Beauvoir, "Must We Burn Sade?" pp. 3–64.

[62] Lacan, "Kant with Sade," p. 71.

[63] See Borch-Jacobsen's discussion of this really impossible distinction between the symbolic and the imaginary, p. 118. He discusses it in terms of Lacan's extension of the Kojèvian dialectic between master and slave into his concept of Oedipus. Again, my argument follows his, if on a very different level, quite closely.

from Lacan's Sade is the spirit in which he is constructed, figured. That is, if the distinction is not as theoretically convincing as Lacan would have it, Lacan's Sade feels different. He is more human than saintly or prophetic. Lacan declared that Sade's drama of potency represents the "senile tragic." That is, he is no more than a two-bit actor in a rather silly melodrama, and he is not "duped by his fantasy."[64] Yet Lacan also asserted that Sade becomes noble by virtue of his senility, by virtue of his refusal to see that he is upholding the law. By virtue of this extreme blindness, Sade's silly "platitudes" come to have a "somber beauty": "This beauty bears witness for us to the experience for which we search behind the fabulation of the fantasy. A tragic experience, for it projects its condition in a lighting beyond all fear and pity."[65] Sade is very blind, and very human, like a neurotic Oedipus. His very neurosis defines his humanity. Along with Bataille and Klossowski, Lacan sought to rethink Sade in terms of his proximity to rather than his distance from humanity. But Lacan's version of Sade's humanity most effectively describes how it is that law-abiding citizens can also be monsters, because he is most explicitly concerned to demonstrate to what extent the very logic of the law makes us who we are (constitutes us through repression).

Thus, depending on whom one listens to, Sade is hard as stone (as an unwitting executioner) or a hard moralist in the Kantian sense (which means of course that one is hard for somebody else's good, as the philosopher of the bedroom always insisted). But again, finally, what distinguishes the hard man of imaginary illusions from the hard moralist who has learned and now himself preaches a good lesson? Both embody the predicament of a modern "man" who has to live in a world in which he has no ground to stand on but a law whose foundation can never be known, which is already constituted as the law, and thus in which his "true" desire, his "true" self, can be articulated only as an (albeit legal) lie.

Sadomasochism and the Self

Thus, surrealism began a long process by which Sade was given back his humanity. But what is the meaning of that restoration?

---

[64] Lacan, "Kant with Sade," p. 65.
[65] Ibid., p. 73.

How do we account for the specific construction of his humanity? I have argued that Sade's sadomasochism became a metaphor of the self from surrealism through Lacan. In order to account for Sade's rehabilitation, I have argued as well that it was part of an effort to place desire at the center of what Susan Suleiman calls a "project of cultural subversion,"[66] effected by the surrealists but made possible by a broader medical attempt to redefine the normal self in terms of heretofore unacceptable perverse sexual impulses. But to maintain that the self was ontologically rooted in the libido (whose cultural representation itself shifts) begs the question of what the relationship between the self and the libido is, and what determines that relationship and its permutations.

In order to account for one prewar permutation, I have maintained that Bataille's, Klossowski's, and Paulhan's concepts of the self represented the subversion of conventional boundaries between normality and perversion implicit in the surrealists' conflation of the self with Sade's sadomasochistic pleasure. They used the logic implicit in this articulation of Sade's sadomasochism—that pleasure has no reference except the punishment that produces it—to figure a self that is always already repressed and hence whose truth is other, beyond symbolization. Sade's writing now no longer represented a glorious and tragic, if natural and healthy, masculinity but a wounded, fragile manhood, an impossible desire to be selfless. Writing is a bloody, messy business whose genesis is dependent upon an unspeakable experience of pain and self-doubt. From the surrealists through Klossowski (though it can be extended to Lacan), the image of a neurotic father burdened by his own authority, tormented as well by his unfulfilled dreams and aspirations, an image fashioned after Sade, became the central metaphor for the production of culture. That image refigured identity in terms of a new kind of selfhood rooted paradoxically in a desire for selflessness, in a death wish. It is already implicit in the tragic masculinity constructed by the surrealists and was fully developed in the interwar years into a father Georges Bataille called terrible and yet magnificent, a patriarch in decline who nevertheless incarnated—whose decline is paradoxically the condition of—authority, a man who is not a degenerate, a pervert, a stately

---

[66] Susan Rubin Suleiman, *Subversive Intent: Gender, Politics, and the Avant-Garde* (Cambridge: Harvard University Press), pp. 74–77.

sadomasochist, or an iconoclast but a terribly fragile revolutionary whose aggression is ultimately turned inward.

If fatherhood therefore remained the fundamental condition of authorship, its authority no longer derived from a potent virility. The father's identification with the executioner, with authority, is instead expressed as a desire for self-punishment. As Leo Bersani puts it in another context, "Given the limitation of our effective power over the external world, it could be said that the curbing of aggressiveness offers the only realistic strategy for satisfying aggressiveness."[67] If for the surrealists Sade's criminal works were metaphors of an essential and heretofore repressed self, for Bataille, Paulhan, and Klossowski, they were metaphors for a self, to repeat, whose essence was released only when its desires were repressed; they were the products of an author who "cured" himself of his obsessive desire by nurturing his pathology. Though they didn't employ this term, these authors used Sade's self as a metaphor for what Ellie Ragland-Sullivan interprets as an "unsymbolized Imaginary [self] . . . [that] stands between him and metaphorical death: corporal and perceptual fragmentation."[68] Sade's masochistic desire now replicated that "neurosis of self-punishment" which Lacan claimed structured the (imaginary) self.[69]

This concept of the self as an illusion, like Lacan's concept of the imaginary, also marked a refusal of the attempts of medical men and the surrealists to establish a normative, essential self or, in this case, to normalize Sade—a refusal to make him submit to the lessons of good hygiene. Much as Lacan listened to Aimée—and in the process revolutionized psychoanalytic thought—they sought to listen to what others could not hear Sade say. And the construction of a new, tragic virility also echoed Lacan's critique and resurrection of patriarchy, his father in decline. After all, fatherhood remained the fundamental condition of authorship even as the conventional concept of virility was undermined, for what, we might ask, were the implications of *this* rehabilitation of Sade for Rose Keller?

Bataille noted that "in an official statement, Rose Keller spoke of

[67] Leo Bersani, *The Freudian Body* (New York: Columbia University Press, 1986), p. 23.
[68] Ragland-Sullivan, p. 150.
[69] Lacan, *Ecrits: A Selection*, pp. 28–29.

the appalling cries which accompanied [Sade's] orgasm."[70] Bataille was not concerned with Keller; he wanted to accentuate Sade's marginality, his extremity, isolation, and violence, and therefore his humanness. Klossowski's discussion of Sade's misogyny, we recall, was all about how Sade strove to be a man he could never be. As long as Sade's self was the absolute metaphor of selfhood (as was, we recall, Lacan's paternal imago), Rose Keller fared no better in Bataille's and Klossowski's writings than she did in the surrealist rehabilitation of Sade. For the surrealists Keller did not count, because they conflated the self with Sade's self and hence so-called normal desire with Sade's desire—in other words, they assumed that what Sade desired Keller also desired. For Bataille, Paulhan, and Klossowski she did not count because they too conflated the self with Sade's self. In their work the pleasure of the self was seen as always bound up with its repression. Keller's pain, like Sade's, was thus always also her pleasure.

The prewar attribution of Sade's compulsion to write to his desire to be a victim was thus the consequence of an effort to listen, born of writers' identification with Sade's paradoxically privileged marginality. After the Second World War, their emphasis was no longer on Sade's outsider status, on the lucidity that rendered him incapable of serving the very society he wanted to serve. In other words, Sade was no longer a tragic man whose silence paradoxically asserted the claims of existence in a reified world. Instead, he seemed to herald the *triumph* of that kind of instrumental rationality. He embodied the logical consequences of an imperative to be the law to which one at the same time necessarily, categorically, submits.[71] It is in this bleak world that Kant meets Sade. It is here too that Lacan's Sade joins Bataille's and Klossowski's in an ever-deferred quest for death, for absolute mastery.

In the past two chapters I have tried to account for the regulatory fictions that governed this reconstruction of Sade. I have sought to demonstrate how and why Sade's sadomasochistic self came to be a metaphor in sexual and textual terms for a new concept of the self: one whose ontological basis is sexual, one that is nonreferential, that has no discernible origins except the law that constitutes it

---

[70]Bataille, *Literature and Evil*, p. 97.

[71]For an interesting discussion of "Kant with Sade," see John Rajchman, "Lacan and the Ethics of Modernity," *Representations* 15 (Summer 1986), 42–56.

through repression. But this law—the law of a reified, alienated, instrumental culture—is precisely the one whose legitimacy Bataille sought to challenge. In this challenge, he can be linked to, but also provides an alternative to, Lacan's vision of self-formation. But this challenge is yet another story, which will require a rather lengthy prelude.

PART THREE

HEADLESSNESS

Nowadays it is usually the man who wants to be vamped, to be KNOWN.
—D. H. Lawrence, *Studies in
Classic American Literature, 1924*

In a recent feminist psychoanalytic study of sexual dominance, Jessica Benjamin argues that masochism is a form of self-affirmation, a means by which the masochist's real pleasure is known. This paradox operates through an elaborate masquerade. Because masochists experience pleasure as pain, they have their pleasure while pretending not to have it; they get to be "bad, wanton, reveling in . . . debasement" and are punished for it at the same time. Benjamin puts it this way: "The torture and outrage to which [the masochist] submits is a kind of martyrdom. . . . her desire to be known is like that of the sinner who wants to be known by God."[1]

This masquerade, as I have argued, is replicated in the way writers interpreted Sade's desire to subvert literary convention; like the masochist's pleasure, Sade's subversive desire is fulfilled only when thwarted. What is unusual about this reconstruction of Sade as masochist is that he is a man. Benjamin's entire book, like many

[1] Jessica Benjamin, *The Bonds of Love: Psychoanalysis, Feminism, and the Problem of Domination* (New York: Pantheon, 1988), p. 60.

feminist studies of sexuality which rightly reject the view of masochism as false consciousness, is an attempt to explore why and
how masochism constitutes a specifically female—indirect, guilt-
ridden—means of appropriating and negotiating power. But what
happens when *men* are masochists and how do gender relations
shift (or do they) when it is men who seek their pleasure in pain?
How could one figure a manhood of which masochism would be
the defining and even ennobling characteristic rather than a pathological lapse into femininity? What is striking about the interwar
writers that concern us is the extent to which they redefined male
identity in masochistic terms. That is, men did not literally become masochists, but the nonreferentiality of the self characteristic of masochism—that the self is known only when repressed—came to constitute masculinity.[2]

We have seen how this conception works in Lacan and in readings of Sade, and in relation to three emblems of male authority:
the scientist, the father, and the writer. In this section, I want to
look again at how the male writer is compromised. In order to do
so, I link the celebration of perversion in interwar France to its
literary proponents—the surrealists. Whereas in other modernist
movements the interwar emphasis on the erotic and the perverse
compromised the self, in France the literary equation of sexual and
criminal deviance with the truth of the self led to a masochistic
model of self-dissolution. The greatness of the work came to reside
no longer in the author's criminality but in his desire to be
punished for his crime.

In the following chapters, then, I seek to account once again for

---

[2] There has been much recent interest in male masochism—or rather in rethinking subjectivity in terms that are masochistic (and inevitably male). Many of these
studies reiterate patriarchal gender norms also implicit in Bataille's and Lacan's
concept of the subject even as they seek to subvert them. They are implicitly
indebted to a specific set of cultural terms in which women do not really figure or
figure only as metaphors for the "gaps" or interstices men refuse to acknowledge in
themselves. See, for example, Leo Bersani, "Is the Rectum a Grave?" in *AIDS:
Cultural Analysis, Cultural Activism*, ed. Douglas Crimp (Cambridge: MIT Press,
1989), 197–222; Deleuze, pp. 9–138. For a different kind of discussion of the link
between the enactment and denial of castration and aesthetic production, see
Charles Bernheimer, *Figures of Ill Repute: Representing Prostitution in Nineteenth-
Century France* (Cambridge: Harvard University Press, 1989), esp. pp. 234–65. And
for a fascinating analysis of male masochism that does not fall into any of these
categories, see Kaja Silverman, "Masochism and Male Subjectivity" *Camera
Obscura* 17 (1988), especially p. 62.

the specificity of this link between "great" art and what Bataille called "headlessness"—the condition of being, like Sade, a "conscience without a head," as Klossowski called it.[3] Apart from Bataille's particular predispositions, how do we account for this overwhelming desire to be guilty which characterized Bataille's model of authorship? Why is it that a glorious, ecstatic self-loss became so fundamental to literary creation? Or to be more specific, how did the notion of a masochistic self-loss that is not a romantic self-sacrifice but a *masquerade* of self-sacrifice become a requirement for literary greatness?

Like Sade, as we shall see, the author was conceived as wanting to be a victim, and his writing was conceived as driven by that desire. And, like Sade, the modern author was also compelled, by social upheaval—here the specter of fascism. In keeping with the analysis of the self thus far, I am not using masochism to refer to Freud's death instinct, to the primordial drive he contrasted with the libido, but rather as a metaphor for a desire for self-annihilation which can never be realized. Chapter 6 discusses how the surrealists and others linked the greatness of literature to the writer's deviance or criminality. Chapter 7 analyzes how and why Bataille linked literary greatness to the writer's desire to be punished. It attempts to explain how the writer's masochism comes to symbolize and shape a new concept of the self and hence, to the extent that notions of selfhood define how texts are produced and interpreted, of literary production, of the text's "truth."

[3] Klossowski, *Sade, mon prochain* (1947), p. 161.

Chapter Six

Writing and Crime

In *Discipline and Punish,* Michel Foucault referred to the romantic doubling of monstrosity and beauty as the "aesthetic rewriting of crime," the transposition "to another social class [of] the spectacle that had surrounded the criminal."[1] Beginning in the late eighteenth century, he argued, crime was no longer the symbol of one social class avenging itself against the injustice of another, but represented individual greatness; in other words, the criminal act was a gesture aimed at escaping bourgeois mediocrity, the mark of an individual's superiority. Criminals were no longer little men but great ones. In Matthew Lewis's gothic novel *The Monk,* the criminal is a noble, religious, and charismatic man whom no one suspects and whose compulsion to crime simultaneously horrifies the reader and increases the monk's stature. Although he must lose in the end, his willingness to use the most immoral means to attain his ends, his abuse of his position and power, and most of all his susceptibility to the subterranean forces that drive him to crime, in fact elevate his nature above the mediocre. Crime thus came to be seen not just as an assault on social order but as an art, and only the greatest men (here women do not figure) could be artists.

There is another distinction implicit in this reading of crime as an aesthetic, one to which Jean Paulhan referred in his preface to *Justine:* the contrast between the "inoffensive appearance" of a

---

[1] Foucault, *Discipline and Punish,* pp. 68–69.

criminal and the evil of his real, criminal soul.[2] The criminal's real nature is superior to that of ordinary mortals precisely because it is hidden, because the criminal doesn't show it off; his reserve distinguishes him from the pauper who has nothing to hide, nothing to be reserved about. In the late nineteenth century especially, the criminal was an aristocrat in spirit if not in blood, which meant above all that he was never so crude as to give himself away, but was discreet, refined, reserved, and mysterious. Thus, writers admired the sadists Sade and Gilles de Rais, but not the equally criminal Joseph Vacher or Jean-Baptiste Troppmann.[3] Although neither Rais nor Sade proved particularly reserved or particularly mysterious, their noble origins guaranteed or supported an elaborate fantasy about their noble characters. If the criminal's "fixed eyes and dilated pupils" indicated what lay below the surface, his "sweet smile" always obscured the cruelty of his soul.[4]

In the course of the nineteenth century not just crime but all that crime symbolizes (perversion, aberration, illness) became a requirement for literary greatness. The writer was reconceived as a metaphorical criminal, an outlaw, a man who cultivated separateness, who held himself, like the dandy, above the crowd. This image of the great writer represents the literary transposition and appropriation of that late nineteenth-century conception of the criminal I sketched out in Part One: an individual who is fundamentally different, marked.[5] The writer too was by nature differ-

---

[2] New literary genres—and here I am thinking in particular of the gothic—devoted to exploring and dissecting evil, to analyzing more specifically the relationship between evil and human passion, developed in the late eighteenth and early nineteenth centuries and testified to a desire to evaluate the underside of reason, to know what lay beneath the conventional appearance of the evildoer. But though I am focusing here on their analysis of the criminal and his motives, these genres also represent an obsessive desire to know the victim. The scopophilia of that cold, analytical strain of romanticism exemplified by Edgar Allan Poe, the images of violated, dismembered (and primarily female) bodies common to gothic literature, and the detailed, obsessive, and prurient newspaper narratives about crime and criminals all testify to what D. H. Lawrence called Poe's desire to "dissect" his lover Ligeia. See Praz, p. 186.

[3] Both were late nineteenth-century murderers. Vacher killed several people, cut their throats and mutilated their cadavers; Troppmann was accused of murdering and mutilating a family. Both were guillotined.

[4] See Sabine Baring-Gould, *The Book of the Werewolves* (London: Smith, Elder, 1865), pp. 209–10. He borrows this description of Gilles de Rais from Paul Lacroix.

[5] For a discussion of the ties between degeneracy theory, naturalism, and the Decadent imagination, see Jean Pierrot, *The Decadent Imagination*, trans. Derek Coltman (Chicago: University of Chicago Press, 1981), pp. 45–55.

ent—hypersensitive, given to sickness, instability, and impulse. But this difference is a sign of superiority, not inferiority, and the mark, when it can be seen (as in the case of illness, of dilated pupils and fixed eyes) indicates, paradoxically, something that is hidden and inaccessible.

Every Man Is a Criminal

In the interwar years criminal and sexual deviance—and I will henceforth use crime as a metaphor for all that was other, nonrational, violent, and so forth—came out of hiding. On the one hand, there was simply more interest in the criminal, in the other. The criminal was no longer the discreet nobleman of high-culture novels but was instead to be found everywhere. As we have already seen, psychoanalysts found criminality lurking in the unconscious, and doctors and sexologists insisted that perversion was compatible with a normal disposition. Finally, avant-garde thinkers, and the surrealists in particular, sang the virtues of crime and of all that bourgeois society deemed other.

And yet because crime was suddenly to be found everywhere, it was also hard to find, meaning it became—to use a loaded but appropriate word—"banal."[6] To be sure, Fascists' attempts to literalize national boundaries in blood represented efforts to draw the boundaries between self and other anew, to give the other a visible face, to designate criminals clearly. But precisely where boundary drawing is frantic there must be the threat of boundary dissolution, and it is on this dissolution that I want to focus. For whereas Fascists had a quite clear idea of who was a criminal, by the interwar years the image of the criminal had in fact become increasingly blurry. The nineteenth-century criminal had murdered in the dark, and the crime had forced him out of obscurity, shed light on his soul. By the interwar years, however, the crime was less likely to occur in sordid places; it had moved inside, into bourgeois interiors in particular. The criminal's tools were as likely to be average household items heretofore associated with female and hence "cowardly" criminals—an oven, a shower, kitchen utensils—as an

[6]I am of course referring to Hannah Arendt's writings on Adolf Eichmann, in which she coined the phrase, "the banality of evil." *Eichmann in Jerusalem* (New York: Penguin, 1975).

unwieldy, jagged knife.[7] The male criminal no longer possessed the mystical aura of the marked man; instead, he had the ambiguous attraction of an individual both fascinating and pitiful because so apparently ordinary.

Take, for example, the French criminal Henri Landru, executed for the murder of several women in 1922 after one of the most publicized criminal trials of the early twentieth century. In search of easy money, Landru, a respectable businessman with a wife and family, placed personal adds in all the local papers looking for wealthy single or widowed women whom he would court, promise to marry, and then murder. He kept meticulous files of all the responses he received, systematically organized according to the woman's probable economic resources. When Landru was arrested in 1919 after several complaints of missing persons set police on his trail, investigators found nothing but some bones and a closet full of women's clothing. An anonymous popular painting from about 1920 depicts Landru in his kitchen (where he supposedly burned the bodies of his victims) immaculately dressed in a suit with a bowtie and calmly eating the body of a woman with a fork and knife. It represents precisely the conflation of murder with the everyday which was perceived to characterize many of the most gruesome crimes after the war.

The meticulousness of his crimes, the premeditation that took the form of planning a daily schedule, and Landru's capacity to live a double life as family man and murderer—all these qualities were specific to narratives about crime after the war: to those about Dr. Marcel Petitot, who turned his office into a veritable torture chamber and murdered his clients with the very instruments of his profession, or of Violette Noizières, who tried to murder her parents (and did murder her father) by giving them poison she claimed was a drug prescribed by the doctor. And what was shocking about the Papin sisters, whom we have already encountered, was that absolutely nothing in their countenance would have allowed anyone to predict their murderous behavior. This problem, after all, lay behind the debates about how to attribute criminal responsibility which began in the nineteenth century and continued after the war. Here it is the ordinariness of extraordinary criminals that

---

[7] The Italian positivist Lombroso had argued that women became prostitutes and committed infanticide because such crimes were weak and cowardly and hence specifically feminine.

characterizes both their horror and their mystery. That is, in contrast to the nineteenth-century crime, which revealed the "real" monstrosity lurking beneath an apparently sweet soul, the modern crime marks precisely the impossibility of distinguishing in any clear way between the ordinary person and the monster. We have already seen this shift occur in reference to Sade, when Paulhan noted that what was troubling about Sade's reason was that it was both rational and nevertheless beyond the comprehension of any normal individual.

This same dissolution of boundaries characterized the shift from the noble, marked or different and hence superior, nineteenth-century writer to an avant-garde writer whose greatness lay (paradoxically) in what he had in common with other people. In surrealist work, this revelation of crime, this discovery of the other in the self, democratized the way to greatness, and to literary greatness in particular. Whereas nineteenth-century writers had conceived crime as a gesture of the truly great, the surrealists construed it as a potential that existed in everyone. We may recall that during this period, thinkers reconstructed Sade as Everyman. So, although the surrealists were heirs of a literary imagination from Dostoevsky through Gide which conceived criminal gestures as *actes gratuits*, as grand existential gestures, they also conceived crimes, like Sade's literary crimes, as the revelation of a real nature possessed by all human beings. Pathology was not a sign of the superiority of certain individuals but a metaphor for the potential of the human imagination in general, not the mark of a true artist but a consequence of the state's and society's repression of his or her art, his or her true self. Pathology, if you will, was normalized.

The surrealists thus also saw crime as a subversive and hence affirmative gesture that demolished rather than confirmed or erected hierarchies between the great and the ordinary. Thus, the Papin sisters, after having mutilated their employer and her daughter, emerge from the scene of the crime, in Paul Eluard and Benjamin Peret's depiction, "armed with a song of Maldoror's." Or René Crevel declares: "The beauty of certain assaults on moral convention or on life itself is that they mark with all their violence the monstrosity of laws, the constraints that create monsters."[8]

---

[8] Paul Eluard and Benjamin Peret, untitled article, *Le Surréalisme au service de la Révolution* 5 (1933), 27–28; René Crevel, "Note en vue d'un psycho-dialectique," *Le Surréalisme au service de la Révolution* 5 (1933), 50.

The surrealists thus celebrated and defended famous criminals, including the Papin sisters and Violette Noizières, because they saw them as victims. They also celebrated madness. In 1925 the group rallied against the psychiatric establishment and against Henri Claude in particular for stigmatizing, labeling, and confining madmen, whom the surrealists recast as prisoners. Breton celebrated the "purest intuition" and the "miracles" he believed described his mad friend, a woman who eventually became the subject of his famous surrealist novel *Nadja*.[9] This is not the place to discuss the surrealists' concept of the feminine—it has been done quite thoroughly by others—though it is important to signal the extent to which, in their perception, the other was gendered feminine. I am less interested in the feminine per se—how it was represented, the consequences of this representation for the surrealists' concept of women's emancipation, and so forth—than in how the feminine was used to reformulate masculine identity. Thus, while the surrealists tended to celebrate female criminals, women were primarily vehicles for the exploration of male selfhood, for the vicarious transgression of boundaries.[10]

Surrealists did not conceive crimes as testimony to criminals' distance from humanity, as expressions of reserve or alienation, but rather (as they had with Sade) to their humanness. Maurice Heine's analysis of a famous necrophiliac, Sergeant Bertrand, represents an extreme example of this kind of interpretation of crime. Heine, we recall, was a surrealist fellow traveler who devoted his life to the works of Sade. He was fascinated by other criminals as well. He had written a piece titled "Tableau de l'amour macabre," a medico-legal compendium detailing the gruesome deeds of many criminals and including an analysis of Sergeant Bertrand.[11]

[9] André Breton, *Nadja*, trans. Richard Howard (New York: Grove Press, 1960), p. 114.

[10] See Mary Ann Caws, "Ladies Shot and Painted: Female Embodiment in Surrealist Art," in Susan Suleiman, ed., *The Female Body in Western Culture* (Cambridge: Harvard University Press, 1985), pp. 262–87; Mary Ann Caws, Rudolf Kuenzli, Gwen Raaberg, eds., *Surrealism and Women* (Cambridge: MIT Press, 1991); Susan Gardner, "Dora and Nadja: Two Women in the Early Days of Psychoanalysis and Surrealism," *Hecate* no. 2 (January 1976), 23–39; Xavière Gauthier, *Surréalisme et sexualité* (Paris: Gallimard, 1971); Rosalind Krauss, "Corpus Delicti," *October* 33 (Summer 1985), 31–72; Bethany Ladimer, "Madness and the Irrational in the Work of André Breton: A Feminist Perspective," *Feminist Studies* 6 (Spring 1980), 175–95; Suleiman, *Subversive Intent*, pp. 20–32, 99–110, 141–79. Krauss is the only author who defends the surrealists against feminist criticism.

[11] The essay was never published. It was scheduled to appear in *Acéphale* but was finally rejected because of its length. See letters from Heine to Leo Malet, July 16,

Bertrand was arrested in 1849 for violating female corpses in various cemeteries, including Père Lachaise. In contrast to nineteenth-century accounts,[12] Heine's version did not portray Bertrand as pathologically depraved; it presented him as the "incarnation of one of those predestined heroes of the romantic period":

> Present from a young age, though always repressed, [Bertrand's] sadism was expressed in a less criminal manner in his zoophilia and also found an attenuated expression in necrophilia. Even though Bertrand was not fully conscious of it, he became a necrophiliac perhaps in order to avoid becoming a murderer. Is this not the intimate drama concealed behind the insistence with which he attested to his joviality, his amenability, his gentleness? Is this not the inexplicable dimension of his psychology which projects [on the legal case] the shadow of premeditation which so troubled [Dr.] Lunier? It is there that the human solution to this enigma resides.[13]

Repudiating Krafft-Ebing's analysis of Bertrand as pathological, as well as other nineteenth-century accounts of the case in which the sergeant's necrophilia was explained as a depraved impulse, Heine transformed Bertrand's perversion into a human solution. If Bertrand was a pervert, his perversion also embodied in a tragic and beautiful way what it means to be human: to overcome one's desire to hurt others.

The idea that the cause of Bertrand's perversion should also be its cure is odd. That is, his necrophilia is sadistic and yet also represents an unconscious impulse to repudiate his murderous, sadistic instinct; it becomes the source of his gentleness, his amenability, in short, his humanness. What Heine seems to be saying is that while crime is instinctive, it also distinguishes human beings from creatures that live solely by instinct; it is the origin of the unconscious, imaginative drives that make human beings human. Now Bertrand was not, like that other famous sadist over whom so much surrealist ink had been spilled, a writer. But his crime, like that of the Papin sisters, was "beautiful," not because it marked

---

1939, and Heine to Guy Levis-Mano on October 12, 1938, Bibliothèque Nationale, ms. 24397. The latter is quoted and partially reprinted in Bataille, *Oeuvres complètes* 2:674.

[12] See especially Krafft-Ebing, *Psychopathia sexualis;* and Baring-Gould, *Book of Werewolves,* p. 140.

[13] Heine, *Recueil de confessions,* pp. 269–70.

him as superior to other men but because it affirmed what he had in common with them. Crime thus did not mark individuals off from one another or demarcate between them, did not distinguish great from little people, but defined their common humanity.

Instead of marking criminal nature, as happened in the nineteenth century, this celebration of and fascination with crime made it disappear. That is, criminals' real natures were no longer confirmed by their behavior or their body; their perversity was no longer "there" to be revealed by a crime or—to suggest a parallel with the analogous shift previously outlined—by perspicacious scientists. Criminal nature was no longer distinct from the nature that characterized the vast community of civilized human beings. The criminal's crime was thus no longer evidence that he or she was a being apart—whether that distinction was valorized or not— but instead confirmed his or her humanity.

The surrealists thus defined what it meant to be human in terms of a dissolution of the boundaries between humanness and deviance and hence in terms of a confusion between self and other which was in keeping with other revolutions in the human sciences—in psychoanalysis, sexology, ethnography. But while the surrealists sought to democratize the road to greatness in politics—they did, after all, affiliate themselves with the Communist party in 1930—as avant-garde writers and painters they sought above all to revolutionize literary practice. It was this effort to apply "political" theory to literary practice, among others, that inspired Jean-Michel Heimonet to observe that during those years in France it became "increasingly difficult to distinguish between art and violence—between art and death."[14] Heimonet did not reiterate the nineteenth-century insistence that crime is an art; he wanted to convey to what extent art itself became infused with politics, with violence, to what extent crime conceived as art no longer emphasized the boundaries between seen and unseen (between the criminal's appearance and his or her soul), between great and ordinary people, but testified to their dissolution. It is fitting that a struggle for democracy should begin by dissolving distinction, but it is not clear precisely how dissolving the distinction between crime and art would translate into a democratic literary practice, or what democracy in such a context might mean. How, then, did the conflation of crime and art during the interwar years

[14]Heimonet, *Politiques de l'écriture*, p. 102.

dissolve the boundary between self and other? And what was the meaning of that conflation?

The Art of Crime

The surrealists conceived the writer as a metaphorical criminal because he struggled to illuminate crime, to bring it out of the dark, out of hiding. He called a spade a spade. He chose not to celebrate aristocratic reserve, to romanticize the veil concealing the criminal soul, but to shred the veil and proclaim crimes out loud. Above all, he rejected aristocratic reserve and bourgeois hypocrisy in favor of a return to what the surrealists conceived as authenticity: as a real or true self long left stagnant under the weight of bourgeois norms.

In literary practice, this quest for authenticity, for the unleashing of crime understood as repressed otherness, took two main forms: the aesthetic techniques of "convulsion" and automatic writing. The surrealist writer sought through art to recover the hidden, repressed criminal or other in himself and in the world—hence André Breton's famous phrase in *Nadja* (1928): "Beauty will be convulsive or will not be at all."[15] The surrealists conceived crime as the transgression of taboos, the release of a desire that, as they saw it, constituted the origin of art. Through art the creator returned to something once lost. "The soul rediscovers itself in a luminosity where finally its members relax," wrote Antonin Artaud, "there where the barriers of the world seem infinitely destructible." In the sensation of shredded flesh and shattered boundaries, limits are transgressed: art represents the "recovery of a complete and permeable state."[16] It represents the recovery of a truth that a century of bourgeois culture had muted—the paradoxical recovery of the self in the unbinding of subjectivity.

In surrealist aesthetics, writing conceived as crime, or what Jean Paulhan, we recall, referred to as "terror," thus led back to authenticity. Terror—and Paulhan meant to evoke the Terror of 1793—as method was characterized by an explosion of old meanings from within, a wrenching of words into a new language that spoke from

[15] André Breton, *Nadja*, p. 160.
[16] Antonin Artaud, "L'Art et la mort," *Oeuvres complètes*, 21 vols. (Paris: Gallimard, 1962), 1:122.

the body, from overfullness, a language rooted in a desire for literary freedom often metaphorically evoked as a desire to "lose one's head." "Language," as Paulhan put it in his denunciation of surrealist method, would thereby be rendered "direct and innocent."[17] Surrealist writers thus eroticized art by merging it with violence, and they reconceived it as the product of a libidinal, primarily sadomasochistic drive that metamorphosed everyday objects, especially the human body. The violent and sensual image of the convulsion was thus central to surrealist method. It was not always literally erotic but its origins were libidinal; it represented a metaphorical lovemaking that shocks, startles, and wrenches apart what Breton called "ready-made realities."[18]

Convulsion as method expressed most fundamentally the revolt of desire against bourgeois morality and effected the translation of unconscious, unwieldy desire into a new aesthetic language capable of undermining received ideas about culture. Through the convulsions created by the coupling of disparate realities, (e.g., Lautréamont's coupling of the umbrella and the sewing machine), contexts considered to be natural or normal were denaturalized and shown to be merely other systems of representation. They were revealed to be but arbitrary sets of artificial cultural arrangements and hierarchies.[19] Surrealism's material was thus not exclusively but primarily the female body, and its technique the transgressive violence of a metaphorical convulsion. Henry Ey thus described the surrealist "attitude" in terms of a "mystique, not a mystification, a mystique of cruelty."[20] And more recently Xavière Gauthier claimed the surrealists "sexualized" language and used perverse images to "decompose" and "disarticulate" the body so as to "transform it into language."[21]

This quest for authenticity was also expressed in another technique, automatic writing, as central to the surrealist critique of culture as the convulsion. It was, as Maurice Blanchot puts it, "a

[17] Paulhan, *Les Fleurs de Tarbes*, pp. 151–52.

[18] Breton, *Manifestoes of Surrealism*, p. 275.

[19] For a discussion of convulsive beauty as one of the core concepts of surrealism, see Rosalind Krauss, *The Originality of the Avant-Garde and Other Modernist Myths* (Cambridge: MIT Press, 1986), pp. 112–13.

[20] Henri Ey, "La Psychiatrie devant le surréalisme," *EP*, special issue, 4th installment (1948), 17–18.

[21] Gauthier, p. 17.

war machine against reflection and language."[22] In automatic writing the surrealists believed the unconscious was made transparent in words and images expressed "automatically," written down in a kind of aesthetic free association. The surrealists assumed that the unconscious expressed itself directly, not understanding that all manifestations of automatic writing are mediated articulations that have to be deciphered. In *Nadja*, André Breton mocked the psychiatrist Henri Claude and testified both to the failure of psychiatry to understand the mentally ill and to the success of an art inspired by madness; he meant the art produced by automatic writing.[23] In automatic writing literary production represented a transparent and unmediated expression of desire's violence, a stripping away of all the layers of artificial mediation to a pure level of meaning. With the concept of automatic writing, then, surrealism sought to go beyond the material boundaries of literary form, to do away with the mimetic function of language entirely. The surrealists thus condemned the naïveté of those who believed in the innocent relationship between words and things at the same time as they proposed a new means of attaining that kind of innocence, a "zero-degree" of culture.

The Perfect Crime

Other writers inspired by both surrealism and psychoanalysis also brought crime out of hiding. Short-lived journals such as Bataille's *Documents* published an array of images that the surrealists themselves found repugnant because they represented an absolutely antiromantic vision of human violence.[24] These kinds of images appeared in disparate places. A photograph of a Chinese

[22] Maurice Blanchot, *La Part du feu* (Paris: Gallimard, 1949), p. 93.

[23] Breton, *Nadja*, pp. 39–41. See also the 1930 article "La Médecine mentale devant le surréalisme," in *Point du jour* (Paris: Gallimard, 1970), pp. 88–93. Walter Benjamin noted to what extent Najda was but an instrument in bringing Breton closer to a world to which he would not otherwise have had access. Breton, he said, "is closer to the things that Nadja is close to than to her." Walter Benjamin, *Reflections* (New York: Harcourt, Brace, and Jovanovich, 1979), p. 181. Automatic writing also derived from Charcot, Janet, and experiments with hypnotism at the end of the nineteenth century.

[24] See André Breton's criticism of Bataille in *Manifestoes of Surrealism*, pp. 180–86.

man being tortured and flayed alive appeared in Georges Dumas's *Traité de psychologie* and inspired Bataille's metaphysical musings.[25] Pierre-Jean Jouve also used it as a vehicle for the main character's self-discovery in his novelistic account of psychoanalysis.[26] Beginning in 1920, the psychoanalytically oriented Groupe d'Etudes Philosophiques et Scientifiques pour l'Examen des Idées Nouvelles, founded by the analyst René Allendy, sponsored conferences about irrational forces that escape scientific explanation. Such discussions were often published in the *Revue Française de Psychanalyse*, which included in its 1934 edition a series on "magic thought" to which I have once referred.

In 1937 René Allendy, Bataille, Michel Leiris, and the analysts Adrien Borel and Paul Schiff formed the Société de Psychologie Collective, whose aim, according to Bataille, was "to study the role of psychological factors, and particularly unconscious ones, in social facts; to converge research heretofore undertaken in isolation in diverse disciplines."[27] Though the collective was short-lived, it stayed together long enough to publish a two-part article on circumcision which appeared in *L'Hygiène Mentale* in 1938.[28] The article treated circumcision as a ritualized form of castration and made it part of a broader discussion about the otherness embedded in the most routine practices of so-called civilized nations.

Adrien Borel followed Georges Bataille in looking to the atavistic yearnings of the new, fascist man as testimony to the presence of a collective sacrificial desire within so-called civilized people. He was an unorthodox analyst with strong ties to the Société Psychanalytique de Paris and the avant-garde art world. His occult interests placed him at the margins of French psychoanalysis, with René Allendy and a few others, even though he was one of the founders of the SPP and belonged to what Roudinesco dubs the *groupe chauvin*—Angelo Hesnard, Edouard Pichon, and Henri Co-

[25] Georges Bataille, *L'Expérience intérieure* (Paris: Gallimard, 1954), p. 139. Bataille had been shown the photograph by his own analyst, Adrien Borel.

[26] Pierre-Jean Jouve, *Vagadu* (Paris: Mercure de France, 1963); René Spitz, "Vagadu," *RFP* 3 (1934), 566. For a discussion of Jouve's relationship to psychoanalysis, see Roudinesco, *Lacan and Co.*, pp. 94–100.

[27] Bataille, Notes to "Société de psychologie collective," *Oeuvres complètes* 2:444.

[28] Papers from a symposium "La Circoncision," *HM* (May 1938), 73–85, and pt. 2: (June 1938), 89–96. See also Bataille, "Société de psychologie collective," pp. 281–87.

det.[29] He had also psychoanalyzed many members of the dissident surrealist group that met at Raymond Queneau's apartment in the Desnouettes Square, including Bataille, Leiris, Robert Desnos, Roger Vitrac, and others, and he was closest to Bataille, to whom Borel remained attached his entire life.[30]

Though he did not declare this as his intention, Borel sought to explore the psychic roots of fascism. Thus he was uninterested in its socioeconomic base but wanted to understand the psychological dimensions of fascist power.[31] His 1935 study of the *convulsionnaires* at the Eglise Saint-Médard under the reign of Louis XV was, I think, really an effort to understand the collective psychology of fascism. In that article, Borel tried to explain in psychoanalytic terms the "miracle" occurring at the tomb of a Jansenist deacon named Paris. Men and women who touched the tomb went into convulsions that sent those gathered outside the church into a collective frenzy. The whole episode deeply worried the Jesuit authorities, who were obviously not receptive to the idea that a Jansenist priest might be a saint. What interested Borel, however, was less the ecclesiastical power struggle than the miracle itself. He argued that the miracle unleashed repressed desire in such a way that the spectators did not have to recognize them as their own. They could be passive victims: "The rapprochement around the tomb of the deacon . . . the victims offered up finally by the revelation of the convulsion, numerous victims ready for the worst, defenseless victims doubtless consumed by desire . . . [all this] conspired to provoke a new transformation [of the graveyard into a theater]."[32]

[29] Roudinesco, *Lacan and Co.*, pp. 4, 8–9. This is not to say that Borel was not, first and foremost, a doctor, but that he is best understood as what Roudinesco calls an "occultist." She argues that the occultist emphasis on the spiritual, mystical, and the irrational above the rational demands of science, represented by foreign analysts such as Carl Jung, Wilhelm Reich, and Otto Rank, never penetrated the interior of the SPP. At the same time, Borel's interest in mysticism, art, and the world of dreams and the spirit celebrated by surrealists made him perhaps the most important interwar occultist. It was fitting that near the end of his life he played an older Catholic priest in Robert Bresson's film version of Georges Bernanos's story of a young priest's martyrdom, *Journal d'un curé de campagne*.

[30] Jean Piel, *La Rencontre et la différence* (Paris: Fayard, 1982), p. 116.

[31] For an interesting discussion of French fascism along these lines, see Alice Yaeger Kaplan, *Reproductions of Banality: Fascism, Literature, and French Intellectual Life* (Minneapolis: University of Minnesota Press, 1986), p. 13.

[32] Adrien Borel, "Les Convulsionnaires et le diacre Paris," *EP* no. 4 (1935), 15.

Borel's victims, then, were victims of their own "perverse instincts"; they were neurotics, hysterics, and above all "masochists
avant la lettre" who believed themselves to be overwhelmed by a
transcendent spiritual force. The self-mutilations and tortures the
convulsionnaires inflicted on their own bodies—they dismembered themselves, hurled themselves against walls, and drove nails
through their skin—gave them pleasure, and in this respect their
desires were no different from those of most human beings caught
up in an "ardent crowd":

> We understand better now these particular aspects of collective psy-
> chology in which each person, by the mere fact of being part of a crowd
> and especially of an ardent one, loses his individuality to become
> merely the plaything of emotional currents unleashed by the multi-
> tude. We have seen, in such conditions, the most pusillanimous men
> become heroes animated by a ferocious courage. At Saint-Médard the
> most normal people, once swept up in the fury, and seized by the
> collective enthusiasm, became *convulsionnaires*, and perhaps some-
> times even convulsed and contorted themselves more than the others.

The miracle thus served as a "theater of self-revelation" in which
"profound unconscious tendencies"—the true nature of human-
kind—were revealed.[33] Borel argued that these analyses of collective psychology dissolved the distinctions between normal and
pathological behavior and between male and female behavior,
though he claimed that women made better *convulsionnaires* than
men because of their heightened "nervousness" and "sensitivity."
He insisted that such tendencies were latent in everyone and
would emerge given the right conditions.

In Borel's analysis, the liberation of desire thus has a democratic
effect: It levels distinctions, dissolves boundaries. This desire is by
no means pathological. It doesn't set the *convulsionnaires* off from
normal people but turns normal people into so-called pathological
cases. In so doing, this "collective liberation" of desire dissolves
the distinctions between normality and pathology and, in this particular example, between actor and spectator. Though Borel doesn't
use the word *banal*, one is tempted to say that the self-mutilations
and contortions of the *convulsionnaires* become banal occur-

[33] Ibid., p. 23.

rences, or as Borel himself puts it, "The surprising multiplicity of incidents through which [masochism] manifested itself during these ten years proves in any case the depth of this tendency and also its generality."[34]

Borel, like the surrealists before him, thus defined what it meant to be human in terms of the dissolution of boundaries between pathology—crime or, in Borel's case, the masochistic desire to be wounded—and humanness. And like them, he too sought to recover the authentic, creative self in this quest for a world without boundaries, this desire to have boundaries violated, to be a "plaything" of forces greater than oneself. According to Borel, artistic creation is a privileged state of consciousness in which the true self is recovered in the unbinding of subjectivity. As he argued elsewhere, it is only when the artist plunges into an affective state that he becomes God's equal (a desire Borel linked to infant narcissism). According to Borel, then, Prometheus steals the fire to lose himself in the flame.[35]

Borel thus reinscribed in his own work the paradox at the heart of the surrealist project, the paradox implicit in the "dissolved" boundaries between humanness and criminality. If the true self was to be found in the unbinding of subjectivity, in otherness or crime, then the confounding of the self with its own unraveling was epistemologically complete. Thus, the surrealist quest for an "unmediated unity" between the self and crime had the peculiar effect of dissolving the self.[36] Did not this paradoxical liberation of the true "criminal" self replicate the paradox implicit in the surrealists' liberation of Sade's criminality: that in normalizing Sade they rendered his crimes unreal, made them disappear, made them, as it were, banal? It does seem that this well-intended democratization of crime (and hence of the road to literary greatness) led to the

---

[34] Ibid.

[35] Borel, "La Pensée magique dans l'art" *RFP* 7 (1934), 76. Borel elaborated his ideas in a series of articles including (with Michel Cénac) "L'Obsession," *RFP* 5 (1932), 586–647; "L'Expression de l'ineffable dans les états psychopathiques," *EP* no. 2 (1934), 35–53; "Le Symptôme mental: Valeur et signification," *EP* no. 1 (1947), esp. 111.

[36] Charles Taylor has noted the proximity of surrealism and Italian futurism, which adhered to Mussolini's Fascists. Both desired an "unmediated unity": in futurism (and fascism) between the world and the will, in surrealism between the ego and nature. *Sources of the Self* (Cambridge: Harvard University Press, 1989), p. 471.

absolute leveling of all distinctions. But now it was impossible to tell precisely what drove a writer to be a writer, what made him distinct, so that the writer disappeared without leaving a trace (at least nothing that could be distinguished from anyone else's remains). How in fact could literature be saved from banality, from a lack of distinction, without repudiating a democratic impulse? How could literature avoid elitism (the writer's superiority), on the one hand, and suicide (banality), on the other?

Chapter Seven

Returning to the
Scene of the Crime

In 1929–1930, a group of intellectuals, some of them disaffected surrealists, published a tract titled *Un Cadavre*, in reference to a 1924 surrealist pamphlet of the same name which had
mocked the pompous funeral rites of Anatole France. Supposedly it
was Bataille's idea to include a portrait of Breton as Jesus, with a
crown of blood-stained thorns around his head. The depiction suggested that though the surrealists' literary "crimes" were meant to
dissolve distinctions, Breton in fact fancied himself above the
crowd. It reflected the increasing dissonance within the French
avant-garde and the increasing resentment toward Breton, whose
popelike status was made official when he excommunicated
Robert Desnos, Antonin Artaud, and Bataille from the movement
in 1929.

But Bataille meant to do more than simply call attention to
Breton's lofty status when he portrayed him as Jesus. He wanted to
demonstrate to what extent Breton had succumbed to the logic of
cultural appropriation. If Breton acted as if he were another son of
God, then he had turned his putative renunciation of distinctions
(his outsider or criminal status) into a distinction. That is, in trying
to be true to the crimes that would level distinctions, Breton had in
fact distinguished himself so much that his crime was eventually
applauded, paid for. It was written up no longer in the scandal
sheets but in the columns of art reviews. In 1938, notes Denis
Hollier, "surrealism experienced a success free of scandal," and its

subversive history ended as surrealists "signed paintings, books, and checks like ordinary artists."[1]

Thus, as Bataille saw it, by the very effort to put himself above the crowd, Breton rendered himself banal, an ordinary artist. As the example of Breton demonstrates, when writers proclaim their criminality, when they take a position in relation to the market, they already accept a certain market value. The ineluctability of this logic perhaps explains why Bataille had a penchant for secret societies, which, as one critic has pointed out, constitute distinctions that cannot be seen.[2] In a very late work on the sadist Gilles de Rais, Bataille wrote that crime "is a fact of the human species . . . but it is especially its secret aspect, the impenetrable aspect. . . . Crime hides itself, and that which escapes us is the most horrible." And yet, he goes on, "the nobility of Rais is not a sweet nobility; instead, it "announces the monster."[3] But how exactly can nobility announce a crime (a monster) that at the same time remains hidden? Whereas the surrealists' attempts to announce crime finally hid it, now Bataille's texts both hide and proclaim it. This chapter is about how Bataille reconceived art in terms of a crime announced and yet hidden, how he used crime as a metaphor for literary production. Specifically I want to explore how he reconceived the relationship between literary production and crime, or, more precisely, unconscious desire. But in order to account for Bataille's paradoxical insistence on a rather noisy secrecy, and hence his refusal of cultural appropriation, we must define more precisely his relationship both to surrealism and to fascism.

Elevations

Bataille and those around him appreciated the extent to which surrealism had "underscored the absurdity of the bourgeois world," but they repudiated what Bataille called the surrealists' "Icarian naïveté"—their illusion that they were subversive outsiders, when

[1] Hollier, College of Sociology, p. ix.
[2] For a discussion of secret societies in the work of Roger Caillois, which is also helpful in thinking through Bataille, see Denis Hollier, "Mimesis and Castration, 1937," October 31 (Winter 1984), 13–15. Also Roger Caillois, "Orders, Secret Societies, Churches," in Hollier, College of Sociology, pp. 145–56.
[3] Georges Bataille, Le Procès de Gilles de Rais (Paris: Pauvert, 1972), pp. 11, 47.

"every sentence [Breton] writes situates them *above*."[4] In trying to seize the self in its authenticity, the surrealists merely erected another one above the old, superimposing new values on old ones; bourgeois rebels are nothing if they are not, in spiritual terms, upwardly mobile. The concern the bourgeois rebel shows for the oppressed does not make him a brother in struggle but rather elevates him above the crowd. In Bataille's unflattering portrait, bourgeois rebellions are about self-fashioning, about image, and hence are motivated not by a real desire to change the world but by a desire to see oneself as a noble soul. But whereas real nobles, remember, are discreet—they hide—this quest for nobility is ultimately a quest for attention:

> In December 1929, M. Breton did not hesitate to make himself ridiculous by writing that "the simplest surrealist act consists of dashing down into the street, pistol in hand, and firing blindly, as fast as you can pull the trigger, into the crowd." That such an image should present itself so insistently to his view proves decisively the importance in his pathology of castration reflexes: such an extreme provocation seeks to draw immediate and brutal punishment. But the worst is not to be subject to reactions of this order (which no bourgeois rebel, it goes without saying, could have avoided); the *literary* use to which they are put is much more significant. Others instinctively know how blocked impulses are to be taken into account. The surrealists employ them in literature, in order to attain the displaced and pathetic grandeur that ridicules and strips them of relevance.

Bourgeois rebels demand a response, a "brutal punishment," to testify to the significance of their gestures. But as Bataille noted, "to the loss of a head there is no . . . reply."[5]

Thus, if this desire for recognition has subversive potential—a real desire to risk one's head—it aspires too high, manifests itself in what Bataille called a "will to poetic agitation" which seeks to change the world by transposing it into heaven. Didn't Sade's world, as the surrealists conceived it, become surreal and hence dreamlike, a place, like heaven, that exists nowhere but in the

---

[4] Bataille, "The Old Mole and the Prefix *sur* in the Words *Surhomme* and Surrealist," *Visions of Excess*, p. 42.

[5] Ibid., pp. 39, 43.

mind it freed? Wasn't it true that the surrealists themselves were self-styled martyrs trying to go to heaven—that is to say, above the world—and hence could their art be criminal without finally expelling the crime, without cleansing the writer's soul? Surrealist literature—and this was what Bataille meant when he decried the literary use to which the surrealists put their blocked masochistic impulses—betrayed the writer's original criminal purpose: He loses his head not in the service of crime but in order to get to heaven.

In the very act of writing about crime, then, crime is quite literally expelled, repented. As Bataille stated in reference to the surrealists' worship of Sade, "In the most favorable cases, the author of *Justine* is in fact thus treated as any given foreign body; in other words, he is only an object of transports to the extent that these transports facilitate his excretion (his peremptory expulsion)." In the surrealists' anal-retentive psyches, Sade has only the "use value" of excrement: "For the most part, one most often only loves the rapid (and violent) pleasure of voiding this matter and no longer seeing it."[6] When crime tries to be an art, the thrill of subversion becomes indistinguishable from the thrill of cleansing the soul.[7]

In Bataille's view, fascism also ended up turning its adherents into martyrs. In contrast to many of his contemporaries, Bataille recognized and sought to analyze fascist power—as Borel did after him—in psychological rather than in socioeconomic terms. His interest in the psychic, religious, and emotional yearnings implicit in fascist politics was part of a broader critique of the "instrumental reason" that he believed characterized capitalism and parliamentary democracy.[8] It is important to note in this regard that parliamentary democracy had been discredited in France during the interwar years by both the Left and the Right, though the immediate reference for Bataille's essay was Hitler's rise to power. The Stavisky Affair exposed corruption in government; the Popular Front, squeezed between the demands of its constituents and the pressures of business interests, had failed to fulfill its promise and

[6]Bataille, "The Use Value of D. A. F. de Sade (an Open Letter to My Current Comrades)," in *Visions of Excess,* p. 92.

[7]But this is not a cleansing that is infinitely deferred, that requires the perpetuation of crime, as in Klossowski's analysis of Sade. It is instead a cleansing that is completely confounded with subversion.

[8]Bataille, "The Notion of Expenditure," in *Visions of Excess,* pp. 116–29.

had not even come to the aid of the Spanish republicans; the French Right's motto was "Better Hitler than Blum."

Bataille's interest in fascism was thus most fundamentally an interest in how the other was embedded in so-called civilized cultures. That is, as Allan Stoekl has argued, it was no longer enough to "glorify Sade or the Papin sisters and posit a purely fantasmatic gratuitous act: the order of the day was how to consider violence and ecstasy *in* society and political formations."[9] Fascism rendered this kind of analysis all the more urgent. A year after Bataille's essay on fascism was published and some months after fascist rioters clashed with police at the Place de la Concorde, Jean Paulhan asked André Gide why and under what conditions civilized societies might feel the need to wrench themselves apart. Paulhan implicitly linked that need to the other embedded within the self.[10]

In the essay Bataille published in *La Critique Sociale* in 1933, he analyzed fascist power in terms of a renewal of what he called the "heterogeneous" forces of human life, a revision of Emile Durkheim's concept of the sacred. Bataille conceived culture as composed of homogenous and heterogeneous forces. Homogenous forces were those that dominated bourgeois culture and could be defined in terms of use value: "Homogeneity signifies here the commensurability of elements and the awareness of this commensurability: human relations are sustained by a reduction to fixed rules based on the consciousness of the possible identity of delineable persons and situations. . . . Homogeneous society is productive society, namely, useful society." Joining Marx's critique of commodity fetishism to Durkheim's sociology, Bataille thus conceived homogeneity above all as the reduction of human life under capitalism to its economic or useful function, the whole to its parts: "According to the judgment of homogenous society, each man is worth what he produces; in other words, he stops being an existence *for itself*."[11]

To define heterogeneity, Bataille drew on his own reading of anthropologist Marcel Mauss's "Essay on the Gift" (1925), which ana-

[9] Stoekl, "Nizan, Drieu, and the Question of Death," p. 117.

[10] Frederic J. Grover, "Les Années 30 dans la correspondance Gide-Paulhan," *Modern Language Notes* 95 (May 1980), 840.

[11] Bataille, "The Psychological Structure of Fascism," in *Visions of Excess*, pp. 142, 138.

lyzed the ritual of potlatch in primitive societies. In potlatch, a tribal leader offers a gift meant to obligate, humiliate, or defy a rival by virtue of its sumptuousness. Such competition took the form not only of giving but of destroying (one's own) wealth. Bataille modeled his concept of the heterogeneous in modern culture after this ritual offering and "destruction of spectacular wealth" which defied the instrumental reason inherent in capitalist economies. He theorized the heterogeneous as "unproductive expenditure," as an incommensurate excess, the surplus energy of the laborer which capitalist production processes cannot measure. It was thus possible to understand the heterogeneous in positive terms, as a force that exists for itself. "However," Bataille noted, "an explicit understanding of the sacred, whose field of application is relatively vast, presents considerable difficulties. Durkheim faced the impossibility of providing it with a positive scientific definition: he settled for characterizing the sacred world negatively as being absolutely heterogeneous compared to the profane. It is nevertheless possible to admit that the sacred is known positively, at least implicitly." Bataille claimed heterogeneity was "identical to the structure of the unconscious" and that its exclusion from bourgeois culture was analogous to the exclusion of repressed material from the unconscious.[12] Because the bourgeoisie had become slaves to the homogenizing forces of capitalist social relations, heterogeneity was concentrated in the working class, who by analogy were the bourgeoisie's own repressed material. Fascism drew its force from this unconscious, as it were, from the affective dimension of human existence which characterized primitive societies and their symbolic structures.

Because fascism used powerful symbolic rituals both to mobilize the masses and to ground its authority, because it aestheticized politics, to paraphrase Walter Benjamin,[13] Bataille conceived fascism as "one of the numerous forms of royal authority." Like royalty, fascism unites "the heterogeneous elements with the homogenous elements, . . . sovereignty in the strictest sense with the State." He said that fascism was the "sovereign form of sovereignty." It situates its authority "above any utilitarian judg-

---

[12] Ibid., pp. 120–26, 142, 141.
[13] Walter Benjamin, *Illuminations*, trans. and ed. Hannah Arendt (New York: Schocken, 1969), p. 241.

ment," in a charismatic leader who embodies a state that exists for itself. But the state's status as something other, and hence as heterogeneous, merely provides the foundation for a more rigidly imposed homogeneity. Bataille argued that the leader is "exalted," "noble," and "higher." If the heterogeneous nature of the slave is "akin to that of the filth in which his material situation condemns him to live, that of the master is formed by an act excluding all filth: an act pure in direction but sadistic in form."[14] Thus, while the fascist leader taps into emotions that bourgeois culture consigns to the pathological and the irrational, he nevertheless establishes his "strict authority":

> In opposition to the impoverished existence of the oppressed, political sovereignty initially presents itself as a clearly differentiated sadistic activity [one that is not also masochistic]. . . . The differentiation can be more or less complete—individually, sovereigns have been able to live power in part as an orgy of blood—but, on the whole, within the heterogeneous domain, the imperative royal form has historically effected an exclusion of impoverished and filthy forms sufficient to permit a connection with homogenous forms at a certain level.[15]

While the fascist leader appeals to subversive, masochistic desires, he aspires too high, manifests his authority in a pure sadism that reinforces his position above the crowd: He weeds out dissent, subversion, and "filth."

This fascist will to power is thus rooted in a pure heterogeneity[16] that "appears in human terms, to be the noblest—exalted to majesty—pure in the midst of the orgy, beyond the reach of human infirmities." The leader "fulfills the *ideal* of society." He upholds an ideal that is in fact above the world and is therefore ultimately nowhere; it "exists for itself by denying itself."[17] Or the ideal exists only by repressing all that it deems impure. The fascist attempt to unleash the power of the heterogeneous—of deviance, subversion, boundarylessness, and filth—thus becomes indistinguishable from its attempt to purify or cleanse the nation. When crime is raised to

---

14 Bataille, "The Psychological Structure of Fascism," pp. 155, 145, 146.
15 Ibid.
16 For example, "having become the negation of the principle of utility, it refuses all subordination." Ibid., p. 148.
17 Ibid.

the level of art, as in the aestheticized politics of fascism, the thrill of subversion becomes indistinguishable from the necessity of murder.

Self-Loss and Politics

Bataille was interested in the emotions fascism unleashed precisely because they confirmed his belief in the transgressive, antiutilitarian, and hence revolutionary quality of self-loss. Translated into political terms, his celebration of self-loss was not always easy to distinguish from a fascist celebration of self-sacrifice, from the paradoxical self-fulfillment through self-annihilation to which fascist sympathizers such as Pierre Drieu la Rochelle and Henri de Motherlant so often alluded. Much of Bataille's language, from his advocacy of a political strategy called *surfascisme* to his claim that war would restore men to their virility, raised and still raises eyebrows.[18] Rumor even has it that Bataille hoped to stage a public human sacrifice, but that he could not find anyone willing to play the role of executioner.[19]

In 1935 Breton and his followers accused Bataille of being complicitous with fascism, and a couple of years later, in 1937, surrealists claimed that the Collège de Sociologie, founded that year by Bataille, Leiris, and Roger Caillois, had fascist sympathies.[20] In the first instance, these accusations can be traced back to the rivalry between Bataille and Breton which resurfaced in the antifascist group Contre-Attaque, in which they tried to reconcile for a short time. Bataille had thrown his weight behind a strategy that Jean Dautry had rather unfortunately termed *surfascisme*, and Breton and his followers used the word as a pretext to attack Bataille.[21]

The *surfasciste* spectacle—say, a sacrifice—would transcend the mechanized structures of both fascism and liberal democracy by turning the street into a theater. It would lift the people out of their individual selves and suspend them in the embrace of a spiritual

---

[18] Bataille, "The Sorcerer's Apprentice," in *The College of Sociology*, pp. 13–14. See also "Declaration of the College of Sociology on the International Crisis," p. 45.

[19] Roger Caillois, *Approche de l'imaginaire* (Paris: Gallimard, 1974), p. 93.

[20] *Clé* no. 1 (January 1939), 8.

[21] For an account of Contre-Attaque and the origins of *surfascisme*, see Henri Dubief, "Témoinage sur Contre-Attaque (1935–36)," *Textures* 6 (1970), 52–60.

community. "We need to know how to appropriate the arms created by our adversaries," wrote Bataille.[22]

But Bataille conceived the very nature of this spectacle as symbolic; participants transcend themselves by identifying with the
sacrificial victim. They experience an essentially vicarious death,
self-loss, and hence oneness with the community. Thus, as Bataille
conceived it, the spectacle is a simulation of self-loss which feels
real, a mimetic reproduction of an experience that can be experienced only through an imaginary identification with the victim. In
this sense, *surfascisme* as strategy represented an effort to challenge fascism with an "organic antifascist movement" to which
Bataille and other antifascist intellectuals subscribed as an alternative to Soviet-style communism.[23] *Surfascisme* would permit
the kind of self-transgression and affirmation of community characteristic of fascist movements without degenerating into real
murder. It would preclude a fascist celebration of the nation and
hence an ultimately self-destructive erasure of the boundaries between self and other.

The heterogeneous or other can thus be rendered only as art, as
spectacle, through a mimetic gesture that gives expression to its
unassimilable forces while protecting individuals from the inevitable consequences of uncontrolled violence. Nevertheless, the merging of the impulse to create with the heterogeneous *is* inspired by
an attempt to reintegrate art into the body, to blend the stage with
the street. The concept of *surfascisme* thus drew on the aestheticized politics characteristic of fascist ritual: it moves from the
logocentrism of liberal democracy to the iconographic emphasis of
fascism.

In the sense that Bataille failed to provide an unambiguous guide
to political action and insisted on individuals' own complicity in,
or attraction to, the violence they sought to combat, he was "complicitous" with fascism. It is not clear, after all, how his antifascist
strategy could be made concrete except in terms of what we know
from the rumors about his desire to perform public sacrifices. What
is clear, however, is the difficulty of turning a theory of subjectivity
rooted in eroticism and (primarily masochistic) pleasure into a
guide for political action, whose impetus, even if fraught with am-

[22] Bataille, "Vers la révolution réelle," *Oeuvres complètes* 1:421.
[23] Ibid., p. 424.

biguity, must finally be unambiguous.[24] It is thus perhaps not surprising that Bataille's interest in manifestations of the heterogeneous—in myths, rituals, and above all, the restoration of spiritual community in a hopelessly atomized world—left him open to charges of collusion with fascism. "In those days," Hollier notes, "rightly or wrongly, anything less than blind rejection of fascism was taken for complicity, as if even theoretical concern would inevitably constitute a first step toward sympathy."[25]

As I have noted, the surrealists and others on the Left accused the Collège de Sociologie of having fascist tendencies. The founding of the college in 1937 furthered the agenda implicit in Bataille's analysis of fascism. It was conceived as an antidote to surrealism and, more specifically, as a sort of institutionalized counter to the universalist, humanist exposition of "Man" at the Musée de l'Homme in 1936, where Leiris, a writer and ethnographer, worked.[26] While purporting to represent universal man, the exhibit reinforced the conception of so-called primitive man as other, as an exotic display in a museum, to be observed, digested, and appreciated. That is, primitive man remained safely outside rather than embedded in contemporary Western civilization.[27]

The members of the college conceived their function as the study of the sacred in everyday life. That is, they sought to apply Durkheimian sociology and Maussian anthropological theories to the study of modern Western societies and focused on myths, rituals, secret societies, religion, festivals, and so forth. In spite of their differences (and their differences were great) they were committed to exploring the ways in which the other was both embedded in and excluded from the self, how the other was hidden—excluded, repressed, veiled—but did not disappear. The college attracted a large

[24]On this point, see Denis Hollier, "On Equivocation (between Literature and Politics)," *October* 55 (Winter 1990), 3–22; and Bersani, *Culture of Redemption*, pp. 117–22.

[25]Hollier, "Mimesis and Castration," p. 4.

[26]On the juxtaposition of the two, see James Clifford, *The Predicament of Culture: Twentieth-Century Ethnography, Literature, Art* (Cambridge: Harvard University Press, 1987), pp. 139–48.

[27]On the college, see Hollier, *The College of Sociology*; Jean Jamin, "Un Sacré Collège; ou, Les Apprentis sorciers de la sociologie," *Cahiers Internationaux de Sociologie* 68 (January–June 1980), 5–30; Marina Galletti, "Masses: A Failed Collège?" *Stanford French Review* (Spring 1988), 49–63.

number of intellectuals, including Jean Paulhan, Pierre Klossowski, Alexandre Kojève, and even Walter Benjamin.

The college's founders were not fascists. In fact, most of them
were active antifascists. I do not mean that there was no proximity
between their interests and fascism. There was, as I have suggested
in regard to Bataille, and it should be explored. But that exploration
must distinguish carefully between different constructions of the
dissolution of the boundary between self and other.[28] Proximity, in
other words, should not necessarily be considered cause for indict-
ment but instead should perhaps lead to a careful assessment of
how effective or subversive a politics based (in Bataille's case) on
the necessity of self-loss can be, to an assessment of the limits of
certain kinds of critiques of instrumental reason. Or it might lead,
on another level, to a reassessment of how we define politics itself.[29]

Whether Bataille's thought is problematic on this level or not is a
complicated question the dimensions of which would require a
separate treatment. Suffice it to say that what Bataille said about
both surrealism and fascism was that each in a different fashion
turned crime into art at the expense of crime itself—that is, both
conflated crime with the unbinding of the self, with self-sacrifice.
The desire to be above, in other words, was inseparable from a
desire for self-destruction, for death. When crime and art are confounded so completely that crime is art, then, if we follow
Bataille's line of reasoning, criminal subversion can be accounted
for only as the desire to be martyred, to expel or be punished for the
crime. For Bataille, "to the loss of a head there can be no reply," but
how does one live without a head?

[28] The relationship between Bataille and fascism has been addressed primarily
through an analysis of his concept of sovereignty. For example, Martin Jay has
written of this in an unpublished paper, "The Reassertion of Sovereignty in a Time
of Crisis: Carl Schmitt and Georges Bataille"; and see Hollier, "On Equivocation,"
pp. 12–15.

[29] The debate about the relationship between certain philosophical positions and
fascist politics has recently been ignited by the controversies around Martin
Heidegger and Paul de Man. Subtler connections are drawn between poststructuralism and right-wing politics (or at least a politics of complacency) by Nancy
Fraser in her discussion of the "French Derrideans." Nancy Fraser, Unruly Practices: Power, Discourse, and Gender in Contemporary Social Theory (Minneapolis:
University of Minnesota Press, 1989), pp. 69–92.

Literature and Punishment

Bataille constructed an image of writing as a paradoxical decapitation that precipitates a return to the scene of the crime, in which the utilitarian and moral purposes of the guillotine are reconceived as self-sacrifices *that make crime and literature possible.* According to Bataille, the guillotine does not represent the finality of justice so much as an "eternal return" of culpability, the self-punitive drive of a masochism ever unsatisfied (to which there is never a satisfactory reply): "The 'eye of the conscience' and the 'woods of justice' incarnate eternal recurrence, and is there any more desperate image for remorse?" Decapitation—any self-mutilation for that matter—is thus the necessary precondition for any literary undertaking, which is perhaps why Bataille mourned the intractability of his own "philosopher's head."[30] It is perhaps not surprising, in this regard, that Bataille chose the name Henri Troppmann, that of the brother of the celebrated criminal decapitated in 1871, as his pseudonym for *W.C.* or that the "hero" in *Le Bleu du ciel,* a masochist and necrophiliac, bears the same name.

Thus, in Bataille, literature is born of a wound that does not heal. This notion is supported by Bataille's method of healing his personal wounds. In response to his brother Martial's distress over Bataille's purported misrepresentation of their parents in an interview with *L'Express* in 1961, Bataille begged forgiveness on grounds that he had suffered from depression:

> I want to tell you this [he wrote his brother]: what happened to me nearly fifty years ago still makes me want to tremble, and I'm not surprised that at that time I was not able to find another way of helping myself than by expressing myself anonymously. I was cared for by a doctor [the psychoanalyst Adrien Borel] (my state being serious) who told me that the means that I employed, in spite of everything, were the best I could find.[31]

Many of Bataille's books, including *W.C.,* which he burned, and *L'Histoire de l'oeil* (*Story of the Eye*), were indeed written pseudonymously, the first, as I said, under the name Troppmann,

---

[30] Georges Bataille, *Story of the Eye* (London: Penguin, 1979), p. 76, 75.
[31] Bataille, Notes to *Histoire de l'oeil, Oeuvres complètes* 1:644.

the second under the name Lord Auch. Pseudonymity, he later claimed, "is the transgression of all language."[32] It is this transgression, this paradoxical strategy in which the author silences himself, which structures Bataille's oeuvre. Because it is written pseudonymously, his work constitutes the presence of an author who is absent; it loses its point of reference and unravels, occupying a space between presence and absence—between writing (authorial intentionality) and silence (into which the author has slipped). Writing, in this sense, is a form of self-mutilation, a slip of the pen in which the author effaces himself while remaining present. And insofar as the author remains an ever-elusive presence he is, metaphorically speaking, mutilated.

The notion that writing pseudonymously functions as a psychoanalytic cure seems odd from this perspective, for it confounds the cure and the pathology. Yet, as Bataille's interpretation of Van Gogh suggests, self-mutilation inspires rather than diminishes creation; it is the gesture that separates the painter who makes a contribution to art history from the painter who, like Van Gogh, "paints the bloody myth of human existence." Thus Van Gogh's self-mutilation generated an "explosion" of sunlight in his paintings, a mesmerizing light of such intensity that it blinds, burns the eyes out—hence the "close association between the solar flower obsession and the most exasperated torment becomes all the more expressive when the heightened fancy of the painter sometimes leads to the representation of the flower as withered and dead." Bataille argued that Van Gogh's painting was thus the metaphorical equivalent of the artist's self-mutilation—his sacrifice. It was a "throwing oneself out of oneself," a glorious enucleation that made vision possible, that freed the artist to "offend polite society" with a "love that refused to take anything into account and in a way spat in the faces of all those who have accepted the elevated and official idea of life that is so well known."[33] The sun, like Van Gogh, like art, must "die," transposed into a withered sunflower at the same time as it retains its inspirational force.

When Bataille began to write about Van Gogh's self-mutilation, his psychoanalyst Adrien Borel referred him to a clinical study

---

[32] Bataille, Notes to *Madame Edwarda*, ibid., 3:493.

[33] Bataille, "Sacrificial Mutilation and the Severed Ear of Vincent Van Gogh," *Visions of Excess*, pp. 63, 67, 70–71.

Borel and his colleagues had published in the *Annales Médico-Psychologiques* in 1924. Bataille claimed that this study of one Gaston F., another self-mutilator, only confirmed his own interpretation of Van Gogh. Gaston F.'s self-mutilation—he had bitten off his finger—similarly had no explicable motive, and after extensive psychiatric examination, the young man was confirmed to have been in full possession of his reason (and here we should recall the mystery of unmotivated crime explored in Chapter 1). His self-mutilation seems to have been a form of self-sacrifice by which he attempted to cure himself, to "vanquish a feeling of inner powerlessness." Gaston F.'s act was a way, as he put it himself, of "getting out of this state." The authors of the case study confirmed this assessment. They concluded that such apparently pathological behavior was Gaston's way of "readapting to the environment," reflecting a struggle between the pull of an interior, affective life and the necessity of adjusting to the demands of reality.[34]

Such a potentially "useful suicide," as Gaston called it,[35] this pathological gesture reconceived as a cure, suggests a paradoxical notion of utility in which uselessness becomes useful: A mutilated hand leads to the discovery of a new inner power—for Gaston, the renewal of his artistic talents—in an endless play of normality and pathology which dissolves into a cure that is always a form of pathology. It is precisely because the cure (the purpose of self-mutilation) sought by Gaston F., by Van Gogh, and by Bataille himself does not conform to any conventional notion of utility and is in fact purposeless within a rational or utilitarian economy that the disease cannot be diagnosed or its motivation explained in traditional psychiatric terms. Such a self-mutilation remains outside the limits of scientific explanation, which needs to establish some verifiable relationship between cause and effect. Yet the origins of self-mutilation perpetually elude rational explanation because, as with criminality, they are to be found not in any utilitarian motive, but in a desire to be wounded, in a pathology, like *autopunition*, that is always already a cure.

Likewise, decapitation only simulates sacrifice. As pseudonyms are simulacra of authors, and as the withered sunflower is a sim-

---

[34]Ibid., p. 259. See also Henri Claude, Adrien Borel, Gilbert Robin, "Une Automutilation révélatrice d'un état schizomaniaque," *AMP* (March 1924), 334–38.
[35]Claude, Borel, Robin, "Une Automutilation révélatrice," p. 334.

ulacrum of the sun, crime, the drive to the guillotine, is only the simulacrum of a cure. Writing, too, is the simulation of a cure, generated by the violence of a self-mutilation that wounds in order to heal.

Therapy

After writing his first novel, *Story of the Eye,* Bataille sought to decode it with the aid of psychoanalysis. In 1925 he had been driven to Adrien Borel's couch by his obsessions, in particular a propensity to necrophilia. He claimed that his analysis "had a decisive result; it ended in August 1927 after the mishaps and failures with which I had long struggled [had been resolved]."[36]

Remember that Borel had encouraged Bataille to write as a means of working through his obsessions, and indeed, *W.C.* was a product of this analysis, as were *Story of the Eye* and its autobiographical supplement, *Coincidences.* Bataille claimed that the supplement was a psychoanalytic exercise employed to decode the meaning concealed in the obscene images of *Story of the Eye.* He stated that he "began writing with no precise goal, animated chiefly by a desire to forget, at least for the time being, the things I can be or do personally."[37] In a reversal of psychoanalytic practice, he defined symbolic transformation as essential to the cure, or at least to the garnering of psychoanalytic knowledge. Hence Bataille claimed that he could restore his memories to life only by "transforming them and making them unrecognizable, at first glance, to my eyes, solely because during that deformation they acquired the lewdest of meanings."[38]

Story of the Eye, like much of Bataille's work, is filled with "obscenities" and "perversions." But how exactly did writing about perversion "cure" Bataille of his perversion? How did transforming his memories serve a revelatory function, and what are the implications of this logic for literary production? How, then, did Bataille conceive the relationship, decoded in *Coincidences,* between his unconscious desire and his novel? Or to put it in more

---

[36] Bataille, "Notice autobiographique," *Oeuvres complètes* 7:460.
[37] Bataille, *Story of the Eye,* p. 64.
[38] Ibid., p. 74.

conventional psychoanalytic terms to which Bataille himself alluded, how did he resolve or not resolve his Oedipus complex?

In the oedipal drama, the son is terrified of the paternal prohibition of the mother, and his terror is symbolized by castration anxiety. The son's attachment to his mother and his ambivalence toward his father reach such an intolerable peak of intensity that he introjects the father and hence identifies with him. Yet in *Coincidences* Bataille never clarifies precisely what his feelings were for his mother. He does not mention incestuous desire, at least not for her. We do know that in *W.C.*, the work he claimed to have burned, Bataille declared that he had masturbated before his mother's corpse.[39] Furthermore, Denis Hollier reminds us that Bataille is, after all, the author of *Ma Mère*, a novel in which the mother and her female lover offer the son a thorough sexual education.[40]

But if there is evidence to suggest that Bataille had an incestuous attachment to his mother, his own account suggests something different: "However, the very contrary of most male babies, who are in love with their mothers, I was in love with my father."[41] Bataille in fact sexualizes his father, who is blind, syphilitic, and sadistic: "This [beating] has the effect of reminding me that my father being young would have wanted to do something atrocious to me with pleasure."[42] In Bataille's eyes, however, his father's sadism does not diminish but empowers him, distinguishes him from the run of the mill and makes him desirable. Above all, Bataille remembers, with a mixture of pleasure and terror, or more precisely, a terror that is experienced as pleasurable, the punishments his father inflicted on him when he was a boy. Speaking of a dream whose associations he tried to decipher, Bataille wrote: "Terrors of childhood spiders etc. linked to the memory of having my pants down on my father's knees. Kind of ambivalence between the most horrible and the most magnificent." Or another memory: "I'm something like three years old my legs naked on my father's knees and my penis bloody like the sun. This for playing with a hoop. My father slaps me and I see the sun."[43]

[39] Ibid., p. 76.
[40] Denis Hollier, "Bataille's Tomb: A Halloween Story," *October* 33 (Summer 1985), 102.
[41] Bataille, *Story of the Eye*, p. 72.
[42] Bataille, "Dream," *Visions of Excess*, p. 4.
[43] Ibid.

Thus, once again we are confronted with the ambiguity of the paternal imago, its function as center of prohibition and sublimation. Here, Bataille's ambivalence reiterates the ambivalence characteristic of the entire oedipal drama—that the father is at once the object of rivalry (and love) and of sublimation. But what were the implications of this oedipal dilemma for Bataille's concept of writing? We recall that Lacan, confronted with the same dilemma, sought to "save" father and son from the consequences of imaginary identification by diminishing the natural foundation of the father's authority in favor of what he later called a symbolic one. But Bataille was not a psychoanalyst, and unlike Lacan, he was not attempting to challenge the authority of men who sought to save the father at all costs. So what do we make of Bataille's portrait of his father? Does his homosexual, masochistic, ambivalent love for his father render him more perverse than his surrealist counterparts? Or is he just stuck, as Lacan would have it, at an imaginary stage of development?

Recently, Susan Suleiman raised a question about how perverse "perverse" avant-garde work really is. That is, she questions the revolutionary claims of surrealist painters as well as Bataille's "subversive intent." She asks whether their perversity represents a rebellion against the father, whose authority they claim to challenge: "Could one of the underlying fantasies fueling this programmatic avant-garde picture be not the 'straight' Oedipal fantasy of displacing the father and sexually possessing the mother, but its homosexual variant: the fantasy of being sexually possessed by the father? That fantasy is perverse, to be sure. But is it a sign of rebellion against the father?" In other words, avant-garde work looks perverse, but if we explore its origins in terms of the artist's unconscious fantasies, we discover that the rebellion against the "father"—Marcel Duchamps's parody of the *Mona Lisa*, Max Ernst's parody of Parmigianino's *Madonna of the Long Neck*—veils a real "fascination with the phallus."[44] That rebellion disguises a repudiation of the mother's perceived castration and hence a resumption of the phallic position in the artist's very effort to denounce it. Both Duchamps's *Mona Lisa* and Ernst's *Blessed Virgin Chastizing the Infant Jesus before Three Witnesses* are blasphemous—Duchamps paints a moustache on the *Mona Lisa*, Ernst

---

[44] Suleiman, *Subversive Intent*, pp. 153, 161.

paints a muscular virgin spanking the infant Jesus. At the same time, these women represent "phallic mothers" because they rebel against the father while repudiating the mother's femininity.

The surrealists were thus ultimately, if unconsciously, complicitous with patriarchal norms. "Could it be," asks Suleiman, "that the son's rebellion, whether 'straight' or 'perverse' and no matter how outrageously innovative on the level of artistic practice, is always in the last analysis, phallocentric—and to that extent in alliance with the father and repudiating the mother?"[45] Breton's expression of distaste for male homosexuality gives power to Suleiman's argument that the surrealists may indeed have repressed (in other instances) their real adherence to gender norms.[46] Other feminist commentators have reached the same conclusion about the surrealists' "subversion" of patriarchal conventions. It is more difficult to make this argument about Bataille, however, since he was contemptuous of what he saw as the surrealists' refusal of perversion. Remember that he criticized the surrealists' idealist effort to elevate the perverse to the status of art, thereby expelling the perversity from perversion and compromising their subversive intent.

Unlike the surrealists, who celebrated *l'amour fou*—the summit of true, heterosexual, monogamous love—Bataille uninhibitedly announced his perverse, because fundamentally homosexual, pleasure and its unconscious origin. Whereas the surrealist's ambiguous attitude toward castration can be decoded in works that are "subversive" of patriarchal norms, Bataille embraced ambiguity, declared his perverse love for his sadistic father proudly and provocatively. But is he truly subversive because he "says it all," because he refuses to idealize perversion and hence expel it? And if not, if both Bataille and the surrealists reiterated paternal authority, how can we account for the distinction between their quite different models of literary production?

To begin, we can look at how Bataille explained the genesis of *Story of the Eye*. In spite of his father's sickliness, Bataille insisted that he took this pathological and yet noble man as a role model.

---

[45] Ibid., p. 161.
[46] André Breton et al., "Recherches sur la sexualité," *La Révolution Surréaliste*, March 15, 1928, pp. 32–40. Many of his comrades, including Jacques Prévert and Pierre Unik, joined Breton in his opinion. Raymond Queneau, however, did not share their revulsion.

Bataille identified with his father, who laid down the law not by incarnating moral order but by destroying it.[47] In a well-known episode from *Coincidences*, Bataille recounted that while his mother and the doctor attending his father were in the next room, his father cried out, "Doctor, let me know when you're done fucking my wife!" "For me," Bataille claimed, "that utterance, which in a split second annihilated the demoralizing effects of a strict upbringing, left me with something like a steady obligation, unconscious and unwilled: the necessity of finding an equivalent to that sentence in any situation I happen to be in: and this largely explains *Story of the Eye.*"[48]

As Suleiman interprets this passage, the father "reveals to the son that the mother's body is sexual. . . . The recognition of the mother's body as female and desirable [is] a recognition forced on the son by his blind but still powerful father." The paternal dictate at once reveals and sublimates the mother's sexualized body, and this body comes to haunt Bataille's work, to constitute the "source of the narrator's pornographic imagination." The text is thus the metaphorical equivalent of the mother's body, which "in its duplicity as asexual maternal and sexual feminine, is the very emblem of the contradictory coexistence of transgression and prohibition, purity and defilement." The text is a metaphor of the mother's duplicitous body to the extent that it expresses both the son's fear of and his desire to transgress the paternal prohibition. In so doing, it represents a "confrontation between an all-powerful father and a traumatized son—staged across and over the body of the mother."[49]

The text in this view thus does not "release" the sexualized maternal body—the other—as the surrealists hoped it would, but instead sublimates it. Like the introjection of the father through which the boy both compensates for and renounces his desire for the mother, the novel—the "pornographic imagination"—remembers and yet renounces or immobilizes desire, forgets or sublimates

[47] It is interesting to note that Klossowski in his psychoanalytic study of Sade claimed that Sade identified with "the father of the family who destroys the family." As I have argued, this pattern is central in Lacan, the reception of Sade, and now in Bataille, albeit in different ways. See Klossowski, "Eléments d'une étude psychanalytique," p. 466.

[48] Bataille, *Story of the Eye*, p. 73.

[49] Suleiman, *Subversive Intent*, pp. 85, 87.

it. The mother is but an emblem, then, for the struggle between
father and son in which the father's law, as it were, triumphs.
Writing marks the passage through which the boy becomes a man.
If Bataille's claim that writing cured him of his obsessions is placed
in this context, then writing made him "whole" again, made him a
man, by repressing identification with the mother. Thus, the text
is only apparently feminized, only apparently born of an alliance
between mother and son.

But Bataille's text does not simply reinforce the father's law; it
reinforces the law in *new terms*. After all, the father upholds the
law by destroying it. That is, Bataille's writing is allied with the
father, but the terms of that alliance shift. Bataille remains, to be
sure, a man, but a different sort of man; he remains heterosexual,
but he is a straight man with a twist. Bataille's repudiation of
castration is not that clear-cut, that neatly sublimated. But I don't
want to argue that his work is more perverse than the surrealists'
simply because he writes about necrophilia, or about lovemaking
in the midst of manure (*Story of the Eye*) or in cemeteries (*The Blue
of Noon*). Bataille's literary obsessions are not unmediated expressions of desire but displacements that symbolize repressed desire, like dreams. Thus, his work is not about the mother but about
how the son copes with the paternal prohibition.

Bataille's case is complicated because he did love his father and
thus (if we are to follow Freud) identified with his "castrated"
mother. But he does not, as Freud argued in "A Child Is Being
Beaten," replace his unconscious fantasy about being beaten
(which functions as a regressive substitute for being loved) by his
father with a conscious fantasy of being beaten by his mother
(Duchamps's and Ernst's phallic mothers)—this in order to defend
against homosexual desire. In Bataille, we recall, it is not the mother who appears as other, as castrated, as the site of fear and desire,
but the syphilitic, sadistic, and blind (in Freudian terms, castrated)
father.[50] In fact, what is significant about Bataille's account of his
childhood (and hence of the unconscious genesis of the text) is that
it is characterized not by a rivalry over the mother, as Hollier
himself notes, but by the son's desire to be beaten—to be loved—

[50]Note that Suleiman remarks that the father is "blind but still powerful" but
does not find the description irreconcilable with a traditional oedipal reading. It is
surprising that she does not, since in Freudian terms, blindness symbolizes castration.

by his father, to "see the sun." In short, as Bataille made quite clear, the object of his desire is less the mother than the horrible, sadistic, authoritarian father who lays down the law by destroying it. Thus, the *father* is the site of both otherness *and* the law, prohibition and sublimation.[51]

Borch-Jacobsen argues that this sort of scenario in fact best describes Lacan's version of Oedipus, that in Lacan the object of rivalry is not the mother but the "phallic object that he [the boy] would like to be."[52] Thus, the identification that would make Bataille a man is, paradoxically, also the identification that revives the aggressive ambivalence immanent in the son's relation to the primary object of identification—here, the father. In Bataille (as we have already seen in Lacan's analysis of the excessive superegos) the Oedipus complex, which is normally desexualized if properly resolved, is thus resexualized. The father does not facilitate the sublimation of pleasure (by prohibiting the son's desire through the castration complex) but guarantees manhood by promising repression *as* pleasure (which is why Bataille's father at once upholds and destroys the law). In other words, he guarantees manhood, paradoxically, through an eroticized castration. In this reading, *Story of the Eye* is not a sublimation of the son's desire for and terror of the mother's sexualized body but rather a reenactment of the father's punishment, over and over again, in any situation Bataille happened to be in.

The son is thus born guilty: "My father having conceived me when blind (absolutely blind), [castrated] I cannot tear out my eyes like Oedipus." There is no relief from guilt; because there is none, Bataille claimed that even as he tried to "escape his destiny" by "abandoning his father," he himself ended up blind and abandoned: "Today I know I am 'blind,' immeasurable, I am man 'abandoned' on the globe like my father at N."[53] Here, then, Bataille rejected the surrealists' conflation of the self with perversion or deviance or

---

[51] I am extending Denis Hollier's argument in "Bataille's Tomb." At the end of that article he makes some suggestive remarks about the relationship between Bataille and his father which I have used to begin this interrogation of Bataille's unconscious. He draws a parallel between the Commander figure in *The Blue of Noon*, the proletariat Bataille (ambiguously) champions, and Bataille's father. In his analysis, Bataille ends up being the bourgeois who wants to be castrated (punished) by the proletariat, in an unconscious reenactment of his own childhood dreams.

[52] Borch-Jacobsen, p. 221.

[53] Bataille, *Story of the Eye*, pp. 77, 78.

with the castrated other—the mother. The mother in particular, as I have shown, does not represent the other or the true self. Bataille's pleasure has no reference other than the repression that constitutes it. I think this is what Hollier means when he claims that the father does not "quell" desire but "stamps the son with the violence of his own sexuality." The oedipal drama is not one in which sexuality is quelled; rather, it is constituted through an identification with the blind father. The text is thus born of the father, who "conceives the son blind."[54]

In this new version of literary production, the novel is born at the juncture between unconscious desire and the father's law. Because unconscious pleasure cannot be differentiated from the repression that constitutes it, that pleasure can be known, paradoxically, only when it is repressed. In Bataille, writing—the compulsion to castration, to alliance with the mother—no longer represents the sublimated other; it symbolizes an other, an unconscious, that cannot be symbolized, that is always already written. The text is thus born of an eroticized castration that the writer simulates again and again.

The Cure

Bataille thus worked out his concept of literary production within the framework of surrealist aesthetics and through his repudiation of/complicity with fascist politics. It was structured by the contradictory attempt, common to both surrealism and fascism in different ways, to retrieve the self by unbinding it.[55] Bataille asked whether the self could be preserved from annihilation without betraying its desire for self-loss, its pleasure; whether literature could be the site both of repression (sublimation, projection, displace-

[54] Hollier, "Bataille's Tomb," p. 101. Hollier notes too that in Bataille, "it is also because castration now no longer incurs punishment for some anterior sexuality, that it constitutes the ordeal through which the body is introduced to the regime of sexuality" (p. 102).

[55] For a discussion of how this paradox is common to all forms of modernism, see Taylor, pp. 456–93. The French surrealists, of course, articulated it differently from, say, the German expressionists or the Italian futurists. For one, they were far more interested in criminal deviance as a metaphor for the self.

ment, and so on) and of subversion (self-loss or transcendence, the explosion of limits), or prohibition *and* transgression.

Bataille took the surrealists' conflation of prohibition and transgression, of the self and the criminal other, as a starting point from which to draw new boundaries. He reconceived those boundaries in terms of a paternal prohibition that was always pleasurable or in terms of a cure that was always pathological, a pathology that always operated as a cure. The criminal, the syphilitic, blind, and sadistic father, and the automutilator, Gaston F., Van Gogh, the writer, were not metaphors for our deeper or other being, as they had been for the surrealists; they were metaphors for an otherness that had ceased to be referential, that was always already symbolized.

Bataille painted a stunning portrait of the Oedipus complex in which the dilemma of having to be a man one can never be results in a dialectic of self-punishment (taking pleasure in repression) through which the self is constituted. But Bataille, in spite of his proximity to Lacan, went a step further than the psychoanalyst. If we were to imagine a conversation between Bataille and Lacan, we could hear Bataille saying: Don't try to pretend the father is not castrated; don't make maturity or sexual identity conditional upon an illusion of having a phallus; don't try to create an artificial and wholly illusory symbolic father who would be distinguished from those real castrated and neurotic ones; don't insist on props you yourself know are nothing but props, an insight to which your entire theory of the imaginary attests. And finally, don't imagine that the world will fall apart if the father doesn't have a phallus. Castration and virility are not at all incompatible: Manhood is the impossibility of ever being a whole man.

But how can the paradox of a man who is both castrated and virile be lived if he doesn't succumb to the illusion that he has a phallus? How could Bataille identify with the father Lacan claimed was in decline, weak, neurotic, and authoritarian, without going mad? How could one imagine a moment when one might be another and be or experience one's self (the nonsymbolic or "true" self that is always already deferred, lost forever)? In short, how can the dialectic of self-punishment, the constituent moment of selfhood, be lived as anything other than a perpetual drive to crime?

In Bataille, as we have seen, the desire to be guilty results not in crime but in adherence to the father's law. It does so because the law is already defined in terms of a castration (Bataille's blind father); the law is itself always guilty. The law does not punish transgression but *constitutes* sexuality as a prohibited transgression; the law is in fact a tautology for the son's transgression. Transgression is thus lived as the law (we recall that Bataille's father upheld the law by destroying it); the loss of the self is lived as the constituent moment of selfhood. The self no longer resists or rivals the law, for it is born guilty.

The self does not have to pass from a primary to a secondary identification, because it lives its desire to be an-other as the law, lives its pleasure as repression. It can't see its reflection in the mirror because it is born blind, because it is already castrated, already beyond being tempted by the seductive image in the mirror. The dialectic of self-punishment (the desire to be guilty which suspends guilt) is not lived as pathology, regression, or arrested development but as the very constitution of civilized man. It is as if Bataille at once took away the prop holding up the symbolic father and yet refused to do away with the necessity of fathers. This is not to say that Bataille's concept of self-formation and Lacan's imaginary are identical. Whereas Lacan looked to a secondary identification to move beyond a dialectic of self-punishment and so eventually effected a rigid (and, as I have suggested, theoretically unconvincing) separation of the imaginary and the symbolic, Bataille theorized how to live repression as pleasure without going mad.[56]

For Bataille, the father is upright only to the extent his back is bent, a visionary to the extent he can't see, but he is, quite significantly, a father. Bataille now uses the term *virility* not for the man who follows the rules or even the man who nobly breaks them but for the tragic man who refuses to become but one of the parts of the great machine in whose image a rational, productive society fashions itself. In other words, the virile man is he who refuses our culture's definition of what it means to be whole. His wholeness (his manhood) is paradoxically linked to an experience of trans-

[56] Later in his life Lacan seemed to abandon the self to its own nothingness. For a persuasive discussion of this development in the late Lacan, see Borch-Jacobsen, pp. 218–39. For a brief account of the differences between Lacan and Bataille, see Francis Marmande, *Georges Bataille politique* (Lyon: Presses Universitaires de Lyon, 1985), pp. 104–5.

gressing limits rather than of containment within boundaries that would demarcate his being. But where do women figure in this scheme of things? For if a woman is already not whole, as culture has defined her, as Lacan called her, and as Bataille paradoxically conceived her plentitude, if she already has the status Bataille's tragic man unwittingly aspires to, how could her renunciation of wholeness be subversive? Wouldn't her so-called lack affirm rather than challenge cultural norms of female subjectivity? No wonder, perhaps, that the subject in question for Bataille as well as Lacan, is necessarily exclusively male.[57]

Thus, as Bataille demonstrated, escaping from one's (male) head is not so easy. Because the moment at which the self experiences itself as loss (as mutilated, punished, castrated) is also the moment at which it is constituted as a self, or more precisely, as a man. Hollier suggests a (parodical) analogy with Lacan:

[Bataille's] article "Architecture" describes it as an essential stage in the process leading from animal to human as a sort of anthropological mirror stage that might be called, in a parody of Lacan's title, "the architecture stage as formative function of the We" (of man's social imago). In this sense, even though he seems to denounce the repression exercised over man by architecture, Bataille's real point of intervention is the catachresis requiring that man only take form with architecture, that the human form as such, the formation of man be embedded in architecture.[58]

Repression is thus the very condition of pleasure.

[57] See Elizabeth Grosz's critique of Julia Kristeva on these grounds. Kristeva implies that the avant-garde artist is necessarily male. Grosz, pp. 164–65.
[58] Denis Hollier, "Bloody Sundays," *Representations* 28 (Fall 1989), 79.

Conclusion

This book has attempted to account for the process by which a repressed otherness became the structuring principle of male subjectivity, of a new split subject. In Bataille and Lacan (particularly the Lacan of the interwar years covered by this book), the self has been decentered, but it has not been relocated in an "other" awaiting liberation (as in surrealism) or abolished. The self is conceived in catachretic terms: It is a deliberately paradoxical figure, structured by internal contradictions, eternally different within itself. For this reason Bataille has been seen as a predecessor to poststructuralism. Lacan's use of catachresis, furthermore, undercuts his structuralist insistence on the transcendence of the phallus and makes it difficult to deem him simply a structuralist, to reduce his work to a formalist doctrine.

But this concept of the subject is most fundamentally indebted to a rearticulation of the relationship of sexuality to culture and to aesthetics, to what both Bataille and Lacan formulated in different ways as the law (hence Sade and Freud figure prominently in this account). At the same time, there is some friction between the parts of this book, generated by the differences between Lacan and Bataille. After all, Lacan constructs a self that becomes phallic and upright through a process of splitting, whereas Bataille constructs a self that is always already split (in his imagery, castrated). In Lacan, the self is at once symbolized and lost; in Bataille the self "lives itself as a loss," meaning that it is caught up in a paradoxical mobility that can never be frozen, petrified by a gaze in the mirror. So what, then, do they have in common?

In historical terms, the split subject is the product of a link between sexuality and the self first developed by Freud, mediated here by postwar crises as they were interpreted by French psychoanalysts and surrealists, and extended and transformed by Lacan and Bataille. That is, in both Bataille and Lacan, the self is indisputably and fundamentally constituted in and through desire rather than reason or morality. But in contrast to Freud or to Bataille's surrealist predecessors, their formation of the self is inseparable from what John Rajchman has called a love of the law: The writer and the psychoanalyst are driven by the pursuit of a truth that can be known only when repressed and punished, and hence, they are driven, inevitably, by an (unconscious) desire to *be* punished.[1] For this reason, I have used the nonreferentiality of the self implicit in masochism—in which desire is generated when repressed—as a metaphor for a self whose "truth" Bataille and Lacan located in its repression.

Both Bataille and Lacan thus formulated a self that the law constitutes as an irretrievable other. As Rajchman has pointed out, the truth can no longer be found in narrative unity and closure (in a cure); it lies beyond narrative. It is why he can link Lacanian ethics to modernity, to the concept of an aesthetics that is "in love" with fragmentation and dissolution, for which love—no longer about duty, obligation, or happiness—finds its privileged expression in sexuality, in sexuality as a metaphor for "trauma, otherness, and unspeakable truth."[2]

But how, more specifically, do we account for this love of the law, this unspeakable pleasure that in Bataille and Lacan came to define the self? The concept of an arrested drive to self-annihilation is more than a combination of Kojève, Hegel, and Freud, more than an extrapolation of the master-slave dialectic (though of course it is that, too). First of all, Bataille and Lacan read these thinkers through a set of mutually reinforcing quests for spiritual renewal. The mental hygiene movement, psychoanalysis, and surrealism sought to rehabilitate the deviant in the name of revitalizing the

---

[1] Rajchman, p. 53. I think this remark is true of Lacan because he never made clear how secondary identification desexualizes repression, never clarified the differences between the symbolic and the imaginary from what Borch-Jacobsen calls the "perspective of truth" (p. 118).

[2] Rajchman, p. 53.

national or the human spirit, albeit with different concepts of spirituality in mind.

I do not want to suggest these movements were identical. Rather, they were symmetrical. In Part One, I argued that French psychoanalysts pursued a project of cultural renewal that was hard to distinguish from a broader program of social sanitation endorsed by left- and right-wing thinkers alike, including socialists and eugenicists. Even though he twisted psychoanalytic method in another direction, couched in a moral rather than medical vocabulary, the fascist Edouard Pichon pursued the same hygienic goals as his counterparts. In other words, French analysts did, as Roudinesco and others have argued, deviate from Freud's teachings. But those deviations, in particular their assimilation of a model of mental hygiene, outlined herein, account for their originality (or, in any case, their specificity).

The similarities between the psychiatric and the surrealist rehabilitation of Sade also make this symmetry evident. In Part Two, in discussing Sade, I sought to demonstrate how that rehabilitation cut across those diametrically opposed medical and avant-garde discourses, thereby establishing grounds on which Bataille and Lacan might meet. And finally, Part Three ventured a bit farther afield to suggest that surrealism and fascism were both characterized by a desire for unmediated unity between self and other which sanitized the self, which at once drew from and negated the affective dimension of human existence.

I have argued that psychiatrists, psychoanalysts, and surrealists articulated in specific terms the dissolution of the spatial symbolism and its corollary valences which doctors, writers, and others used (in common with all of Western metaphysics) to structure human identity—high and low, self and other, and so on. Psychiatrists, psychoanalysts, and surrealists impeded and expressed the dissolution of the boundaries between normal and deviant and reason and desire implicit in the Great War's intensification of anxieties about identities of all sorts. In their analogous projects to normalize or rehabilitate deviant identities, they thus laid the foundation for the undoing of identity, for what I have called the unraveling or unbinding of the self.

This book tells the story of how that dialectic became increasingly explicit in analysts' and surrealists' efforts to renew the self, finally becoming identical with the structure of subjectivity in the work of Bataille and Lacan. Thus, in their attempts to nurse the self back to health, to rehabilitate criminals—including so-called deviant women, Sade, and outlaw writers—analysts and surrealists theorized the self as an other, at once fixed and eroded, explained and inexplicable, present and uncannily absent. In identifying the self as other, then, they also unraveled it. Hence autopunition, the equal but always different man, and scotomization at once explained the deviant's motivation and obscured its source. Sade's crimes, real and metaphorical, were explained by explaining them away, by transforming his crimes into "normal" behavior, into the very force of his reason. Surrealists, too, rehabilitated criminals only to purge them of their criminality. Even fascists tapped into so-called deviant longings for boundary dissolution, only to draw the most absolute boundaries.

Bataille and Lacan opposed what they saw as the normalizing tendencies of these various attempts to rescue the now "other" self. For Bataille, as we have seen, the surrealists' rehabilitation of Sade was as hygienic as psychiatrists' efforts to steer deviants in the right direction. And Lacan believed psychoanalysts wanted to purge the self of its affective dimension, to sanitize it in the interests of social order. Both Lacan and Bataille nevertheless participated in the self-renewal of the interwar years, but they did not rescue the self by bringing it out of hiding. Instead, *they tried to save it by defining the other (true or real) self as a (now irretrievable) other.* In so doing, they conflated the dialectic implicit in analysts' and surrealists' efforts to discover and rehabilitate the self (the dialectic whereby the self's rescue leads to its unraveling) with the very structure of subjectivity.

For example, they both countered the self-destructive tendencies of fascism, its authoritarian, eroticized suppression of the (other) self, by theorizing a father figure who represented both the law and its unarticulated presuppositions. That is, they both reaffirmed the necessary masculinity of the self in its various expert guises—as father, analyst, or writer—while eroding the very foundations of masculinity and hence of expertise. Again, Bataille's and Lacan's father figures are not the same. Bataille's is always already headless, and Lacan's always already has a head. But as I have maintained, Lacan is perhaps closer to Bataille than we realize. Lacan's symbolic is not necessarily so distinct from Bataille's own reworking of the Oedipal story. Mikkel Borch-Jacobsen has in fact persuasively argued that Lacan, late in his career, theorized a subject who lives his or her own nothingness.[3] And by reference to cultural origins, I have suggested that the stages of development Lacan was to call the imaginary and the symbolic may be read synchronically. Most important, then, in order to save the self both Bataille and Lacan theorized one that is no longer merely "other"—a metaphor for our deeper being, our true self—but is instead an other beyond symbolization.

This concept of the self is therefore very much of its time, and it represents the French expression of a more general European crisis. This self is part of a spiritual renewal, but a decidedly unusual one fashioned after the perceived failures of psychoanalysis and surrealism to give it a place to be itself. It represents the establishment of norms that are instantly called into question, that at once permit and preclude self-expression. In their context, Bataille and Lacan thus sought to "save" all they perceived to be threatened by the hygienic impulses of both right- and left-wing doctors and even writers, including criminality, sexuality, and madness.

This formation of the self links Bataille and Lacan in spite of their differences and establishes the presuppositions on which poststructuralist thought would later be built. Of course, it would be anachronistic to call either Bataille or Lacan a poststructuralist, a label whose origins must be sought in the work of Martin Heidegger and Friedrich Nietzsche, among other thinkers. But French poststructuralism is also rooted in these culturally specific calls to renew political and theoretical opposition to the status quo, and above all in the *ambiguity* of that renewal. For the self that Bataille and Lacan saved cannot be symbolized or articulated, even as it calls into question the authority of what is being said.

The ambiguity that structures the decentered subject thus silences the other self it purportedly rescues: self-renewal becomes inseparable from a silencing of the self. This formulation of the decentered subject, of a self whose truth, as Bataille said, is "beyond any imagining,"[4] thus rescues the so-called other self by defining it as the unarticulated presupposition of all thought and

---

[3] Borch-Jacobsen, p. 239. Borch-Jacobsen has argued that by the end of his life, Lacan "finally reworked the rigid opposition between the symbolic and the imaginary, recognizing in the latter the capacity to reveal the truth of the subject in its abyssal non-being." (p. 237).

[4] Bataille, *Story of the Eye*, p. 80.

culture. But as I have suggested, this radical position now only conflates the dialectic implicit in the failed efforts of French interwar movements to rescue the other with subjectivity itself. Or to put it another way, the self Bataille and Lacan conceived is conflated with the process by which it is produced, so that the self and its history are one and the same thing. For this reason the historical and cultural presuppositions on which the self was founded must remain beyond question even as they are perpetually called into question. This conflation between historical product and process perhaps accounts for why so much poststructuralist thought returns to "history"—calls all truths radically into question by insisting that their meaning is always other, always deferred—and makes history impossible to write.

By analyzing in historically specific terms how the very relationship between self and other was formulated by Bataille and Lacan, I have sought to make explicit the presuppositions on which the decentered self in France was founded. A truly radical questioning of the categories of self and other would have to discard those presuppositions (for example, about the gendering of the other) that give self and other their cultural meaning. I do not mean that we should ressurrect the liberal, humanist self, but that we call the categories of self and other into question from a point of view we have only begun to imagine. In this book, then, I have not argued for or against the self-dissolution implicit in the construction of some forms of modern (and now postmodern) subjectivity but suggested that neither alternative will do, that it might be possible to be for and against self-dissolution at the same time. That is the legacy of Bataille and Lacan.

Selected Bibliography

Abbreviations

AML   *Annales de Médecine Légale, de Criminologie, et de Police Scientifique*
AMP   *Annales Médico-Psychologiques*
EC   *Etudes Criminologiques*
EM   *L'Esprit Médical*
EP   *L'Evolution Psychiatrique*
HM   *L'Hygiène Mentale*
RFP   *Revue Française de Psychanalyse*

Primary Sources

Alexander, Franz, and Hugo Staub. *Le Criminel et ses juges.* Paris: Nouvelle Revue Française, 1934.
Allendy, René. *La Justice intérieure.* Paris: Denoël and Steele, 1931.
——. "Le crime et les perversions instinctives." *Crapouillot* (May 1938), 8–12.
Alméras, Henri d'. *La France devorée par les poux.* Paris: Collections des Frondeurs, 1933.
Apollinaire, Guillaume. *L'Oeuvre du marquis de Sade.* Paris: Bibliothèque des Curieux, 1909.
Armand, Ernest. *La Revision de la morale sexuelle.* Paris: L'En Dehors, 1930.
Balkis. *Pages curieuses du marquis de Sade.* Paris: Les Bibliophiles Libertins, 1928.
Balthazard, Dr., and Eugène Prevost. *Une Plaie sociale.* Paris: A. Maloine, 1912.
Bataille, Georges. *L'Expérience intérieure.* Paris: Gallimard, 1954.
——. *Literature and Evil.* Trans. Alastair Hamilton. New York: Urizen Books, 1973.

——. *Oeuvres complètes*. Paris: Gallimard. Of the 12 volumes published to date, I made most use of the first nine:
1. *Premiers écrits, 1922–1940*. Paris: Gallimard, 1970.
2. *Ecrits posthumes, 1922–1940*. 1970.
3. *Oeuvres littéraires*. 1971.
4. *Oeuvres littéraires posthumes*. 1971.
5. *La Somme athéologique, 1*. 1973.
6. *La Somme athéologique, 2*. 1973.
7. *L'Economie a la mesure de l'univers; La Part maudite; La Limite de l'utile; Théorie de la religion; Conférences, 1947–1948*. 1976.
8. *L'Histoire de l'érotisme; Le Surréalisme au jour le jour; Conférences, 1951–1953; La Souveraineté*. 1976.
9. *Lascaux; ou, La Naissance de l'art; Manet; La Littérature et le mal*. 1979.
——. *Le Procès de Gilles de Rais*. Paris: Pauvert, 1972.
——. *Story of the Eye*. London: Penguin, 1979.
——. *Visions of Excess*. Trans. and ed. Allan Stoekl. Minneapolis: University of Minnesota Press, 1985.
Beauvoir, Simone de. "Must We Burn Sade?" In D. A. F. Sade, *The 120 Days of Sodom and Other Writings*, trans. Austryn Wainhouse and Richard Seaver. New York: Grave Press, 1966.
Béliard, Octave. *Le Marquis de Sade*. Paris: Laurier, 1928.
Bion, René. *La Nature féminine et le féminisme*. Lyon: Chronique Sociale de France, 1927.
Bizard, Léon. *La Vie des filles*. Paris: Grasset, 1934.
Bloch, Iwan [Eugen Duehren, pseud.]. *Le Marquis de Sade et son temps*. Paris: A. Michalon, 1901.
Bonmariage, Sylvain. *La Seconde vie du marquis de Sade*. Lille: Mercure de Flandre, 1927.
Borel, Adrien, and Gilbert Robin. *Les Rêveurs éveillés*. Paris, 1925.
Bourdon, Dr. J. R. *Perversions sexuelles*. Paris: Editions Internationales, 1931.
Breton, André. *L'Amour fou*. Paris: Gallimard, 1976.
——. *Anthologie de l'humour noir*. Paris: Pauvert, 1972.
——. *Manifestoes of Surrealism*. Trans. Richard Seaver and Helen R. Lane. Ann Arbor: University of Michigan Press, 1972.
Brousson, Jean-Jacques. *Les Nuits sans culottes*. Paris: Flammarion, 1930.
Bureau, Paul. *L'Indiscipline des moeurs*. Paris: Blond and Gay, 1921.
Cabanès, Dr. Augustin. *Le Cabinet secret de l'histoire*. Paris: Albin Michel, 1925.
Caillois, Roger. *Approche de l'imaginaire*. Paris: Gallimard, 1974.
Camp, Maxime du. *Paris: Ses organes, ses fonctions, et sa vie dans la seconde moitié du XIXe siècle*. Vol. 4. Paris: Hachette, 1873.
Camus, Albert. *The Rebel*. New York: Knopf, 1957.
Canguilhem, Georges. *The Normal and the Pathological*. Trans. Carolyn R. Fawcett. New York: Zone Books, 1991.
Chable, Dr. Robert. *Education sexuelle et maladies vénériennes*. Neuchâtel: Editions Forum, 1921.
Chavigny, Paul. *Psychologie de l'hygiène*. Paris: Flammarion, 1921.

———. *Sexualité et médecine légale*. Paris: J. B. Baillière et Fils, 1939.

Claude, Henri. *Psychiatrie médico-légale*. Paris: G. Doin, 1932.

Debordes, Jean. *Le Vrai Visage du marquis de Sade*. Paris: Editions de la Nouvelle Revue Critique, 1939.

Desthieux, Frédéric-Jean. *Scandales et crimes sociaux*. Paris: La Pensée Française, 1924.

Escande, Dr. Frank. *Le Problème de la chasteté masculine au point de vue scientifique*. Paris: Librairie J. B. Baillière et Fils, 1919.

Fély, Pascal. *Les Princesses de Cythère*. Paris: Jean Fort, 1920.

Fiaux, Louis. *Enseignement populaire de la moralité sexuelle*. Paris: F. Alcan, 1908.

Flake, Dr. Otto. *Le Marquis de Sade*. Trans. Pierre Klossowski. Paris: Grasset, 1933.

Frappa, Jean-José. *Enquête sur la prostitution*. Paris: Flammarion, 1937.

Freud, Sigmund. *Civilization and Its Discontents*. New York: Norton, 1961.

———. *The Freud Reader*. Ed. Peter Gay. New York: Norton, 1989.

———. *General Psychological Theory*. New York: Macmillan, 1963.

———. *Inhibitions, Symptoms, and Anxiety*. New York: Norton, 1959.

Freud, Sigmund, and René Laforgue. "Correspondance, 1923–1937." *Nouvelle Revue de la Psychanalyse* 15 (Spring 1977), 235–314.

Ginisty, Paul. *La Marquise de Sade*. Paris: E. Fasquelle, 1901.

Goncourt, Edmond de, and Jules de Goncourt. *La Femme au XVIIIe siècle*. Paris: Flammarion, 1982.

Good, Paul. *Hygiène et morale*. Paris: Editions Je Sers, 1931.

Hamel, Maurice, and Charles Tournier. *La Prostitution: Enquête*. Nice: Palais Marie-Christine, 1927.

Heine, Maurice. *Le Marquis de Sade*. Paris: Gallimard, 1950.

———. *Recueil de confessions et observations psychosexuelles*. Paris: Editions du Terrain Vague, 1957.

Hermant, Abel. *Les Confidences d'une aïeule*. Paris: Editions de France, 1933.

Hesnard, Angelo. *Traité de sexologie normale et pathologique*. Paris: Payot, 1933.

Hirschfeld, Magnus. *Perversions sexuelles*. Paris: Editions Internationales, 1931.

———. *Le Tour du monde d'un sexologue*. Paris: Gallimard, 1938.

Hollier, Denis, ed. *Le Collège de sociologie*. Paris: Gallimard, 1979.

———. *The College of Sociology*. Trans. Betsy Wing. Minneapolis: University of Minnesota Press, 1988.

Inman, Georges. *Voyages au pays des déments*. Paris: Editions des Portiques, 1934.

Javelier, André. *Thèse pour le doctorat en médecine: Le Marquis de Sade et les "Cent-vingt Journées de Sodome" devant la psychiatrie et la médecine légale*. Paris: Librairie le François, 1937.

Klossowski, Pierre. *Sade, mon prochain*. Paris: Seuil, 1947 and 1967.

———. *Sade, My Neighbor*. Trans. Alphonso Lingis. Evanston, Ill.: Northwestern University Press, 1991.

Kojève, Alexandre. *Introduction to the Reading of Hegel's Phenomenology of*

Mind. Assembled by Raymond Queneau. Ed. Allan Bloom. Trans. James Nicols, Jr. New York: Basic Books, 1969.

Krafft-Ebing, Richard von, trans. *Psychopathia sexualis*. Paris: E. Laurent and Sigismund Csapo, 1931.

Kun, Jean. *Les Principales Imperfections du code pénal*. Paris: Editions Domat-Monchrestein, 1933.

Kyrkos, Evangèle. "Les Causes de la criminalité juvénile." Thèse, University of Rennes. 1931.

Lacan, Jacques. "Au-delà du principe de la réalité." *L'Evolution Psychiatrique* 3 (1936), 67–86.

——. *Les Complexes familiaux dans la formation de l'individu: Essai d'analyse d'une fonction en psychologie*. Paris: Navarin, 1984.

——. *De la psychose paranoïaque dans ses rapports avec la personnalité*. Paris: Seuil, 1980.

——. *Ecrits*. Paris: Seuil, 1966.

——. *Ecrits 1*. Paris: Seuil, 1970.

——. *Ecrits 2*. Paris: Seuil, 1971.

——. *Ecrits: A Selection*. Trans. Alan Sheridan. London: Tavistock, 1977.

——. *Feminine Sexuality*. Trans. Jacqueline Rose. New York: Norton, 1985.

——. *The Four Fundamental Concepts of Psychoanalysis*. Trans. Alan Sheridan. London: Penguin, 1979.

——. "Hiatus irrationalis." *Le Phare de Neuilly* 3–4 (1933), 37.

——. "Kant with Sade." Trans. James B. Swenson, Jr. *October* 51 (Winter, 1989), 55–75.

——. *The Language of the Self: The Function of Language in Psychoanalysis*. Ed. and trans. Anthony Wilden. Baltimore: Johns Hopkins University Press, 1968.

——. "Motifs du crime paranoïaque: Le Crime des soeurs Papin." *Minotaure* 3–4 (1933), 25–28.

——. "Le Problème du style et la conception psychiatrique et les formes paranoïaques de l'experience." *Minotaure* 1 (1933), 68–69.

——. *Le Séminaire I: Les Ecrits techniques de Freud*. Paris: Seuil, 1975.

——. *Le Séminaire II: Le Moi dans la théorie de Freud et dans la technique de la psychanalyse*. Paris: Seuil, 1978.

——. *Le Séminaire III: Les Psychoses*. Paris: Seuil, 1981.

——. *Le Seminaire VII: L'Ethique de la psychanalyse*. Paris: Seuil, 1986.

Lacroix-Dupouy, Marie-Thérèse. "Les Services ouverts dans les asiles." Thèse, University of Paris, 1926.

Laforgue, René, and Angelo Hesnard. "Les Processus d'autopunition en psychologie des névroses et psychoses, en psychologie criminelle, et en pathologie générale. *Revue Française de Psychanalyse* 4 (1930–31), 3–84.

Laforgue, René, René Allendy, Raymond de Saussure, and Edouard Pichon. *Le Rêve et la psychanalyse*. Paris: N. Maloine, 1926.

Larouche, Ivan-Claude. *Prestigue du crime*. Paris: Société Parisienne d'Edition, 1946.

Laure [Colette Peignot]. *Ecrits*. Paris: 10/18, 1978.

Laurent, Emile. *Sadisme et masochisme*. Paris: Vigot Frères, 1903.

Lefebvre, Charles. *La Famille en France*. Paris: Marcel Giard, 1920.

Leiris, Michel. *L'Age d'homme*. Paris: Gallimard, 1939.

Lély, Gilbert. Prologue to D. A. F. Sade, *Morceaux choisis*. Paris: Seghers, 1948.

Lorrain, Jean. *La Maison Philibert*. Paris: Librairie Universelle, 1904.

Margueritte, Victor. *Prostituée*. Paris: Bibliothèque Charpentier, 1907.

Mialane, Lucien. *La Criminalité juvénile*. Paris: Les Presses Modernes, 1921.

Minkowski, Eugène. *La Schizophrénie: Psychopathologie des schizoïdes et des schizophrènes*. Paris: Payot, 1927.

Mondor, H. *Les Avortements mortels*. Paris: Masson, 1936.

Moreau de Tours, Dr. Paul. *Des aberrations du sens génésique*. Paris: Asselin, 1880.

Morel, Genviève. "Les Tueuses d'enfants." Thèse, University of Nancy, 1927.

Mounier, Emmanuel. *Manifeste au service du personnalisme*. Paris: Editions Montaigne, 1936.

Paulhan, Jean. *Les Fleurs de Tarbes*. Paris, 1941.

——. "The Marquis de Sade and His Accomplice." In D. A. F. Sade, *Three Complete Novels: Justine, Philosophy in the Bedroom, Eugénie de Franval, and Other Writings*. New York: Grove Press, 1965.

Pauvert, Jean-Jacques, ed. *L'Affaire Sade*. Paris: Pauvert, 1963.

Perceau, Louis [Louis Helpey, pseud.]. *Le Marquis de Sade et le sadisme*. Sadopolis: Imprimé spécialement pour l'auteur et quelques amis, n.d.

Pichon, Edouard, and Jacques Damourette. *Des mots à la pensée: Essai de grammaire de la langue française*. 7 vols. Paris: D'Artrey, 1911–50.

Planhol, René de. *Les Utopistes de l'amour*. Paris: Garnier Frères, 1921.

Quint, L. Pierre. *Le Comte de Lautréamont et Dieu*. Marseilles: Les Cahiers du Sud, 1929.

Richard, Gaston. *L'Evolution des moeurs*. Paris: Gaston Doin, 1925.

Sade, D. A. F. *Correspondance inédite*. Ed. Paul Bourdin. Paris: Librairie de France, 1929.

——. *Three Complete Novels: Justine, Philosophy in the Bedroom, Eugénie de Franval, and Other Writings*. New York: Grove Press, 1965.

——. *The 120 Days of Sodom and Other Writings*. Trans. Austryn Wainhouse and Richard Seaver. New York: Grove Press, 1966.

St. Paul, Dr. G. *Thèmes psychologiques: Invertis et homosexuels*. Paris: Vigot Frères, 1930.

Saleilles, Raymond. *L'Individualisation de la peine*. Paris: Felix Alcan, 1898.

Sarfati, Salvador. *Essai médico-psychologique sur le marquis de Sade*. Lyon: BOSC Frères, 1930.

Siau, Jacques. *La Prostitution devant la loi, la morale, et l'hygiène*. Lyon: BOSC Frères, 1931.

Teutsch, Dr. Robert. *Le Féminisme*. Paris: Société Française d'Editions Littéraires et Techniques, 1934.

Toulouse, Edouard. *La Question sociale*. Paris: Editions du Progrès Civique, 1921.

Tournier, Claude [Dr. Marciat, pseud.]. "Le Marquis de Sade et le sadisme." In *Vacher, l'éventreur, et les crimes sadiques*, ed. Dr. Alexandre Lacassagne. Lyon: A. Storck, 1899.

Vachet, Dr. Pierre. *La Psychologie du vice*. Paris: Librairie Blond et Gay, 1930.
Verger, Henri. *L'Evolution des idées médicales sur la responsabilité des délinquents*. Paris: Flammarion, 1923.
Villette, Armand. *Du trottoir à St. Lazare*. Paris: Editions Henry-Parville, 1925.
Voivenel, Paul. *Les Belles-mères tragiques*. Paris: Renaissance du livre 1927.
Wieth-Knudsen, Dr. K. A. *Le Conflit des sexes dans l'évolution sociale et la question sexuelle*. Paris: Marcel Rivière, 1931.
X, Jacobus. *Le Marquis de Sade devant la science médicale et la littérature moderne*. Paris: Charles Carrington, 1901.
Yocas, Panagiote. *L'Influence de la guerre européenne sur la criminalité*. Paris: Jouve, 1926.

Secondary Sources

Arac, Jonathan, and Barbara Johnson, eds. *The Consequences of Theory*. Baltimore: Johns Hopkins University Press, 1991.
Bayle, Jean-Loubet del. *Les Non-conformistes des années trentes*. Paris: Seuil, 1969.
Benjamin, Jessica. *The Bonds of Love: Psychoanalysis, Feminism, and the Problem of Domination*. New York: Pantheon, 1988.
Benvenuto, Bice, and Roger Kennedy. *The Works of Jacques Lacan: An Introduction*. New York: St. Martin's Press, 1986.
Bercherie, Paul. "The Quadrifocal Oculary: The Epistemology of the Freudian Heritage." *Economy and Society* 15 (February 1986), 23–68.
Bernheimer, Charles. *Figures of Ill-Repute: Representing Prostitution in Nineteenth-Century France*. Cambridge: Harvard University Press, 1989.
Bernstein, Richard, ed. *Habermas and Modernity*. Cambridge: MIT Press, 1985.
Bersani, Leo. *The Culture of Redemption*. Cambridge: Harvard University Press, 1990.
——. *The Freudian Body*. New York: Columbia University Press, 1986.
Blanchot, Maurice. *Lautréamont et Sade*. Paris: Editions de Minuit, 1949.
——. *La Part du feu*. Paris: Gallimard, 1949.
——. "The Main Impropriety." In *Literature and Revolution*, ed. Jacques Ehrmann. Boston: Beacon Press, 1970.
Borch-Jacobsen, Mikkel. *Lacan: The Absolute Master*. Trans. Douglas Brick. Stanford: Stanford University Press, 1991.
Bowie, Malcolm. *Freud, Proust, and Lacan: Theory as Fiction*. Cambridge: Cambridge University Press, 1987.
Butler, Judith. *Gender Trouble: Feminism and the Subversion of Identity*. New York: Routledge and Kegan Paul, 1990.
——. *Subjects of Desire: Hegelian Reflections in Twentieth-Century France*. New York: Columbia University Press, 1987.
Carter, Angela. *The Sadeian Woman*. New York: Pantheon, 1978.
Case, Sue-Ellen, ed. *Performing Feminisms: Feminist Critical Theory and Theatre*. Baltimore: Johns Hopkins University Press, 1990.

Castel, Robert. *L'Ordre psychiatrique: L'Age d'or d'aliénisme.* Paris: Editions de Minuit, 1976.

Caws, Mary Ann, Rudolf Kuenzli, and Gwen Raaberg, eds. *Surrealism and Women.* Cambridge: MIT Press, 1991.

Certeau, Michel de. *Heterologies: Discourses on the Other.* Minneapolis: University of Minnesota Press, 1986.

Clément, Catherine. *The Lives and Legends of Jacques Lacan.* New York: Columbia University Press, 1983.

Clifford, James. *The Predicament of Culture: Twentieth-Century Ethnography, Literature, Art.* Cambridge: Harvard University Press, 1988.

Corbin, Alain. *Women for Hire: Prostitution and Sexuality in France after 1850.* Trans. Alan Sheridan. Cambridge: Harvard University Press, 1990.

Culler, Jonathan. *On Deconstruction.* Ithaca: Cornell University Press, 1982.

Davidson, Arnold I. "Sex and the Emergence of Sexuality." *Critical Inquiry* (Autumn 1987), 17–48.

Deleuze, Gilles. *Masochism: Coldness and Cruelty.* Trans. Jean McNeil. New York: Zone Books, 1989.

Derrida, Jacques. *Of Grammatology.* Trans. Gayatri Chakravorty Spivak. Baltimore: Johns Hopkins University Press, 1976.

——. *The Post Card: From Socrates to Freud and Beyond.* Trans. Alan Bass. Chicago: University of Chicago Press, 1987.

——. *Writing and Difference.* Trans. Alan Bass. Chicago: University of Chicago Press, 1978.

Descomes, Vincent. *Modern French Philosophy.* Cambridge: Cambridge University Press, 1980.

Donzelot, Jacques. *The Policing of Families.* New York: Pantheon, 1979.

Dor, Joel. *Introduction à la lecture de Lacan, I: L'Inconscient structuré comme un langage.* Paris: Denoël, 1985.

Dubief, Henri. "Témoinage sur Contre-Attaque (1935–36)," *Textures* 6 (1970), 52–60.

Dworkin, Andrea. *Pornography: Men Possessing Women.* New York: Putnam, 1981.

Ehrmann, Jacques, ed. *Literature and Revolution.* Boston: Beacon Press, 1967.

Ellenberger, Henri. *The Discovery of the Unconscious: The Evolution of Dynamic Psychiatry.* New York: Basic Books, 1970.

Felman, Shoshana. *Jacques Lacan and the Adventure of Insight: Psychoanalysis in Contemporary Culture* Cambridge: Harvard University Press, 1987.

——. *Writing and Madness: Literature, Philosophy, Psychoanalysis.* Ithaca: Cornell University Press, 1985.

Felski, Rita. *Beyond Feminist Aesthetics: Feminist Literature and Social Change.* Cambridge: Harvard University Press, 1989.

Ferdière, Gaston. *Les Mauvaises Fréquentations.* Paris: J. C. Simoën, 1978.

Forrester, John. *The Seductions of Psychoanalysis: Freud, Lacan, and Derrida.* Cambridge: Cambridge University Press, 1990.

Foucault, Michel. *The Birth of the Clinic: An Archaeology of Medical Perception.* Trans. A. M. Sheridan Smith. New York: Vintage, 1975.

———. *Discipline and Punish*. Trans. Alan Sheridan. New York: Vintage, 1979.

———. *Histoire de la folie à l'âge classique*. Paris: Gallimard, 1972.

———. *The History of Sexuality*. New York: Vintage, 1980.

———. *I, Pierre Rivière, Having Slaughtered My Mother, My Sister, and My Brother....* Lincoln: University of Nebraska Press, 1975.

———. *Madness and Civilization: A History of Insanity in the Age of Reason*. London: Tavistock, 1979.

Fraser, Nancy. *Unruly Practices: Power, Discourse, and Gender in Contemporary Social Theory*. Minneapolis: University of Minnesota Press, 1989.

Gallop, Jane. *The Daughter's Seduction: Feminism and Psychoanalysis*. Ithaca: Cornell University Press, 1982.

———. *Intersections: A Reading of Sade with Bataille, Blanchot, and Klossowski*. Lincoln: University of Nebraska Press, 1981.

———. *Reading Lacan*. Ithaca: Cornell University Press, 1985.

———. *Thinking through the Body*. New York: Columbia University Press, 1988.

Gauthier, Xavière. *Surréalisme et sexualité*. Paris: Gallimard, 1971.

Gilbert, Sandra, and Susan Gubar. *No Man's Land: The Place of the Woman Writer in the Twentieth Century*. New Haven: Yale University Press, 1988.

Gilman, Sander. *Difference and Pathology: Stereotypes of Sexuality, Race, and Madness*. Ithaca: Cornell University Press, 1985.

———. *Disease and Representation: Images of Illness from Madness to AIDS*. Ithaca: Cornell University Press, 1989.

Goldstein, Jan. *Console and Classify: The French Psychiatric Profession in the Nineteenth Century*. Cambridge: Cambridge University Press, 1987.

Gorer, Geoffrey. *The Life and Ideas of the Marquis de Sade*. Westport: Greenwood Press, 1978.

Grossman, Atina. "The New Woman and the Rationalization of Sexuality in Weimar Germany." In *Powers of Desire: The Politics of Sexuality*, ed. Ann Snitow, Christine Stansell, and Sharon Thompson. New York: Monthly Review Press, 1983.

Grosz, Elizabeth. *Jacques Lacan: A Feminist Introduction*. New York: Routledge, 1990.

Habermas, Jürgen. *The Philosophical Discourse of Modernity*. Cambridge: MIT Press, 1987.

Harsin, Jill. *Policing Prostitution in Nineteenth-Century Paris*. Princeton: Princeton University Press, 1985.

Heimonet, Jean-Michel. *Politiques de l'écriture: Bataille/Derrida: Le Sens du sacré dans la pensée française du surréalisme à nos jours*. Chapel Hill: University of North Carolina Press, 1987.

Hirsch, Arthur. *The French New Left: An Intellectual History from Sartre to Gorz*. Boston: South End Press, 1981.

Hollier, Denis. *Against Architecture: The Writings of Georges Bataille*. Cambridge: MIT Press, 1989.

———. "Bataille's Tomb: A Halloween Story." *October* 33 (Summer 1985), 73–102.

———. "Bloody Sundays." *Representations* 28 (Fall 1989), 77–88.

———. "On Equivocation (between Literature and Politics)." *October* 55 (Winter 1990), 3–22.

———. "Mimesis and Castration, 1937." *October* 31 (Winter 1984), 3–15.

———. "La Tragédie de Gilles de Rais au 'Théâtre de la cruauté.'" *L'Arc* 44 (1971), 77–86.

Horkheimer, Max, and Theodor Adorno. *The Dialectic of Enlightenment.* London: Verso, 1979.

Hunt, Lynn, ed. *The New Cultural History.* Berkeley: University of California Press, 1989.

Jaeger, Marcel. *Le Désordre psychiatrique: Des Politiques de la santé mentale en France.* Paris: Payot, 1981.

Jameson, Fredric. "Imaginary and Symbolic in Lacan: Marxism, Psychoanalytic Criticism, and the Problem of the Subject." In *Literature and Psychoanalysis: The Question of Reading: Otherwise,* ed. Shoshana Felman. Baltimore: Johns Hopkins University Press, 1977.

Jardine, Alice. *Gynesis: Configurations of Woman and Modernity.* Ithaca: Cornell University Press, 1985.

Jauss, Hans Robert. *Towards an Aesthetic of Reception.* Minneapolis: University of Minnesota Press, 1982.

Julien, P. *Le Retour à Freud de Jacques Lacan.* Paris: Littoral, 1985.

Juranville, Alain. *Lacan et la philosophie.* Paris: Presses Universitaires Françaises, 1984.

Kaplan, Alice Jaeger. *Reproductions of Banality: Fascism, Literature, and French Intellectual Life.* Minneapolis: University of Minnesota Press, 1986.

Kelly, Michael. *Modern French Marxism.* Baltimore: Johns Hopkins University Press, 1982.

Krauss, Rosalind. *The Originality of the Avant-Garde and Other Modernist Myths.* Cambridge: MIT Press, 1986.

Lacan avec les philosophes. Paris: Albin Michel, 1991.

LaCapra, Dominick, and Steven Kaplan, eds. *Modern European Intellectual History: Reappraisals and New Perspectives.* Ithaca: Cornell University Press, 1982.

Laplanche, Jean, and J. B. Pontalis. *The Language of Psychoanalysis.* Trans. Donald Nicholson-Smith. London: Hogarth Press, 1973.

Laugaa-Traut, Françoise. *Lectures de Sade.* Paris: Armand Colin, 1973.

Leland, Dorothy. "Lacanian Psychoanalysis and French Feminism: Toward an Adequate Political Psychology." *Hypatia* 3 (Winter 1989), 81–103.

Lemaire, Anika. *Jacques Lacan.* Trans. David Macey. London: Routledge and Kegan Paul.

Macey, David. *Lacan in Contexts.* London: Verso, 1988.

McLaren, Angus. *Sexuality and Social Order: The Debate over the Fertility of Women and Workers in France, 1770–1920.* New York: Holmes and Meier, 1983.

MacMillan, James. *Housewife or Harlot: The Place of Women in French Society, 1870–1940.* Sussex: Harvester Press, 1981.

Marmande, Francis. *Georges Bataille politique.* Lyon: Presses Universitaires de Lyon, 1985.

Mehlman, Jeffrey. *Legacies of Anti-Semitism in France.* Minneapolis: University of Minnesota Press, 1983.

Murard, Lion and Patrick Zylberman. "De l'hygiène comme introduction à la politique expérimentale, 1875–1925," *Revue de Synthèse* 55 (July–September 1984), 313–41.

Mordier, Jean-Pierre, *Les Débuts de la psychanalyse en France, 1895–1926.* Paris: Maspéro, 1981.

Nye, Robert. *Crime, Madness, and Politics in Modern France.* Princeton: Princeton University Press, 1984.

——. "Degeneration and the Medical Model of Cultural Crisis in the French Belle Epoque." In *Political Symbolism in Modern Europe: Essays in Honor of George Mosse,* ed. Seymour Drescher et al., 19–41 (New Brunswick: Transaction Press, 1982).

O'Brien, Patricia. "Crime and Punishment as Historical Problem." *Journal of Social History* 4 (Summer 1978).

——. *The Promise of Punishment.* Princeton: Princeton University Press, 1982.

Orfall, Ingrid. *Fiction érogène à partir de Klossowski.* Stockholm: CWK Gleerup, 1983.

Pefanis, Julian. *Heterology and the Postmodern: Bataille, Baudrillard, and Lyotard.* Durham: Duke University Press, 1991.

Perrier, François. *Voyages extraordinaires en translacanie.* Paris: Lieu Commun, 1985.

Piel, Jean. *La Rencontre et la différence.* Paris: Fayard, 1982.

Praz, Mario. *The Romantic Agony.* Oxford: Oxford University Press, 1970.

Poster, Mark. *Existential Marxism in Postwar France.* Princeton: Princeton University Press, 1975.

Ragland-Sullivan, Ellie. *Jacques Lacan and the Philosophy of Psychoanalysis.* Chicago: University of Illinois Press, 1987.

Rajchman, John. "Lacan and the Ethics of Modernity." *Representations* 15 (Summer 1986), 42–56.

Richman, Michèle. *Reading Georges Bataille: Beyond the Gift.* Baltimore: Johns Hopkins University Press, 1982.

Roth, Michael. *Knowing and History: Appropriations of Hegel in Twentieth-Century France.* Ithaca: Cornell University Press, 1988.

——. *Psycho-Analysis as History: Negation and Freedom in Freud.* Ithaca: Cornell University Press, 1987.

Roudinesco, Elisabeth. *La Bataille de cent ans: Histoire de la psychanalyse en France.* Vol. 1. Paris: Ramsay, 1982. Vol. 2. Paris: Seuil, 1986.

——. *Jacques Lacan and Co.: A History of Psychoanalysis in France, 1925–85.* Trans. Jeffrey Mehlman. Chicago: University of Chicago Press, 1990.

——. "M. Pichon devant la famille." *Confrontations* 3 (Spring 1980), 209–226.

Roustang, François. *Un Destin si funeste.* Paris: Editions de Minuit, 1976.

——. *Lacan: De l'équivoque à l'impasse.* Paris: Minuit, 1986.

Scheidhauer, Marcel. *Le Rêve freudien en France, 1920–1926.* Paris: Navarin, 1985.

Schneider, William H. *Quality and Quantity: The Quest for Biological Regeneration in Twentieth-Century France.* Cambridge: Cambridge University Press, 1990.

Schneiderman, Stuart. *Jacques Lacan: The Death of an Intellectual Hero.* Cambridge: Harvard University Press, 1983.

Sichère, Bernard. *Le Moment lacanien*. Paris: Grasset, 1983.

Silverman, Kaja. "Histoire d'O: The Construction of a Female Subject." In *Pleasure and Danger: Exploring Female Sexuality*, ed. Carole Vance, pp. 320–49. Boston: Routledge and Kegan Paul, 1984.

Smirnoff, Victor. "De Vienne à Paris: Sur les origines d'une psychanalyse à la française." *Nouvelle Revue de Psychanalyse* 20 (Autumn 1979), 13–58.

Smith, Joseph, and William Kerrigan, eds. *Interpreting Lacan*. New Haven: Yale University Press, 1983.

Smock, Ann. *Double Dealing*. Lincoln: University of Nebraska Press, 1986.

Stoekl, Allan. "Nizan, Drieu, and the Question of Death." *Representations* 21 (Winter 1988), 117–45.

———. *Politics, Writing, Mutilation: The Cases of Bataille, Blanchot, Roussel, Leiris, and Ponge*. Minneapolis: University of Minnesota Press, 1985.

———, ed. *On Bataille*. New Haven: Yale University Press, 1990.

Sturrock, John, ed. *Structuralism and Since*. Oxford: Oxford University Press, 1979.

Suleiman, Susan Rubin. *Subversive Intent: Gender, Politics, and the Avant-Garde*. Cambridge: Harvard University Press, 1990.

Surya, Michel. *Georges Bataille: La Mort à l'oeuvre*. Paris: Librairie Séguier, 1987.

Taylor, Charles. *Sources of the Self*. Cambridge: Harvard University Press, 1989.

Theunissen, Michael. *The Other: Studies in the Social Ontology of Husserl, Heidegger, Sartre, and Buber*. Cambridge: MIT Press, 1984.

Turkle, Sherry. *Psychoanalytic Politics*. Cambridge: Harvard University Press, 1981.

Tytell, Pamela. *La Plume sur le divan*. Paris: Aubier, 1982.

Wright, Gordon. *Between the Guillotine and Liberty: Two Centuries of the Crime Problem in France*. Oxford: Oxford University Press, 1983.

Zizek, Slavoj. *The Sublime Object of Ideology*. London: Verso, 1989.

Index

Abortion, 59, 61, 66–67, 69, 71
Acéphale, 42n, 171–72, 184
Adorno, Theodor, 183
Alexander, Franz, 34, 39–41
Alienism, 21, 24–25, 29–30, 99
Allendy, René, 11, 32, 37, 39, 108, 112, 216
Ambrosino, Georges, 171
Amiaux, Mark, 123
Anti-Semitism, 12, 114
Apollinaire, Guillaume, 138n, 155, 159, 162
Armand, Ernest, 131
Artaud, Antonin, 213, 221
Automatic writing, 213–15. *See also* Surrealism
Autopunition, 3, 36–41, 121, 197, 249; in Bataille, 234, 243–44; in Freud, 37–39; in Lacan, 45–48, 53–57, 90–91, 194
Avant-garde movements, 8, 11, 42, 108, 159, 202, 207, 209, 212, 216, 221, 237, 245, 248

Bachelard, Gaston, 11n
Balzac, Honoré de, 166
Barbey d'Aurevilly, Jules, 154, 160
Baruk, Henri, 29–30, 99
Bataille, Georges, 42–43, 105, 125, 170, 199, 203, 216; autopunition in, 234, 243–44; and fascism, 171, 224–231, 242; and heterogeneity, 225–27, 229–30; and homogeneity, 225–27; and Lacan, 1–9, 243, 246–

251; and masochism, 227, 229, 232; oedipal story in, 236–45, 249; and pseudonymity, 232–33; and psycho-analysis, 232–33; on Sade, 172, 183, 187–90, 194–98; and surrealism, 42n, 170–72, 221–24, 228, 230–31, 241–43, 249; transgression in, 190, 228, 239, 243–45. *See also* Identification
Beauvoir, Simone de, 183, 194
Béliard, Octave, 138, 144, 148
Benjamin, Jessica, 201–2
Benjamin, Walter, 184, 215n, 226, 231
Bercherie, Paul, 12n, 13n, 56, 86n, 102
Bergson, Henri, 3–4, 12n
Bersani, Leo, 197
Binot, René, 134n
Bion, René, 75
Bizard, Léon, 69–70
Blanchot, Maurice, 7, 179n, 189, 214–15
Bleuler, Eugen, 100–4, 106, 109
Bloch, Iwan [pseud. Eugen Duehren], 127, 128n, 129–30, 142n
Bonaparte, Marie, 11, 35–39, 41, 56, 79–80, 83, 86; and analysis of Madame Lefebvre, 35–39, 41–42
Bonmariage, Sylvain, 148n, 158n, 165
Bonnafé, Lucien, 30
Bonneau, Alcide, 143
Borch-Jacobsen, Mikkel, 48n, 89n, 93, 119, 188–89n, 194n, 241, 247n, 249–50

Borel, Adrien, 11, 102–7, 109, 216–20, 224, 232–35
Bourdin, Paul, 140, 162
Breton, André, 33n, 42n, 162–63, 168, 171–72, 210, 213–15, 221–23, 228, 238. See also Surrealism
Brousson, Jean-Jacques, 139, 145–46, 148n, 151
Bureau, Paul, 69, 71, 76
Butler, Judith, 1

Cabanès, Augustin, 139
Caillois, Roger, 49n, 228
Calbairac, M. G., 26, 72
Camus, Albert, 189–90
Canguilhem, Georges, 11n
Carter, Angela, 182
Cartesianism, 1, 3–4, 7, 12–13
Castration, 76, 81, 96, 115, 117, 189n, 236–38, 240–44, 246. See also Oedipal scenario
Cénac, Michel, 108
Chable, Robert, 74, 77
Charpentier, René, 27
Chavigny, Paul, 78
Claude, Henri, 26, 42, 99, 102–7, 109, 210, 215
Clérembault, Gaston de, 42
Codet, Henri, 12, 39, 83, 109, 216
Collège de Sociologie, 172, 176n, 228, 230
Constitutionalism, 43–45, 102–7
Convulsion, 213–14, 217–19. See also Surrealism
Corbin, Alain, 69
Courbon, Paul, 26–27
Crevel, René, 209
Criminal motivation, 32–41, 43–48, 51–55
Criminal responsibility, 18–20, 22, 24–29, 31, 33, 35–36, 40

Dali, Salvador, 43
Dandyism, 149, 152, 158n, 160, 162, 190
Dautry, Jean, 228
Deconstruction, 2
Degeneracy theory, 17–18, 60–62, 99–100, 104n, 128, 142
Deleuze, Gilles, 188n
Delirium, 43–44, 53, 105, 120
Dementia, 25, 27–28, 99–101, 103
Demi-fou, demi-folie, 19, 31

Derrida, Jacques, 2, 6
Desbordes, Jean, 138, 144, 147n, 151, 167
Descaves, Lucien, 65, 127
Desire, 108–13; in Freud, 14, 41; in Lacan, 5, 45, 49–50, 52, 54, 57, 88, 91, 96, 119–20, 190–97, 247
Desnos, Robert, 217, 221
Desthieux, Frédéric-Jean, 22
Donzelot, Jacques, 20, 31, 76, 78, 79n
Du Camp, Maxime, 124
Duchamps, Marcel, 237–38, 240
Duehren, Eugen. See Bloch, Iwan
Dumas, Georges, 99, 216
Dupouy, Roger, 22–24
Durkheim, Emile, 225–26
Dworkin, Andrea, 146n

Ecole Française de Psychanalyse, 114
Ecole Freudienne de Paris, 114
Ellis, Havelock, 129, 130n, 131
Eluard, Paul, 162–64, 209
L'Encéphale, 11–12, 99
Enlightenment, 18n, 174, 190
Ernst, Max, 237–38, 240
Eroticism, 90, 128, 131, 139, 166, 202, 214, 229, 241–42
Escande, Frank, 77–78
Eugenics, 72n, 78, 248. See also French Eugenics Society
L'Evolution Psychiatrique, 25, 109, 113
Ey, Henri, 102, 104n, 214

Fascism, 63, 91–92, 171–72, 203, 207, 216–17, 219n, 224–31, 242, 248–49
Felman, Shoshana, 118
Female sexuality: deviance and, 58–61; efforts to control, 59–60, 74–79. See also Prostitution
Feminism, 59, 64; perceptions of feminists, 81–82, 84, 91; theory and criticism, 97n, 120, 146n, 182n, 201–2, 238, 245. See also Garçonne, la; Gender roles; New Woman, the
Ferri, Enrico, 31n
Flake, Otto, 140, 142n, 148, 166–68
Flaubert, Gustave, 143, 153–54
Fleuret, Fernand, 138n, 158n
Foucault, Michel, 1–2, 6, 31, 54n, 189n, 205
French Eugenics Society, 23
Freud, Sigmund, 4, 13–14, 25, 105,

108–12, 159, 162, 190, 240, 247; on
the death instinct, 38–39, 54, 209;
desire in, 14, 41; on ego formation,
46–48, 50–51; French reception of,
12, 33n, 35, 43; and Lacan, 7, 14,
86–87, 89, 191; narcissism in, 14,
47, 88; on neurosis, 37–39, 41, 114;
Oedipus complex in, 38, 85–88,
115; on psychosis, 41, 114; reality
principle in, 47, 50–51, 93; on self-
punishment, 37–39. See also Identification
Functionalism, 12–13n, 15n, 46, 52,
74–86, 99, 106

Garçonne, la, 63, 68, 70–71, 83. See
also Gender roles; New Woman, the
Gauthier, Xavière, 214
Gender roles, 74, 91; women's chal-
lenges to, 59, 63–67, 70–73, 81–82,
84. See also Garçonne, la; New
Woman, the
Genil-Perrin, G., 20, 34–35
Gide, André, 77n, 209, 225
Gilman, Sander, 60, 100
Ginisty, Paul, 147, 155
Goldstein, Jan, 19
Goncourt, Edmond and Jules de, 149,
153–54
Good, Paul, 75, 78
Gourmont, Remy de, 143
Grossman, Atina, 69, 74
Guiraud, Paul, 25–26, 33, 39

Habermas, Jürgen, 2, 3n, 4
Hegel, G. W. F., 4–5, 48n, 49–50, 177,
247
Heidegger, Martin, 3n, 5, 50, 231n,
250
Heimonet, Jean-Michel, 212
Heine, Maurice, 129, 130n, 136–37,
140, 146, 151–53, 164–65, 167, 190;
and analysis of Sergeant Bertrand,
210–12
Henriot, Emile, 144
Hermant, Abel, 155, 158–59
Hesnard, Angelo, 11–12, 36–39, 41,
79, 82, 132–34, 216
Heterogeneity, 225–27, 229–30
Hippocrate, 137
Hirschfeld, Magnus, 129–30, 132
Hollier, Denis, 57n, 184, 221–22, 230,
236, 240–42, 245

Homogeneity, 225–27
Homosexuality, 37, 45, 60–61, 76–
77n, 81–82, 84, 89–90, 95, 129,
135, 237–38, 240. See also Lesbianism
Husserl, Edmund, 3, 5
Huysmans, Joris-Karl, 154

Identification: in Bataille, 229, 239–
41, 243–44; in Freud, 45, 47, 83, 88;
in Lacan, 15, 48, 50, 51n, 57, 87,
89n, 90–93, 96, 115, 247n
Imaginary, the, 13–15, 46, 51–57,
90–96, 119, 244, 247n, 250
Infanticide, 59, 61, 66–67, 71–72,
208n
Inman, Georges, 30
International Psychoanalytic Association, 13n, 114

Jacobus X, 127–29
Jameson, Fredric, 14
Janet, Pierre, 12, 99, 102, 129, 142,
215n
Janin, Jules, 138–39, 142–43, 147,
193n
Jardine, Alice, 120
Javelier, André, 144, 166
Jay, Martin, 49, 119n, 231n
Jouissance, 178, 185, 191–92
Journal de Psychologie, 49, 99
Jouve, Pierre-Jean, 216

Kant, Immanuel, 190–91
Keller, Rose, 140–46, 148n, 168,
197–98
Kierkegaard, Søren, 171
Klossowski, Pierre, 5, 9, 125, 170–78,
183–90, 194–98, 203, 224n, 231,
239n
Kojève, Alexandre, 5, 7, 49–52, 56,
177n, 231, 247
Kraeplin, Emil, 100, 103
Krafft-Ebing, Richard von, 127, 129,
159, 211
Kristeva Julia, 245n

Lacan, Jacques, 13, 27, 37, 41–48, 51–
54, 125, 170, 239n; on autopunition, 45–48, 51, 53–57, 90–91, 194;
and Bataille, 1–9, 243, 246–51; desire in, 5, 45, 49–50, 52–54, 57, 88,
91, 96, 119–20, 247; the Imaginary

Lacan, Jacques (*cont.*)
  in, 13–15, 46, 51–57, 90–96, 119,
  244, 247n, 250; and language, 15,
  52, 96–97, 113–20; mirror stage of,
  48–52, 86–87, 96, 193; on misrecognition, 48–51, 53, 56, 118; on
  narcissism, 14, 48, 88, 91, 96; on
  neurosis, 54, 90, 92, 116–17; on the
  oedipal scenario, 86, 95, 115, 194n,
  237, 241; on paranoia, 43–48, 51–
  53, 58; phallus in, 15n, 96–97, 115–
  16, 193–94, 237, 243, 246; the Real
  in, 13–15, 52–53, 115, 118–19; on
  Sade, 190–95, 198; the Symbolic in,
  13–15, 92–97, 114–20, 193, 244,
  247n, 249–50; on the unconscious,
  14–15, 98, 117–20. *See also* Identification
Lacroix-Dupouy, Marie-Thérèse, 21n,
  27
Laforgue, René, 11, 36–39, 41, 79–83,
  85, 107–12
Landru, Henri, 208
Language, 5n, 6–7, 100–101, 111,
  188n; and avant-garde writers, 179,
  185–86, 214–15; and Lacan, 15, 52,
  96–97, 113–20; and Edouard
  Pichon, 84–86, 113–14
Laurent, Emile, 17, 128
Lautréamont, Comte de (Isidore
  Ducasse), 163–64, 214
Le Brun, Annie, 163n
Leiris, Michel, 7, 105, 170–71,
  216–17, 228, 230
Lély, Gilbert, 131, 137, 152, 163, 165,
  167
Lesbianism, 60, 81–82. *See also*
  Homosexuality
Leuba, John, 80, 82–83, 86
Libertinism, 124, 142n, 146, 175–78,
  184–89. *See also* Sade, Marquis de
Ligue Nationale Française d'Hygiène
  Mentale, 20–23, 30n, 34, 72–78,
  99. *See also* Mental hygiene move-
  ment
Loewenstein, Rudolph, 11
Lombroso, Cesare, 31n, 208n
Lorrain, Jean, 149–50n

McLaren, Angus, 59, 61n
Magnan, Valentin, 18
Man, Paul de, 231n
Marciat, Dr. *See* Tournier, Claude
Margueritte, Victor, 63n, 64, 68n

Marx, Karl, 49–50, 225
Masochism, 131, 147, 201–3, 218–19,
  247; in Bataille, 227, 229, 232;
  in Freud, 38–39; and Sade, 125,
  177–78, 180–84, 197
Masson, André, 42, 170
Matuschka, Sylvestre, 32
Mauss, Marcel, 225–26
Mental hygiene movement, 8, 20–23,
  73–80, 98–107, 247–50. *See also*
  Ligue Nationale Française
  d'Hygiène Mentale
Merleau-Ponty, Maurice, 5, 52
Minkowski, Eugène, 101–02
Minotaure, 42, 49n, 137
Modernism, 1, 202
Montreuil, Renée de, 147–48
Mordier, Jean-Pierre, 7, 33n
Morel, Bénédict-Auguste, 17–18, 100
Morgenstern, Sophie, 37
Mounier, Emmanuel, 172

Nacht, Sacha, 80
Narcissism, 111, 219; in Freud, 14,
  47, 88;
  in Lacan, 14, 48, 88, 91, 96
Natalism, 72–73
Negative dialectic, 5, 49–50
Neurosis, 79–81, 83–84, 89, 106, 195;
  in Freud, 37–39, 41, 114; in Lacan,
  54, 90, 92, 116–17, 243
New Woman, the, 13, 59, 63–67, 73–
  75, 79, 80, 94. *See also* Garçonne,
  la; Gender roles
Nietzsche, Friedrich, 3n, 5
Nodier, Charles, 159
Noizières, Violette, 208, 210
Nouvelle Revue Française, 137, 178
Nye, Robert, 17n, 18

Odier, Charles, 11, 40, 56, 81–82
Oedipal scenario, 41; in Bataille, 236–
  45, 249; in Freud, 38, 85–88, 115;
  in Lacan, 86–93, 95, 115, 194n, 237,
  241

Papin, Christine and Lea von, 32–33,
  37, 43–46, 208–211, 225
Paranoia, 39, 100, 103; in Lacan, 43–
  45, 48, 51–53, 55
Parcheminey, Georges, 11
Pater, Walter, 165n
Patriarchy, 90; avant-garde artists'

complicity in, 84–85, 197, 238; and the family, 13, 66, 78–79n, 88–97
Paulhan, Jean, 125, 146n, 165–67, 170, 178–84, 194, 196–98, 205, 209, 213–14, 225, 231
Pauvert, Jean-Jacques, 125n, 163n
Pefanis, Julian, 2n
Perceau, Louis, 138–39, 144–45, 147
Peret, Benjamin, 209
Perversion: medical perceptions of, 60, 127, 129–34, 136; and Sade, 124–25, 128, 167, 169, 190; and surrealism, 196, 202, 206–7, 211–12, 214, 235, 237, 241
Pichon, Edouard, 11, 40, 83–88, 91, 93, 95, 107, 110–11, 112–14, 134–35n, 216, 248
Pinel, Phillipe, 18n
Politzer, Georges, 86
Pornography, 146n, 150, 152, 166, 182n, 239
Positivism, 18, 19n, 33–34, 54, 56
Poststructuralism, 1–3, 9, 231n, 246, 250
Praz, Mario, 153–54
Prévert, Jacques, 238n
Prévost, Marcel, 77–78
Prostitution, 20, 28, 60–62, 65–71, 73, 131, 143, 146–47n, 208n
Psychiatry, French tradition of, 8, 12–13, 17–32, 46, 56, 72–79, 98–102, 166–67, 215; relationship of, to psychoanalysis in France, 33–36, 102–9. See also Criminal responsibility; Mental hygiene movement
Psychoanalysis, French tradition of, 4, 7–8, 11–13, 36–42, 79–86, 98, 109–12, 216, 247–50; relationship of, to psychiatry in France, 32–36, 102–9. See also Autopunition; Criminal motivation
Psychosis, 106–7, 109; in Freud, 41, 114; in Lacan, 52, 55–56, 112–21

Queneau, Raymond, 105, 171, 183, 217, 238n

Ragland-Sullivan, Ellie, 51n, 197
Rais, Gilles de, 137–38n, 206, 222
Rajchman, John, 247
Real, the, 13–15, 52–53, 115, 119
Régis, Emmanuel, 12
Restif de la Bretonne, Nicolas, 142, 167

Revue Française de Psychanalyse, 12, 35–37, 102, 216
Rimbaud, Arthur, 163
Robin, Gilbert, 102–7, 109
Romains, Jules, 34, 40
Romanticism, 148, 154, 168, 174–75, 206n, 211
Roth, Michael, 88n
Roudinesco, Elisabeth, 7, 11n, 49–50, 57n, 84, 91n, 109, 113n, 216, 217n, 248
Roussel, Raymond, 163
Roustang, François, 119n

Sade, Marquis de, 8, 123–26, 201, 203, 206, 225, 239n; Bataille on, 172, 183, 187–90, 194–98, 248–49; and fantasy, 124, 151, 164, 168, 178, 181, 191–92, 195; and French Revolution, 124, 148–52, 158, 190; Klossowski on, 173–78, 183–87, 189, 194–98; Lacan on, 190–95, 198; and masochism, 125, 177–78, 180–84, 197; Paulhan on, 178–84, 194, 198; and surrealism, 159–60, 162–70, 172–73, 178–79, 190, 195–98, 219, 223–24. See also Libertinism; Sadism
Sadism, 176–78, 211, 227, 236; in Freud, 38–39; and Sade, 122, 128, 130–31, 135–36, 138, 151–54, 160, 164–68, 191–92
Sainte-Beuve, Charles Augustin, 153
Saleilles, Raymond, 19, 23
Sarfati, Salvador, 130, 139, 146n, 151, 166
Sartre, Jean-Paul, 5, 49n
Schiff, Paul, 22–23, 39, 216
Schizophrenia, etiology of, 13, 98, 100–107, 121
Schneider, William, 23, 67n, 72
Scotomization, 98, 107–14, 119, 121, 249
Sexual difference, 60, 74; efforts to reconstitute, 74–86, 94–97; perceived dissolution of, 71, 74–75, 80, 84, 94–95, 134
Social hygiene movement, 20–21, 23, 65n, 74, 77n
Socialism, 30–31n, 248
Société Française de Psychanalyse, 13n, 114
Société Psychanalytique de Paris, 12, 13n, 36, 114, 216

Société de Psychologie Collective, 216
Sokolnicka, Eugénie, 11–12
Staub, Hugo, 34, 39–41
Stendhal [Marie-Henri Beyle], 153–54, 167
Stoekl, Allan, 7, 225
Subjectivity, 1–10, 13, 120–22, 246–251; in Bataille, 203, 243–44; in Lacan, 50–57, 95–97, 120–21; in Sade, 196–99; in surrealism, 202, 213, 219–20
Suleiman, Susan, 196, 237–39, 240n
Surfascisme, 228–29
Surrealism, 4–5, 8, 238–39, 247–50; and automatic writing, 213–15; and Bataille, 42n, 170–72, 221–24, 228, 230–31, 241–43, 249; and convulsion, 213–14, 217–19; and crime, 207, 209–15, 219–20; and perversion, 202, 237; and politics, 162, 212; and psychoanalysis, 105, 216–20; and Sade, 159–60, 162–70, 172–73, 178–79, 190, 195–98, 219, 223–24. See also Breton, André
Symbolic, the, 13–15, 92–97, 114–20, 193, 244, 247n, 249–50
Swiller, Yvonne Marie, 20

Taylor, Charles, 219n
Telmeyr, Maurice, 164
Teutsch, Robert, 64, 70–71, 76n
Toulouse, Edouard, 20–21, 23, 24n, 73, 76, 129, 134
Tournier, Claude [pseud. Dr. Marciat], 127–29, 147
Transgression: in avant-garde movements, 176, 185, 209–10, 213–14, 219, 243; in Bataille, 190, 228, 239, 243–45
Turkle, Sherry, 12

Vachet, Pierre, 131–32
Van Gogh, Vincent, 233–34
Villiers, Charles de, 149
Vitrac, Roger, 217

Wallon, Henri, 49–51, 56, 86
Wilden, Anthony, 15n
World War I, 4, 63–64, 65n, 66–67, 72–74, 248

Yocas, Panagiote, 67–68, 72

Zola, Emile, 166

Library of Congress Cataloging-in-Publication Data

Dean, Carolyn J. (Carolyn Janice), 1960-
    The self and its pleasures / Carolyn J. Dean.
        p.   cm.
    Includes bibliographical references and index.
    ISBN 0-8014-2660-X (hard : alk. paper). — ISBN 0-8014-9954-2 (pbk. : alk.
paper)
    1. Self—History—20th century. 2. Self (Philosophy)—History—20th
century. 3. Masochism—History. 4. Criminal psychology—
History. 5. Lacan, Jacques, 1901- . 6. Bataille, Georges,
1897-1962. 7. France—Intellectual life—20th century. I. Title.
BF697.D363 1992
155.2'0944'0904—dc20   92-52748